GOVERNORS STATE UNIVERSITY
UNIVERSITY PARK
IL 60466

Treatment Resource Manual for Speech-Language Pathology

3rd Edition

Froma P. Roth
Colleen K. Worthington

THOMSON

DELMAR LEARNING

Australia Canada Mexico Singapore Spain United Kingdom United States

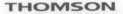

THOMSON

DELMAR LEARNING

Treatment Resource Manual for Speech-Language Pathology, 3rd Edition
by Froma P. Roth, PhD and Colleen K. Worthington, MS

Vice President, Health Care Business Unit:
William Brottmiller

Editorial Director:
Cathy L. Esperti

Acquisitions Editor:
Kalen Conerly

Developmental Editor:
Juliet Steiner

Marketing Director:
Jennifer McAvey

Marketing Coordinator:
Christopher Manion

Editorial Assistant:
Molly Belmont

Project Editor:
Natalie Pashoukos

Art and Design Coordinator:
Christi DiNinni

Production Editor:
Anne Sherman

Library of Congress Cataloging-in-Publication Data
Roth, Froma P.
 Treatment resource manual for speech-language pathology/Froma P. Roth, Colleen K. Worthington—3rd ed.
   p. ; cm.
 Includes bibliographical references and index.
 ISBN 1-4018-4036-1
 1. Speech therapy—Handbooks, manuals, etc.
 [DNLM: 1. Language Therapy—methods. 2. Speech Therapy—methods. 3. Communication Disorders—therapy.] I. Worthington, Colleen K. II. Title.
 RC423.R675 2005
 616.85'506—dc22

                    2005002013

NOTICE TO THE READER

Publisher does not warrant or guarantee any of the products described herein or perform any independent analysis in connection with any of the product information contained herein. Publisher does not assume, and expressly disclaims, any obligation to obtain and include information other than that provided to it by the manufacturer.

The reader is expressly warned to consider and adopt all safety precautions that might be indicated by the activities described herein and to avoid all potential hazards. By following the instructions contained herein, the reader willingly assumes all risks in connection with such instructions.

The publisher makes no representations or warranties of any kind, including but not limited to, the warranties of fitness for particular purpose or merchantability, nor are any such representations implied with respect to the material set forth herein, and the publisher takes no responsibility with respect to such material. The publisher shall not be liable for any special, consequential, or exemplary damages resulting, in whole or part, from the readers' use of, or reliance upon, this material.

*For **Ilana** and **Eli**, each unique and extraordinary, who continue to fill my life with light and infinite delight.*

FPR

*For **Leigh-Anne**, the small miracle who remains the heart of my heart.*

CKW

CONTENTS

PART ONE   PREPARING FOR EFFECTIVE INTERVENTION

CHAPTER 1   The Essential Ingredients of Good Therapy: Basic Skills   3

CHAPTER 2 Information Reporting Systems and Techniques 55

PART TWO PROVIDING TREATMENT FOR COMMUNICATION DISORDERS

CHAPTER 3 Intervention for Articulation and Phonology in Children 87

CHAPTER 7 Intervention for Fluency   263

CHAPTER 8 Intervention for Voice and Alaryngeal Speech   291

CHAPTER 9 Client and Family Counseling   325

LIST OF TABLES

CASE EXAMPLES BY DISORDER

Disorder	Example Profile	Selection of Therapy Targets	Sample Activities	Helpful Hints
Alaryngeal Speech	313	313	314	316
Aphasia	215	215	216	222
	216	217	217	222
	220	220	221	222
Apraxia of Speech	244	244	244	247
	246	246	246	247
Articulation				
Cleft Palate	101	101	101	103
Developmental Verbal Apraxia	111	111	111	112
Functional	93	93, 94	94	99
	95	95	95	99
	97	97	97	99
Hearing Impairment	106	106	107	108
Phonological	116	117	117	121
	119	120	120	121
Dysarthria	233	234	234	239
	235	235	235	239
	236	237	237	239
Fluency	272	272		273
	275	275, 276	275, 276	282
	277	277, 278	278	282
	279	280, 281	280, 281	282
Language				
2–5 years old	150	150	151	154
	152	152	153	154
5–10 years old	171	171	171	181
	177	177	177	181
10–18 years old	184	185	185	195
	191	191	191	195
Voice	301	302	302	307
	304	304	304	307
	305	305	306	307

LIST OF FORMS AND FIGURES

LIST OF FORMS

LIST OF FIGURES

PREFACE

The original purpose of this manual was to provide beginning speech-language pathology graduate students with a practical introductory guide to intervention. It also provided practicing clinicians with a single resource that contains specific therapy techniques and materials for a wide variety of communication disorders. This new edition continues to fulfill these aims and also reflects the changing information and recent advances in the field of speech-language pathology that are essential to address in a text of this kind. Examples include: (a) increased focus on treatment efficacy and evidence-based practice; (b) technological advances such as cochlear implants; (c) the growing diversity of cultural and linguistic backgrounds represented in our client populations; (d) increased responsibility for serving clients with dysphagia; and (e) clearer recognition of the link between oral language and literacy. We have carefully updated each chapter to ensure that the book reflects the most current thinking in research and clinical practice.

Two main factors created the need for a resource of this kind for students. First, speech-language pathology programs across the country are rapidly adopting a preprofessional model of education that eliminates clinical practicum experience at the undergraduate level. Thus, even students with undergraduate degrees in communication disorders are entering graduate school with very little direct knowledge of basic therapy approaches, techniques, and materials. Second, master's programs in speech-language pathology are attracting an increasing number of students with bachelor's degrees in areas other than the hearing and speech sciences. These students enter clinical training without any supporting background. As a result, a genuine need exists for a user-friendly and comprehensive source of effective, practical suggestions to guide beginning clinicians through their first therapy experiences.

Another primary use of this manual is as a textbook for undergraduate and graduate level courses in clinical methods. Traditional textbooks for such courses tend to be largely theoretical in nature and lack practical information on how to do therapy. Thus, instructors are often faced with the task of assembling their own clinical materials to complement the text. One of the aims of this manual is to provide such supplementary information in a single source.

This manual also was written with the practicing clinician in mind. Speech-language pathologists are handling caseloads with a broader spectrum of communication disorders than ever before. This trend is occurring in all clinical settings from hospitals to public schools. Moreover, there has been a dramatic increase in private practice as a service delivery model in the field of speech-language pathology. Many practitioners work independently and may not be able to consult readily with colleagues about the management of communication disorders that are outside their main areas of expertise. This manual can serve as an accessible and reliable source of basic treatment information and techniques for a wide range of speech and language disorders.

The information in this manual is based on existing knowledge about communication disorders and available empirical data, as well as the combined clinical experiences of the authors. It is not intended as a cookbook approach to intervention. The complexities of communication disorders preclude such a parochial approach. The therapy targets and activities we have included are meant to serve as illustrations of basic intervention practice, and only as starting points in the therapeutic process. By their very nature, therapy programs for communication disorders should be designed to accommodate each client's unique strengths and weaknesses as well as individual learning styles.

TEXT ORGANIZATION

The manual is organized into two main sections. The first section covers basic principles of speech-language intervention and information reporting systems. The second section comprises six chapters devoted to therapy strategies for specific communication disorders. Each of these chapters includes a brief description of the disorder, example case profiles, specific suggestions for the selection of therapy targets, and sample therapy activities. These have been designed to illustrate the most common characteristics of a given disorder as well as typical approaches to treatment. Each chapter concludes with a set of helpful hints on intervention and a selected list of commercially available therapy materials. The final chapter offers practical suggestions for beginning clinicians regarding effective client and family counseling skills. Reference tables, charts, and reproducible forms are included throughout the manual.

The focus of this manual is on the most common characteristics and treatment approaches for a given disorder. Unusual or atypical populations are beyond the scope of this book. It is important to remember that a communication difference does not necessarily constitute a communication disorder. Clinicians must give due consideration to cultural variations when determining the communicative status of any individual. This book is written from the perspective of standard American English. The information, procedures, and activities contained in each chapter should be adapted in a culturally appropriate manner.

NEW TO THIS EDITION

This third edition of our book features many changes that serve two main purposes: (a) update material from the previous edition to reflect current knowledge and practices in the field; and (b) respond to feedback and suggestions received from instructors, practitioners, and students. Highlights of the new material contained in this edition include the following:

- Introductory information on legislative issues relevant to speech-language pathology
- Updated ASHA Code of Ethics
- Expanded information on goal selection strategies for articulation and phonological intervention
- Expanded discussion of the efficacy of oral-motor intervention

- Additional information on the characteristics of developmental verbal dyspraxia
- New section on speech-language skills in children with cochlear implants
- Separate chapter on language disorders in children from birth-to-five years includes extensive information on the development of emergent literacy, the roles of the speech-language pathologist, and specific strategies for intervention
- Separate chapter on language disorders in school-age children/adolescents presents new information on the development of reading and writing skills
- New section on swallowing disorders
- Expanded discussion on theories/models of stuttering, approaches to fluency intervention, and recovery issues
- Expanded section on spasmodic dysphonia
- New information on family-centered approaches to counseling
- Expanded coverage of issues relevant to individuals with culturally and linguistically diverse backgrounds
- Updated information on treatment efficacy issues throughout the disorder chapters
- Updated and expanded helpful hints, resources, and recommended readings for each chapter

We hope that the students and clinicians who use this text find it a valuable resource for up-to-date knowledge in the field and for guiding their delivery of evidence-based clinical services.

ACKNOWLEDGMENTS

We thank the many people who have contributed their time, efforts, and talents to the preparation of this revised edition. Enormous appreciation is extended to our colleagues who generously shared with us their insights, expertise, and libraries: Kim Sabourin, Kate Skinker, and Vivian Sisskin. We also want to recognize Jennifer Caruso, Allison MacFarland, and Heidi Corwin, who provided technical support and valuable editorial input. Finally, we thank our husbands, Eddie and Joe, for their support and encouragement, which never wavers throughout the lengthy revision process.

ABOUT THE AUTHORS

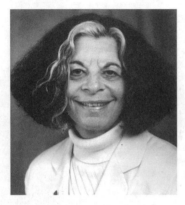

Froma P. Roth

is an Associate Professor in the Department of Hearing and Speech Sciences at the University of Maryland, College Park. She received her bachelor's degree from Hunter College, her master's degree from Queens College, and a doctoral degree from the Graduate Center of the City University of New York. Dr. Roth's current research and clinical interests focus on developmental language and learning disabilities.

Colleen K. Worthington

is the Director of the Speech-Language Clinic in the Department of Hearing and Speech Sciences at the University of Maryland, College Park. She received her bachelor's degree from the University of Maryland and her master's degree from Loyola College, Baltimore. Ms. Worthington's primary professional interests include fluency, phonology and the supervisory process.

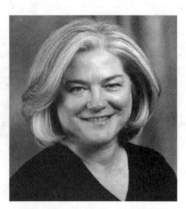

PART ONE

PREPARING FOR EFFECTIVE INTERVENTION

CHAPTER 1

The Essential Ingredients of Good Therapy: Basic Skills

PHILOSOPHY

In the field of communication disorders, the domains of research and clinical practice frequently are regarded as distinctly separate entities. It is true that the aims of the two activities are very different. The main purpose of research is to add to the existing knowledge base in a given area, whereas the ultimate goal of clinical work is to change behavior. However, the two activities also share many common characteristics, and these similarities outweigh the differences. The most fundamental similarity is that both research and clinical practice are scientific processes. Therefore, it is our view that intervention, like research, should be based on the principles of the scientific method. Both research and intervention involve the following:

- Identification of a problem
- Review of existing knowledge regarding the problem area
- Formulation of hypotheses about how to solve the problem
- Manipulation of the independent variable(s)
- Collection and analysis of data
- Formulation of conclusions about the validity of the original hypotheses

Speech and language intervention is a dynamic process that follows a systematic progression. It begins with the diagnosis of a communication disorder and is followed by the selection of appropriate therapy targets. Training procedures are then implemented to facilitate the acquisition of the target behaviors. The intervention process is completed when mastery of these behaviors is achieved. Periodic follow-up is performed to monitor retention and stability of the newly acquired behaviors. Throughout all stages of therapy, advocacy is an important role for the speech-language pathologist. All clinicians should be aware of the Americans with Disabilities Act (ADA, 1990). This federal legislation (Public Law 101-336) prohibits discrimination and ensures equal opportunity in public accommodations, employment, transportation, government services, and telecommunications (see www.ada.gov for more specific information).

The scope of practice in speech-language pathology is delineated by the American Speech-Language-Hearing Association (ASHA, 2001) and is reproduced in Appendix A at the end of this book. Standards for professional and ethical behavior in the field are outlined by the 2003 ASHA Code of Ethics (see Appendix B at the end of this book).

GENERAL PRINCIPLES OF INTERVENTION

Certain basic principles support the concept of effective intervention regardless of client age or disorder. These include:

- Intervention is a dynamic rather than static process in which the clinician continuously assesses a client's progress in relation to established goals and modifies them as necessary.

- Intervention programs should be designed with careful consideration of a client's verbal and/or nonverbal cognitive abilities. Knowledge of a client's level of cognitive functioning is critical to decision-making regarding eligibility for treatment and the selection of appropriate therapy objectives.

- The ultimate goal of intervention is to teach strategies for facilitating the communication process rather than teaching isolated behaviors (to the extent possible).

- Speech and language abilities are acquired and used primarily for the purpose of communication and therefore should be taught in a communicative context. To the extent possible, therapy should occur in realistic situations and provide a client with opportunities to engage in meaningful communicative interactions.

- Intervention should be individually oriented. It should be based on the nature of a client's specific deficits and individual learning style.

- Intervention should be designed to ensure that a client experiences consistent success throughout all stages of the therapy program.

- Intervention is most effective when therapy goals are tailored to promote a client's knowledge one step beyond the current level.

- Intervention should be terminated once goals are achieved or client is no longer making demonstrable progress.

- Intervention practices must be based on scientific evidence.

- Intervention should be sensitive to a client's cultural and linguistic background.

To provide effective intervention for any type of communication disorder, speech-language pathologists must acquire certain essential clinical skills. These skills are based on fundamental principles of human behavior and learning theory. They are the building blocks of therapy and serve as the foundation for all disorder-specific treatment approaches:

- *Programming:* Selection, sequencing, and generalization of therapy targets
- *Behavior modification:* Systematic use of specific stimulus-response-consequence procedures
- *Key teaching strategies:* Use of basic training techniques to facilitate learning
- *Session design:* Organization and implementation of therapy sessions, including interpersonal dynamics
- *Data collection:* Systematic measurement of client performance and treatment efficacy

Successful intervention requires the ability to effectively integrate these five parameters into a treatment program. Appendix 1-A at the end of this chapter provides a checklist of clinician behaviors that correspond to each of the parameters. This checklist can be used by students as a guide for observing therapy sessions or by supervisors for evaluating student clinician performance. The remainder of this chapter is devoted to a detailed discussion of each basic skill area.

PROGRAMMING

Programming involves the selection and sequencing of specific communicative behaviors. New behaviors are introduced and taught in highly structured situations with multiple prompts and maximal support provided by the clinician. Subsequent activities progress through a hierarchy of difficulty and complexity with decreasing support from the clinician. The client demonstrates generalization of each newly learned behavior by using it in novel situations or contexts. The programming process culminates with a client's habitual and spontaneous use of a behavior in everyday speaking and listening situations.

Selection of Therapy Targets

The first step in programming is identification of the communication behaviors to be acquired over the course of the treatment program. These therapy targets are often referred to as **long-term goals**. Initial information about potential therapy targets should be obtained by reviewing the results of previous diagnostic findings. Frequently, assessment data are based, in part, on the administration of standardized tests. These tests typically are designed to sample only one or two exemplars of a given communication behavior. However, a single incorrect response does not constitute a sufficient basis for the inclusion of a behavior as a target in a treatment program. It indicates only a potential area of weakness, which then must be sampled more extensively to determine whether a genuine deficit exists. In addition, it is essential that a clinician consider the client's cultural and linguistic background when identifying potential therapy targets. Speech and language differences arising from dialect usage or a non-English native language do not constitute a communicative disorder. The reader is referred to Appendix C at the end of the book for common characteristics of Black English, Spanish-influenced English, and Asian-influenced English.

This sampling is accomplished through the administration of **pretreatment baselines**. Baselines are clinician-designed measures that provide multiple opportunities for a client to demonstrate a given communicative behavior. A good rule of thumb is to include a minimum of 20 stimuli on each pretreatment baseline. The ratio of correct versus incorrect responses is calculated and the resulting percentage is used to determine whether the behavior should be selected as a therapy target. Many clinicians view a performance level of 75% accuracy or higher as an indication that the communication skill in question is not in need of remediation. Baseline measures that fall below the 75% accuracy level represent potential intervention targets. Ultimately, however, the selection of appropriate therapy targets relies heavily on clinical judgment. Some clinicians believe that behaviors that occur with at least 50% accuracy represent targets with the best potential for improvement. Other clinicians argue strongly that behaviors with much lower baseline rates of accuracy may be the most appropriate choices based on individual client characteristics (e.g., intelligibility level, age, and so on). Often, clients present with several behaviors that qualify as candidates for remediation. In such instances, clinicians typically employ one of two basic strategies to choose among the potential targets: normative or client-specific.

The Normative Strategy. The normative strategy is based on known developmental sequences of communicative behaviors in normally achieving individuals. Therapy targets are taught in the same general order as they emerge developmentally. When two or more potential targets are identified from baseline procedures, the behaviors that occur earliest developmentally would be selected as the first therapy objectives. Following are two examples that illustrate use of the normative strategy:

A 5-year-old child with an articulation disorder produces the following speech sound errors on baseline procedures:

1. /p/ for /f/ as in *p*inger for *f*inger
2. /t/ for /ʃ/ as in *t*ip for *sh*ip
3. /d/ for /dʒ/ as in *d*uice for *j*uice
4. /d/ for /b/ as in *d*oat for *b*oat

Use of the normative strategy guides the clinician to select /b/ as the initial therapy target because normally developing children demonstrate mastery of this sound earlier than the others. According to a developmental progression, /f/ is the next logical target, followed by /ʃ/ and /dʒ/.

A 4-year-old child with a language disorder exhibits the following grammatical errors on baseline procedures:

1. Omission of present progressive tense as in "The boy *play*" for "The boy *is playing*"
2. Omission of the plural marker on regular nouns as in "I see two *bike*" for "I see two *bikes*"
3. Overgeneralization of regular past tense as in "He *runned* down the street" for "He *ran* down the street"

Use of the normative strategy dictates that the first target for therapy is the present progressive form (*is + verb + ing*), because it is the earliest of the three structures to emerge. Developmentally, the plural marker is the next behavior to be targeted, followed by the regular past tense form.

Note: With clients from different cultural/linguistic backgrounds, these grammatical forms may reflect a language difference rather than a language disorder. Therefore, intervention may not be warranted.

The normative strategy tends to be most effective for articulation and language intervention with children. This strategy has less application for adults and disorders of voice and fluency.

A normative strategy for target selection should be implemented with careful consideration of at least two factors. The sample population from which the norms were derived may have been too small to permit valid generalization of the findings to other populations. Moreover, the characteristics of the standardization sample (e.g., ethnicity, gender, socioeconomic status) may differ significantly from those of an individual client. Consequently, it may be difficult to draw direct comparisons between the client's performance and the group norms.

The Client-Specific Strategy. Using the **client-specific** strategy, therapy targets are chosen based on an individual's specific needs rather than according to developmental norms. Relevant factors in the selection of treatment objectives include: (1) the frequency with which a specific communicative behavior occurs in a client's daily activities; (2) the relative importance of a specific communicative behavior to the client, regardless of how often it occurs; and (3) the client's potential for mastery of a given communication skill. This last factor addresses the notion of *stimulability* which is typically defined as the degree to which a client can approximate the correct production of an error pattern on imitation. Following are two examples that illustrate the use of the client-specific strategy:

Mr. Max Asquith, a 52-year-old computer programmer, demonstrates the following speech and language characteristics on pretreatment baseline procedures:

1. Omission of final consonants such as /s/, /k/, and /θ/
2. Distortion of vowels in all word positions
3. Misarticulation of consonant blends such as /br/, /pl/, /fl/, /ks/, and /skw/
4. Omission of the copula forms (*is* and *are*) as in "He sad" for "He is sad"
5. Difficulty with the accurate use of spatial, temporal, and numerical vocabulary
6. Difficulty with subject-verb agreement, especially third person singular constructions as in "He *drink* milk" for "He *drinks* milk"

From the client-specific perspective, initial speech intervention targets could consist of /ks/ and /skw/ because these blends occur in the client's name and therefore constitute a high priority for him. An appropriate initial language target for this client would be vocabulary words that convey number concepts because his position as a computer programmer relies heavily on the use of this terminology.

A 6-year-old child with an articulation disorder exhibits the following speech sound errors on baseline procedures:

1. /θ/ for /s/ as in *th*un for *s*un
2. /g/ for /d/ as in *g*uck for *d*uck
3. /w/ for /l/ as in *w*ight for *l*ight
4. /ʃ/ for /tʃ/ as in *sh*ew for *ch*ew

Using the client-specific strategy, the initial therapy target would be /s/, regardless of developmental considerations. The results of stimulability testing conducted during the diagnostic indicated that this child's ability to imitate /s/ was superior to performance on the other error sounds. In addition, /s/ occurs far more frequently in English than /g/, /w/, and /tʃ/.

Unlike the normative approach, a client-specific strategy can be implemented across a wide range of communication disorders with both pediatric and adult populations. In addition, a combination of the two strategies is often an effective way to approach therapy target selection for children with speech and language impairments.

Sequencing of Therapy Targets

Following therapy target selection and prioritization, programming involves the development of a logical sequence of steps that will be implemented to accomplish each objective. Three major factors determine the progression of the therapy sequence: **stimulus type**, **task mode**, and **response level**. The following outline presents a hierarchy of complexity for each of these factors.

Stimulus Type (nature of input used to elicit target responses)
  1. Direct physical manipulation
  2. Concrete symbols
     - Objects
     - Photographs/colored pictures
     - Black-and-white line drawings
  3. Abstract symbols
     - Oral language
     - Written language

Task Mode (amount of clinician support provided to obtain desired responses)
  1. Imitation
  2. Cue/prompt
  3. Spontaneous

Response Level (degree of difficulty of target responses)[1]
  1. Increase length and complexity of desired response
     - Isolation
     - Syllable
     - Word
     - Carrier phrase (e.g., "I see a _____.")
     - Phrase
     - Sentence
     - Text (conversation, narration)
  2. Decrease latency (actual time) between stimulus presentation and client response

The sequencing process starts with a decision regarding the most appropriate level to begin training on each target behavior. Pretreatment baseline data for

---

[1] This response level hierarchy pertains to oral responses only. Other response types such as gesture, sign, and writing may require alternative hierarchies of difficulty.

a given target are analyzed to determine the entry training level. One rule of thumb that can be used is the following:

If a client obtained a baseline score lower than 50% accuracy, training on that behavior should begin just below the level of difficulty that constituted the baseline stimulus items. If the score was between 50% and 75% accuracy, training can begin at the same difficulty level as the baseline stimuli. For example, a 5-year-old client scored the following on baseline measures for initial /s/: word level = 65%, carrier phrase level = 40%, and sentence level = 30%. In this example, therapy would begin at the word level of difficulty.

Adherence to these procedures generally will result in a progression of targets at the appropriate levels of difficulty. However, there may be occasions when a client does not perform as predicted; a chosen task turns out to be too difficult or too easy for the individual at this time. The clinician must recognize this situation when it occurs and immediately modify the task rather than persisting with the original plan. This modification is known as **branching** and is achieved by increasing or decreasing the difficulty level by one step according to the therapy sequence hierarchies listed previously.

As the client's performance improves and initial training objectives are mastered, the stimulus type, task mode, and response level should be manipulated systematically to gradually increase the difficulty of therapy tasks until final criterion is met for a given target. This criterion level is generally set at 90% accuracy or higher in everyday conversational interactions.

The following sample behavioral objectives illustrate manipulation of each of the three factors.

Behavioral objective: The client will imitatively produce /s/ in the initial position of single words with 90% accuracy while naming 20 photographs.

Modified stimulus type: The client will imitatively produce /s/ in the initial position with 90% accuracy while naming 20 *written* words.

Modified task mode: The client will *spontaneously* produce /s/ in the initial position of single words with 90% accuracy while naming 20 photographs.

Modified response level: The client will imitatively produce /s/ in the initial position of *words in carrier phrases* with 90% accuracy in response to 20 photographs.

Generalization/Carryover

A crucial consideration in programming involves a client's ability to transfer newly mastered communicative behaviors from the clinical setting to the natural environment. Generalization should not be viewed as a distinct event that occurs only in the final phase of the therapy process. Rather, it is an integral part of programming that requires attention from the very beginning. Three main factors can influence the degree to which successful generalization occurs. A variety of **stimuli** (objects, pictures, questions) should be used during therapy activities to avoid learning that is tied to only a small set of specific stimulus items. Similarly, the clinician should vary the **physical environment** (location in room, location in building, real world locations) in which therapy occurs as soon as a new target behavior has been established. This will minimize a client's natural tendency to associate target behaviors with a particular setting. Finally, clinicians should bear in mind that target behaviors frequently become attached to the individual who consistently reinforces them (i.e., the clinician). Therefore, it is important to vary the **audience** (familiar adult, sibling, unfamiliar adult) with whom therapy targets are practiced to maximize the likelihood of successful generalization.

Termination of Therapy

It is difficult to definitively state the point at which intervention services are no longer warranted. At the current time, there are no valid empirical data that can be used to determine appropriate dismissal criteria for any particular communicative disorder. Therefore, it is beyond the scope of this book to indicate realistic time frames for duration of intervention. General discharge guidelines used by many clinicians include: (1) attainment of communication skills that are commensurate with a client's chronological/developmental age or premorbid status, (2) attainment of functional communication skills that permit a client to operate in the daily environment without significant handicap, and (3) lack of discernible progress persisting beyond a predetermined time period. The authors strongly believe that the establishment of reliable treatment outcome measures is critical in the current climate of professional accountability in both the public and private sectors. Within the past few years, the availability of efficacy data has increased significantly for a variety of communication disorders. This information will be presented throughout the book in pertinent chapters.

Formulation of Behavioral Objectives

Once long-term goals and initial treatment levels have been identified, the clinician develops short-term objectives designed to culminate in the achievement of the selected long-term goals. These objectives must be clearly delineated to ensure appropriate and effective intervention programming. A widely used approach to task design is the formulation of **behavioral objectives**. A behavioral objective is a statement that describes a specific target behavior in observable and measurable terms. There are three main components of a behavioral objective:

1. "Do" (action) statement
2. Condition
3. Criterion

The **do statement** identifies the specific action the client is expected to perform. Thus, behavioral objectives should contain verbs that denote observable activity; nonaction verbs should be avoided. List 1 contains examples of verbs that are appropriate for inclusion in behavioral objectives; list 2 is made up of verbs that are unacceptable because they refer to behaviors that cannot be observed.

List 1		List 2	
point	say	understand	know
label	write	think	appreciate
repeat	count	learn	remember
match	vocalize	believe	apply
name	ask	improve	comprehend
tell	elevate	discover	feel

An easy way to check the appropriateness of a verb is to ask yourself, "Will I be able to count (tally) how many times this behavior occurs?" (Mowrer, 1982). For example, consider the following: (1) "to repeat single syllable words" and (2) "to learn single syllable words." Only the first is an appropriate do statement. Number of repetitions can be easily counted, whereas "learning" is a behavior that cannot be directly observed.

The **condition** portion of a behavioral objective identifies the situation in which the target behavior is to be performed. It specifies one or more of the following: when the behavior will occur, where it will be performed, in whose presence, or what materials and cues will be used to elicit the target. Following are common examples of condition statements:

Given the clinician's model

In response to a question

In the presence of three strangers

Given a list of written words

In the home environment

During a job interview

Using pictures

During free play

In the presence of other group therapy members

Condition statements are critical parts of behavioral objectives because clients may demonstrate adequate mastery of a communicative behavior in one situation and yet be completely unable to perform the same behavior under different conditions. For example, a client's ability to perform a do statement, such as "Produce one minute of connected speech without disfluency," is likely to be quite different if the condition statement specifies "talking to a familiar clinician" versus "talking to a potential date."

The **criterion** specifies how well the target behavior must be performed for the objective to be achieved. It can be expressed in several ways, including: percent correct, within a given time period, minimum number of correct responses, or maximum number of error responses. A list of criterion measures typically used in speech-language therapy follows:

90% accuracy

8 correct out of 10 trials

Less than four errors over three consecutive sessions

80% accuracy over two consecutive sessions

90% agreement between clinician and client judgments

Continuously over a two-minute period

A well-formulated behavioral objective allows the client, as well as the clinician, to know exactly what the therapy target is, how it is to be accomplished, and what constitutes successful performance. The following examples illustrate how to formulate behavioral objectives.

Example A

1. Do statement: Verbally segment words into syllables
2. Conditions: Given a written list of 100 multisyllabic words
3. Criterion: With no more than four errors

Behavioral objective: The client will verbally segment 100 written multisyllabic words into their component syllables with no more than four errors.

Example B

1. Do statement: Use a slow rate of speech (four syllables per second)
2. Conditions: Reading single sentences
3. Criterion: With 85% accuracy or better over two consecutive sessions

Behavioral objective: The client will use a slow rate of speech (four syllables per second) with 85% accuracy or higher while reading single sentences over two consecutive sessions.

Example C

1. Do statement: Say /s/ in the initial position of single words
2. Conditions: Given the clinician's model
             Name pictures of animals
3. Criterion: With 90% accuracy

Behavioral objective: Given the clinician's model, the client will say /s/-initial single words with 90% accuracy while naming animal pictures.

Additional examples of behavioral objectives and worksheets are provided in Appendixes 1-B and 1-C at the end of this chapter. Appendix 1-D contains a sample Daily Therapy Plan that illustrates the following components of a single session: behavioral objectives, client data, and clinician comments. (A reproducible copy of the Daily Therapy Plan form is provided in Appendix 1-E, along with a sample form for documenting observation hours in Appendix 1-F.)

BEHAVIOR MODIFICATION

The fundamental purpose of intervention is to either increase desired behavior or decrease unwanted behavior. (The term "behavior" refers to communication targets as well as a client's degree of cooperation and attentiveness.) This is accomplished through application of the principles of behavior modification. Behavior modification is based on the theory of operant conditioning and involves the relationship among a stimulus, a response, and a consequent event (Skinner, 1957). A **stimulus** (or antecedent event) is an event that precedes and elicits a response. A **response** is the behavior exhibited by an individual on presentation of the stimulus. A **consequence** is an event that is contingent on and immediately follows the response. There are different types of consequent events. Consequences that increase the probability that a particular behavior will recur are known as **reinforcement**. Those that are designed to decrease the frequency of a behavior are termed **punishment**.

Types of Reinforcement

There are two basic types of reinforcement: **positive reinforcement** and **negative reinforcement**. Both types are used to increase the frequency of a target response.

Positive Reinforcement. Positive reinforcement is a rewarding event or condition that is presented contingent on the performance of a desired behavior.

Primary. These are contingent events to which a client reacts favorably due to the biological makeup or physiologic predisposition of the individual. Food is the most common example of a primary reinforcer. This type of reinforcer is very powerful and is used most effectively to establish new communicative behaviors (i.e., behaviors not previously present in the client's repertoire). Low-functioning clients often respond well to the basic nature of primary reinforcers. There are known disadvantages of primary reinforcement. First, it can be difficult to present the reinforcement immediately after every occurrence of the target behavior. In addition, this type of reinforcement is susceptible to satiation; that is, it loses its appeal as a reward if presented too often. Finally, skills that are taught using these contingent events are often difficult to generalize outside the therapy setting because primary reinforcers do not occur naturally in the real world.

Secondary. These are contingent events that a client must be taught to perceive as rewarding. This category includes the following subtypes of reinforcers:

Social: This group of reinforcers consists of events such as smiling, eye contact, and verbal praise. It is the most commonly used type of reinforcement in speech-language remediation programs. Social reinforcers are extremely easy to administer after each target response and generally do not disrupt the flow of a therapy session. In addition, this type of contingent response is not very susceptible to satiation (although not totally immune) and does occur in a client's natural daily environment.

Token: This group of reinforcers consists of symbols/objects that are not perceived as valuable in and of themselves. However, the accrual of a specified number of these "tokens" will permit a client to obtain a previously agreed-on reward. Examples include stickers, check marks, chips, and point scores. These reinforcers are generally regarded as very powerful because they are easy to administer contingent on each occurrence of a target behavior and are relatively resistant to satiation.

Performance feedback: This category of reinforcers involves information that is given to a client regarding therapy performance/progress. Many individuals find it rewarding to receive information about the quality of their performance. It is not intended to function as praise and need not be presented verbally. Feedback regarding client performance can be delivered in various formats including: percentage data, frequency of occurrence graphs, numerical ratings, and biofeedback devices. Provision of this type of contingent event decreases a client's reliance on external sources of reinforcement by encouraging the development of intrinsic rewards (i.e., internal satisfaction and motivation) for mastering and maintaining a target behavior.

Negative Reinforcement. An unpleasant event/condition is removed contingent on the performance of a desired behavior.

Escape. This type of reinforcer requires the presence of a condition that the client perceives as aversive. Each performance of the target behavior relieves or terminates this aversive condition, thus increasing the probability that the specified behavior will recur. For example, a clinician might place her hands firmly over a child's hands and remove them only when the child exhibits the target behavior of imitatively producing /s/.

Avoidance. With this type of negative reinforcer, each performance of a target behavior prevents the occurrence of an *anticipated* aversive condition. This contingent event results in increased rates of performance of the desired response on subsequent occasions. For example, a clinician might inform a child that each imitative production of the target /s/ will prevent the imposition of hand restraint.

Use of negative reinforcement is relatively uncommon in the treatment of communication disorders because it repeatedly exposes clients to unpleasant or aversive situations. Use of positive reinforcement is the preferred method for increasing the frequency of desired responses. Positive reinforcement also can improve a client's motivational level and foster an effective interpersonal relationship between clinician and client.

Punishment. An event is presented contingent on the performance of an undesired behavior to decrease the likelihood that the behavior will recur.

Type I. This involves the prompt presentation of an aversive consequence after each demonstration of an unwanted behavior. Examples of this consequence type that might be used in speech-language remediation programming include verbal utterances such as "No!," frowning, or the presentation of bursts of white noise.

Type II. This type of punishment requires withdrawal of a pleasant condition contingent on the demonstration of an unwanted behavior. **Time-out** and **response cost** are the two most common forms used in speech-language intervention. Time-out procedures involve the temporary isolation or removal of a client to an environment with limited or no opportunity to receive positive reinforcement. A modified version can be accomplished by turning the client's chair toward a blank wall in the therapy room or simply withholding direct eye contact from the client for short periods of time. Response cost contingencies occur when previously earned positive reinforcers are deducted or taken back each time the undesirable behavior is demonstrated. This type of punishment can take various forms, including removal of stickers earned for previous correct responses or the partial subtraction of points already accrued by the client earlier in a therapy session. Sometimes, the clinician may choose to give a client several unearned tokens at the beginning of a session or task to institute response cost procedures.

Several factors influence the effectiveness of punishment procedures (adapted from Hegde, 1998):

- Punishment should be delivered after *every* instance of the unwanted behavior.
- Punishment should be presented *immediately* following the undesirable behavior.
- Punishment should occur at the earliest signs of the unwanted behavior rather than waiting until the behavior is full blown.
- Punishment should not be programmed in graduated levels of intensity; this creates the potential for client habituation to the punishing stimulus, thus reducing its effectiveness.
- Punishment duration should be as brief as possible; lengthy periods of punishment call into question the strength of the chosen punishing stimulus.

Punishment procedures should be employed with caution in the therapy setting because there are undesirable effects associated with their use. These may include client anger, aggression, a reluctance to engage in any communicative behavior with the therapist, and the avoidance or actual termination of treatment.

If no contingent consequences occur following a targeted behavior, the frequency of that behavior will gradually decrease and ultimately disappear from a client's repertoire. This phenomenon is known as **extinction** and is used in therapy to eliminate behaviors that interfere with effective communication. Extinction does not occur immediately. In fact, a temporary increase in emission rate may be observed when the behavior is initially ignored. Behaviors that receive reinforcement on a continuous basis are most vulnerable to extinction, whereas those that are only periodically reinforced over a long period of time are least susceptible to this procedure. It is recommended that extinction procedures that are implemented for an undesired behavior (e.g., ignoring crying behavior) be combined with positive reinforcement for the converse behavior (i.e., rewarding noncrying behavior).

Application of all the principles just discussed does not guarantee that a therapy session will run smoothly. The clinician should anticipate the possibility that a client may not pay attention or cooperate with the session plan. This may occur due to a client's developmental level of attention, boredom, frustration, a lack of self-motivation, or a neurological behavior disorder. The clinician must now focus on **behavior management** in addition to behavior modification. In most cases, behavior problems can be managed through the implementation of an additional reinforcement system that (1) addresses only cooperative/attending behaviors and (2) is distinctly separate from the reinforcers delivered for speech-language responses. Most behavior problems can be prevented if the therapy materials are creative, the activities are interesting, and the session is well paced.

Schedules of Reinforcement

Once the appropriate type of reinforcer has been selected for a given client, the clinician must decide how often the reinforcer will be delivered. The two main schedules of reinforcement are **continuous** and **intermittent**.

Continuous Reinforcement. A reinforcer is presented after *every* correct performance of a target behavior. This schedule, sometimes characterized as "dense," tends to generate a very high rate of response. It is most commonly used to shape and establish new communication behaviors. It also can be used when transitioning an already established skill from one level of difficulty to the next (e.g., from word to sentence level). Use of a continuous schedule reduces the risk that a client's production of a target behavior will "drift" from the intended response. The primary disadvantage of this schedule is that behaviors reinforced at such a high density level are very susceptible to extinction. It also may interfere with a client's production of a steady flow of responses.

Intermittent Reinforcement. With this schedule, only some occurrences of a correct response are followed by a reinforcer. Intermittent reinforcement, often termed "lower density," is most effective in strengthening responses that have been previously established. This reinforcement schedule reduces the probability of satiation during treatment and results in behaviors that are extremely resistant to extinction. The four types of intermittent schedules are described as follows.

Fixed Ratio. A specific number of correct responses must be exhibited before a reinforcer is delivered (e.g., every two responses, every ten responses, every 35 responses). The required number is determined by the clinician and remains unchanged throughout a therapy task. This reinforcement schedule generally elicits a high rate of response.

Fixed Interval. Reinforcement is delivered for the first correct response made after a predetermined time period has elapsed (e.g., every 3 minutes; every 50 seconds). The main disadvantage of this schedule is that response rate tends to decline dramatically immediately following presentation of the reinforcer, and therefore a fixed interval schedule may be an inefficient use of therapy time.

Variable Ratio (VR). The number of correct responses required for the delivery of a reinforcer varies from trial to trial according to a predetermined pattern set by the clinician. For example, the pattern might be as follows: after the third response; then after the tenth response; then after the fourth response; then after the seventh response. This pattern of ratios is represented as VR: 3, 10, 4, 7 and would be repeated throughout a therapy task. This schedule tends to be more effective than a fixed ratio schedule because the client cannot predict the seemingly random pattern of delivery and anticipates that every response has an equal chance of being reinforced.

Variable Interval (VI). This schedule is similar to a variable ratio except that the clinician varies the time period required for reinforcement delivery rather than the number of responses. For example, one interval pattern might be as follows: after 3 minutes; then after 10 minutes; then after 1 minute; then after 4 minutes. This pattern is represented as VI: 3, 10, 1, 4 and would be repeated throughout a therapy task.

In general practice, continuous reinforcement is used to establish a new target behavior. Intermittent schedules are introduced in subsequent stages of therapy to promote maintenance and generalization. One rule of thumb is to switch to lower-density intermittent schedules when the target response rate increases 30% to 50% over the original baseline measures.

KEY TEACHING STRATEGIES

Several basic training techniques are commonly used in intervention programs to facilitate the acquisition of communication behaviors. These strategies are used for a variety of purposes and are implemented at different points throughout the remediation process.

Direct modeling: Clinician demonstrates a specific behavior to provide an exemplar for the client to imitate.

Indirect modeling: Clinician demonstrates a specific behavior frequently to expose a client to numerous well-formed examples of the target behavior.

Shaping by successive approximation: A target behavior is broken down into small components and taught in an ascending sequence of difficulty.

Prompts: Clinician provides additional verbal or nonverbal cues to facilitate a client's production of a correct response.

Fading: Stimulus or consequence manipulations (e.g., modeling, prompting, reinforcement) are reduced in gradual steps while maintaining the target response.

Expansion: Clinician reformulates a client's utterance into a more mature or complete version.

Negative practice: The client is required to intentionally produce a target behavior using a habitual error pattern. This procedure is generally employed to facilitate learning by highlighting the contrast between the error pattern and the desired response.

Target-specific feedback: The clinician provides information regarding the accuracy or inaccuracy of a client's response relative to the specific target behavior. This type of feedback contrasts with generalized feedback or consequences.

Direct modeling is the teaching technique most frequently used in the early stages of therapy. It is also employed whenever a target behavior is shifted to a higher level of response difficulty because this type of modeling provides the maximum amount of clinician support. Typically, clinicians augment direct models with a variety of visual and verbal cues to establish correct responses at the level of imitation. Direct modeling also minimizes the likelihood that a client will produce his or her customary error response. Initially, a direct model is provided before each client response.

Once a target behavior is established, continuous modeling should be eliminated because it does not facilitate strengthening or maintaining a target response. Direct modeling can be terminated abruptly or faded gradually. Gradual **fading** can be accomplished in at least two ways. One requires a client to produce multiple imitations for each clinician model (e.g., three imitative responses are required after each direct model). The second method involves the progressive reduction of the length of the behavior modeled by the clinician. For example, the direct model of "The boy is running" is shortened first to "The boy is . . . ," and then to "The boy . . ." while the client's imitative response in all three cases is the production of the complete target sentence, "The boy is running." In general, fading procedures can be initiated once a client is able to produce at least five consecutive correct imitative responses.

In some cases, the stimulus alone is not sufficient to elicit the desired response. **Prompts** are extra verbal and nonverbal cues designed to help a client produce the target behavior. Prompts can be categorized as attentional or instructional. Attentional cues improve performance by focusing a client's concentration on the task at hand. Examples include "Look at me," "Watch my mouth," "Remember to pay attention," or "Are you ready?" Clinicians also can draw attention to a target by modeling the behavior with exaggerated loudness and duration. Instructional cues provide information that is directly related to the specific target behavior being attempted. This may include verbal prompts such as "Remember to elevate your tongue tip at the beginning of each word," "Don't forget to segment your words into syllables if you get stuck," or "Be sure that your answer has at least three words in it." Instructional cues also can be nonverbal such as an index card with the name of the targeted fluency technique written on it, a gesture to indicate that voice loudness should be increased, or drawings that represent the grammatical categories of subject-verb-object.

Some target behaviors are too complex for a client to perform successfully and even the provision of a direct model accompanied by prompts may not elicit a correct imitative response. In such instances, procedures for **shaping by successive approximation** are usually instituted. The simplification of a difficult target into a series of more manageable tasks fosters client success at each step. Each successive step moves progressively closer to the final form of the desired response.

Target-specific feedback is a technique that is useful throughout all phases of the therapy process. It serves three main functions. First, clients benefit from feedback that consists of more than simple accuracy judgments regarding their responses. Target-specific feedback provides precise information about why responses are correct or incorrect (e.g., "Good job!" versus "Good, I didn't see your tongue peeking out when you said, 'Soup'," respectively). Second, use of this strategy tends to maintain a client's awareness of the exact response being targeted without the need for continuous reinstruction during a therapy activity. Finally, this type of feedback assists clinicians in maintaining client focus on the communication behavior being targeted by a given therapy activity. It is a particularly helpful strategy for beginning clinicians who may get too involved in the details or rules of an activity and lose sight of the true purpose of the therapy task.

Negative practice is a strategy intended to enhance a client's awareness of the salient characteristics of his or her error pattern. It is used primarily to illustrate the differences between an "old" response and the intended target. This procedure generally is implemented only after a client demonstrates the ability to produce a given target consistently at the level of imitation. Negative practice is a powerful technique that is best used on a short-term basis. Devoting a significant amount of therapy to client practice on incorrect responses is of questionable value.

In addition to the specific training techniques just discussed, clinicians frequently use the general stimulation procedures of **indirect modeling** and **expansion**. These strategies can be employed at any stage in the therapy process. They provide a client with increased exposure to instances of desirable speech, language, or communication behaviors but are not intended to elicit immediate specific responses. For example, a clinician working with a client on the production of /s/ may implement indirect modeling by including a significant number of /s/-initial words in her off-task comments throughout a session. Expansions are used almost exclusively in language therapy programs and may involve the clinician's interpretation of the client's intended meaning (e.g., Client: "Daddy cookie"; Clinician: "Yes, Daddy is eating the cookie").

Once a target communication behavior has been established in therapy using the techniques specified in the previous section, **homework assignments** can be given to strengthen the response and facilitate its generalization outside the clinical setting. There are certain guidelines for the design and implementation of homework that can increase its effectiveness as an intervention strategy:

- The purpose of homework is to provide the client with practice on an existing skill rather than teaching something new. Therefore, it should focus only on targets that have been solidly established in therapy.

- Homework should be instituted only after a client has demonstrated a basic ability to accurately evaluate his or her performance on a given target.

- To increase the likelihood that homework will be completed, it should be assigned in amounts that are perceived as manageable by a client or family. For example, activities that involve a daily commitment of 5 to 10 minutes may be more effective than those that require 30 to 45 minutes once a week.

- Homework should be assigned on a regular basis throughout the course of therapy.
- Homework assignments should always be accompanied by simple written instructions that specify exactly what the client is expected to do.

SESSION DESIGN

Once therapy targets have been appropriately programmed, the clinician must determine the organizational flow of each therapy session. The first decision to be made is whether treatment will be delivered in an individual or group setting. Session design for both of these formats requires consideration of the basic factors discussed in the sections that follow. Elements that are specific to a group design will be addressed later in this chapter.

Basic Training Protocol

Regardless of disorder type or severity level, all speech and language therapy is carried out using the same basic training protocol. This protocol is the distillation of the therapy process and consists of the following five steps:

(Clinician gives instructions; see Table 1 1)
1. Clinician presents stimulus.
2. Clinician waits for the client to respond.
3. Clinician presents appropriate consequent event.
4. Clinician records response.
5. Clinician removes stimulus (as appropriate).

This sequence represents a single trial for a given target and is repeated continuously throughout a therapy session. The acceptable latency period between stimulus presentation and client response may vary according to disorder type as well as individual client characteristics. It is critical that the consequent event (reinforcement/punishment) follow the response immediately so that the contingent relationship between the two is obvious to the client. For this reason, data recording should not delay the delivery of the consequence.

Task Order

Another important component of session design is the order in which tasks are conducted. Appropriate task order enhances the overall effectiveness of treatment. An ideal progression follows an "easy-hard-easy" pattern. A session should begin with therapy tasks with which a client can be relatively successful without excessive expenditure of effort. This could entail a review of completed homework assignments or nearly mastered targets from a previous session. The central portion of the session should consist of behavioral objectives that are most challenging to the client. The final segment should return to tasks that elicit fairly

| **TABLE 1-1** |
| Guidelines for Effective Instructions |

- Instructions should be worded as clearly and concisely as possible. Long, complicated explanations can be counterproductive to a client's understanding of the intended task. (Beginning clinicians may benefit from writing an actual script of instructions prior to a session.)

- State instructions in the declarative form. Directions that are presented indirectly in the form of requests (i.e., "Would you say /s/ for me?") are pragmatically confusing and understandably may elicit negative replies (i.e., "No" or "I don't want to").

- Be sure to allow clients sufficient time to respond before repeating the instructions. Resist the temptation to repeat instructions or stimuli too quickly because individuals with communication impairments often require increased processing time. Waiting is a strategy that may facilitate correct responses more consistently than repetition of instructions.

- If it becomes necessary to readminister instructions, try to avoid significant reformulation of the original wording. This is particularly important with clients who are language disordered because rewording tends to become a source of confusion rather than clarification.

- The main emphasis of instructions should always be on the targeted behavior rather than on the details of the activity/game being used to elicit the behavior. (This aspect poses particular difficulty for beginning clinicians, who must learn to create the appropriate balance between the amount of time spent explaining elaborate therapy activities versus working on target behaviors.)

accurate performance with minimal effort. This task order increases the likelihood that a given therapy session will begin and end on a positive note. This success-oriented session design promotes high levels of client motivation even during difficult stages of the therapy process.

Dynamics of Therapy

Thus far, this chapter has focused on the technical aspects of intervention. However, the therapy process involves another critical dimension: the dynamics of therapy. Therapy dynamics contribute significantly to session design and include factors such as the clinician-client relationship, work efficiency/pace, materials, and proxemics.

The Clinician-Client Relationship. The nature of the clinician-client relationship influences the success of a therapy program as powerfully as the technical design. One of the most important aspects of the therapeutic relationship is the professional personality of the clinician. Clearly, personal attributes among clinicians vary tremendously. In general, a calm, positive, and firm demeanor is most effective in enhancing clinician-client interaction.

Further, clinicians need to maintain a conscious awareness of their body language, intonation patterns, and social speaking style to prevent client confusion. Body language and voice intonation patterns must be monitored to ensure that they do not conflict with accompanying verbal messages. For example, the message, "You're doing a great job!" may not be perceived by a client as a positive remark if it is delivered without eye contact and in an apathetic tone of voice. Further, the use of overly polite forms of speech should be minimized because they may contradict the message that a clinician intends to convey. For example, beginning clinicians who are reluctant to risk hurting a client's feelings may react to an incorrect response with a big smile, while saying, "Good! Let's try that again!" rather than clearly stating that the attempt was inaccurate.

It is the responsibility of clinicians to adapt their interactive styles (e.g., energy level, humor, talkativeness, vocabulary) to accommodate the comfort level of each client rather than the other way around. It is also important to remember that clients can be easily overwhelmed and intimidated by the excessive use of unfamiliar technical jargon. To maintain a professional yet warm atmosphere, clinicians need to determine on a case-by-case basis the appropriate balance between their use of technical versus more colloquial language forms.

Moreover, clinicians must establish the parameters of the therapeutic relationship from the very first session. This entails an explicit definition of the roles and responsibilities of each partner. This will clearly differentiate the nature of a professional relationship from a personal one. At the beginning of a therapeutic relationship, clients do not always feel comfortable volunteering information about their goals for therapy. Clinicians should make a point of asking clients about their expectations. Whenever possible, clients (and their families) should be active participants in the target selection phase of therapy by identifying the communication behaviors that are the highest priorities in their daily lives.

Clinicians can minimize client anxiety and confusion by providing a clear rationale regarding the purpose of each activity implemented in a therapy session. Intervention tends to be less effective if clients do not understand why they are being asked to perform particular tasks. Further, difficult client questions should be addressed in a manner that allows the clinician to maintain credibility. For instance, instead of responding with "I haven't had that course yet," it is more effective to simply say, "I don't know. I'll do some research on the topic and give you the information at our next session."

Clinicians need to create a balance between responding to and ignoring off-task comments made by clients. Sometimes clients genuinely need to talk about topics that are not part of the clinician's original lesson plan but are important to address (e.g., questions regarding lack of progress, comments concerning family reactions to new communicative behaviors). At other times, off-task comments are meant simply to distract the clinician from a therapy task that a client perceives as difficult or boring.

Ultimately, the success of any therapeutic relationship will be influenced by the clinician's recognition that it is the client, and not merely the disorder, that is the main focus of treatment.

Work Efficiency/Pace. This aspect of session dynamics entails consideration of two main issues. First, every session should be efficiently designed to provide a client with the maximum number of opportunities to practice target behaviors. Second, the pace of each session must be geared to the learning rates and styles of individual clients. A pace that is either too fast or too slow may cause frustration for a client and interfere with successful performance.

Materials. The materials selected for therapy must be appropriate for a client's age, developmental status, language level, and gender. In addition to these criteria, it is important to consider the interest value of therapy materials based on individual client preferences. For example, when selecting materials for a 12-year-old learning-disabled boy who reads at a second-grade level, the clinician must ensure that any stories used in therapy be sufficiently interesting for a preteen, yet be written at a manageable difficulty level. Finally, clinicians should avoid the use of time-consuming and complicated materials or activities. Materials that require lengthy physical manipulation (e.g., cutting, gluing, intricate board games) may negatively affect the efficiency of a session by reducing the amount of time available for client responses.

Proxemics. For the purposes of the present discussion, proxemics involves the spatial arrangement or relationships between the clinician and client(s) within the therapy setting. Proxemics should take into account the spatial factors that affect any social interaction. One of the most important considerations for speech-language pathologists is to determine/estimate a socially acceptable (and, in some cases, culturally acceptable) physical proximity between the clinician and the client. Seating arrangements that are extremely far apart may be perceived by the client as an indication of aloofness or lack of interest on the part of the clinician. In contrast, clients may be very uncomfortable with clinicians who sit too close and invade their personal space. Clinicians may deliberately use proxemics as a strategy to influence client behavior (e.g., reducing impulsive or distractible behavior by sitting very close to a child).

In addition to having social implications, proxemics also influence the effective implementation of certain therapy procedures. For example, monitoring the degree of tongue protrusion for an interdental lisp (i.e., /θ/ for /s/) will be difficult if the clinician cannot see the client's face. On the other hand, a face-to-face seating arrangement may interfere with an activity that requires the clinician and client to read from the same stimulus sheet. Seating arrangements should always be selected based on the goal of a given therapy objective. The three most common sitting arrangements (chair or floor) for conducting individualized therapy are face to face, side by side, and side by side in front of a mirror.

Group Therapy

The use of a group therapy model requires attention to several unique aspects of session design that are not pertinent to individual treatment. Unfortunately, there is a paucity of information on group intervention and even less empirical study of this process in the field of speech-language pathology. However, group therapy is critical to any discussion of session design because it is a frequently used service delivery mode and, in fact, is becoming the dominant model in many therapeutic settings (such as the public schools). Therefore, group therapy is treated as a separate topic in this chapter to provide clinicians with fundamental information on the effective design and execution of these programs.

Clinicians implement a group intervention model for a variety of purposes. Some groups are intended to teach new communication skills at introductory levels. Others are designed primarily to provide clients with practice on skills previously established in individual sessions. Still others have socialization, self-help, or counseling as their main purpose.

The stage of therapy at which group intervention is initiated depends on the purpose of the treatment plan. Some clinicians employ a group model from the very beginning of the therapy process; others use it mainly in the final stages to facilitate carryover. In many cases, a combination of individual and group formats is used throughout all stages of the therapy process.

Group Size. The size of a group will vary depending on its purpose, setting, and age of clients. Groups whose primary purpose is to teach new skills tend to be smaller than those geared for the generalization of previously mastered skills. Group size is also determined by availability of clients in different service delivery settings. Institutions such as metropolitan hospitals and public schools lend themselves more readily to the formation of larger therapy groups than do private practices or small clinics.

Based on the available literature, the recommended group size for children is approximately two to six members (Neidecker, 1987; Weiss, Gordon, & Lillywhite, 1987). Guidelines for adults differ. For example, E. Cooper and C. Cooper (1985) recommend 7 to 12 members for adult stuttering groups. They also caution that groups of fewer than five clients are undesirable for several reasons: (1) personality characteristics of individual group members are more prominent, (2) the absence of a single member can interfere with the group's ability to function, and (3) small groups are more susceptible to domination by a single member.

Group Composition. The primary client characteristics to be considered in the formation of a group are age, gender, disorder type, and disorder severity. Other factors that may be relevant to some groups include intelligence, socioeconomic status, education level, and personality type. As a general rule, the two most important factors are client age and disorder type. Effective groups tend to be relatively homogeneous with respect to one or both of these variables. Clinicians may choose to organize groups in either a closed or open format. Closed groups frequently operate for predetermined time periods and maintain the same membership throughout. In contrast, open groups have revolving membership and accept new individuals whenever space becomes available. One rule of thumb for pediatric groups is that the age or developmental level of the members should be within two or three years of one another because cognitive abilities and social maturity can significantly influence group interaction.

Clinician's Role. The role of the clinician is to function as group leader. Leadership style can be directive or nondirective. A directive style is typically used with groups composed of young children. In addition, it is more common in the early stages of therapy when a group model is being used to teach new communication behaviors. In this role, the clinician sets the agenda, chooses the materials and activities, provides specific instruction, and gives corrective feedback. A nondirective approach is more commonly used in the carryover stages of therapy and with "self-help" groups. In this style, the clinician does not perform a primary teaching function. Instead, group members take charge of session activities, while the clinician serves as a facilitator who oversees rather than directs group interactions. Regardless of style, a group leader is responsible for establishing and maintaining group cohesion, mediating conflicts between members, and ensuring that each member of the group is progressing adequately toward established therapy goals.

Procedures. Several procedures can be used in group settings to maintain the active participation of all members throughout the entire session. In one method, the clinician presents a stimulus and pauses before choosing a particular group member to respond. This strategy increases the likelihood that all members will pay attention and prepare answers to every stimulus in anticipation of being called on. In another strategy, clients can take turns modeling target behaviors for other group members to repeat in unison. Finally, clients can be required to listen, watch, and evaluate the performance of a target behavior by fellow group members.

There are a variety of techniques that clinicians can use to facilitate group interaction. The following examples are applicable to any type of communicative disorder:

- Reinforce client behaviors and comments that are consistent with treatment goals.
- Model the target behaviors/techniques group members are attempting to develop.
- Focus attention and group time on members who are making progress toward established goals.
- Encourage interaction within the group by asking one member to demonstrate a target behavior for the other members.
- Ask open-ended questions that require more than one- or two-word responses.
- Cue a group member to focus on a particular therapy target before she or he begins speaking.
- Restructure comments or topics so they have appeal for all members of the group.
- Use behaviors of individual members to form generalizations that are applicable to the group as a whole.

The delivery of therapy services through a group model has both advantages and disadvantages. The main advantages are as follows:

- Carryover is facilitated.
- Clients stimulate and motivate each other.
- More opportunities exist for natural speaking situations.
- Clients recognize that others have problems similar to their own.
- More occasions exist for clients to engage in critical listening.

- A broader variety of activities and materials can be used.
- The setting provides for socialization and peer interaction.
- Increased opportunities exist to learn by observing others.
- Self-monitoring is encouraged by reducing the client's dependence on the clinician as the sole evaluator of communication behavior.

The primary disadvantages of group intervention include the following:

- Each group member receives less direct attention from the clinician than is given in individual sessions.
- Fewer opportunities exist to address the specific weaknesses of each client, especially when the group is not homogeneous with respect to disorder.
- Clients who are shy, reticent, or of different cultural backgrounds may be reluctant to participate.
- One or two members may become dominant and monopolize the group.
- The group's rate of progress may be too fast for the slowest members and too slow for the most advanced members.

Perhaps the heart of successful group therapy is a clinician's ability to establish and maintain a true group dynamic; otherwise, the sessions merely consist of multiple clients receiving individualized treatment in a group room.

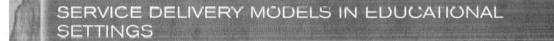

SERVICE DELIVERY MODELS IN EDUCATIONAL SETTINGS

The traditional approach to providing speech-language intervention has been a pull-out model in which a child leaves the classroom and receives therapy in either individual or group sessions. In recent years, there has been a growing trend toward the provision of therapy in a wider variety of service delivery models. Four of the most commonly used models are described below.

Consultative: The clinician acts as a resource for professionals who work directly with a child and parents to help solve problems related to the child's communicative deficit. In this model, the agent of intervention is someone other than the speech-language pathologist (SLP).

Collaborative: The clinician and the classroom teacher share the responsibility for developing speech-language goals for a child and integrating them into the academic curriculum. The goals are implemented primarily by the classroom teacher, although the SLP may occasionally work directly with the child.

Team teaching: The clinician and the teacher share the responsibility for classroom instruction on a regular basis. In this model, a comprehensive program with strong language and academic components can be provided within the context of the classroom.

Self-contained: The clinician alone serves as the classroom teacher and is responsible for developing and implementing all aspects of the curriculum. Classroom activities in all topic areas are specifically designed to promote the development of language skills.

Ultimately, the selection of a particular service delivery model is determined by (1) the needs of a child, (2) the size and composition of a clinician's caseload, and (3) scheduling constraints.

DATA COLLECTION

Speech-language pathologists are accountable for the efficiency as well as the effectiveness of the intervention services they provide. Clients and their families invest valuable time, resources, and effort in the therapy process. The primary mechanism for ensuring clinician accountability is data collection. Information obtained from the data collection process serves two important functions. It allows the clinician to monitor a client's progress from one session to the next. Data collection systems also can be designed to permit documentation of the efficacy of a given treatment strategy. Clinicians need to recognize that "best practices" in service delivery are data driven.

Recording Session Data

Data recording is greatly facilitated by behavioral objectives that are written properly (i.e., in specific and measurable terms). In most cases, data collection difficulties occur because objectives are written in a vague and unclear manner. Following are guidelines for a comprehensive approach to data collection:

1. Appropriate data recording sheets should be designed or selected prior to the onset of a therapy session. (Samples of reproducible data forms and instructions for their use are included in Appendix 1-G at the end of this chapter.)
2. The notation system should provide the type of information that is most relevant to a specific client or disorder. A binary system of "correct" versus "incorrect" is not the only option. Interval scales can be developed to rate responses on a continuum (e.g., degree of correctness or latency of response).
3. The data collection system must allow the clinician to clearly distinguish among imitative, cued/prompted, self-corrected, and spontaneous responses.
4. Once therapy tasks reach the conversational level of complexity, it is often more efficient to use a data recording system that is based on time rather than on total number of responses. For example, it may be easier to document the number of errors per minute rather than identify all occurrences of a target behavior to calculate percentage correct.
5. Reinforcement tokens or stimulus items can be used as an alternative to paper-pencil on-line recording of client responses. One useful approach is

to organize the items/tokens in groups of 10 or 20. Number and percentage of correct responses can be calculated easily by (a) counting the number of unearned reinforcement tokens remaining at the end of an activity or (b) checking the number of stimulus items (e.g., picture cards) that the clinician has placed in a "correct response" versus "incorrect response" pile.

6. Record *every* stimulus-response chain. Even the absence of a response to a particular stimulus should be recorded.

Data collection systems are used to maximize a clinician's effectiveness. It is important to recognize that data yield information regarding a client's status on a particular objective. However, data alone do not identify specific programming changes that may need to be made or how to implement them. These clinical decisions can be made only through a clinician's careful analysis and interpretation of the recorded data.

Probes

Probes are instruments administered periodically throughout treatment to measure a client's progress. They are designed to assess generalization of a trained target behavior (Hegde, 1998). Probes consist of a set of novel stimuli that are equivalent to, but different from, those used for treatment. For example, after teaching the production of initial /s/ with a set of picture cards, the clinician may probe a client's generalization by presenting a new set of unfamiliar pictures to elicit this phoneme (good rule of thumb: 20 stimulus items for each probe).

Probes are similar to baselines in that client responses are elicited without target-specific instruction and do not receive any reinforcement. However, lengthy periods of nonreinforcement may be undesirable for some clients, particularly in the early stages of therapy. Therefore, a **mixed probe** may be instituted, whereby both trained and untrained stimulus items are presented in an alternating sequence. In this procedure, the client continues to receive reinforcement for responses to the trained stimuli.

The findings obtained from probe procedures are used by the clinician to determine the next step in the therapy program. If the predetermined criterion from the behavioral objective has not been achieved, training should continue at the current level. If the criterion has been met, the clinician may choose to shift to a higher level of response complexity in the same target area or move on to a new communicative behavior. Periodic administration of probes is especially important because it minimizes the risk of continuing therapy that is no longer effective or necessary.

Treatment Efficacy/Evidence-Based Practice

Treatment efficacy is a general term that encompasses three basic factors: effectiveness (Does treatment work?); efficiency (Does one treatment work better or faster than another?); and effects (In what ways does treatment alter behavior?). For certain communicative disorders, such as those involving voice and fluency, the definition of successful treatment should account for subjective variables (e.g., client feelings, willingness to communicate) as well as objective variables (e.g., number of stuttered words, maintenance of specified optimal pitch).

In the context of clinical intervention, the most typical approach to data collection is the following single subject design: pretreatment baseline of a target → treatment → posttreatment baseline of the same behavior (in which the baseline measures are identical to one another and different from the treatment items). The information obtained from this data collection method is useful in documenting the amount of change or progress for a specific client. However, it does not address treatment efficacy in that this design does not permit the clinician to determine whether the intervention itself was responsible for the observed change.

To more adequately document the efficacy of treatment, a **multiple baseline** design can be implemented. A simple multiple baseline procedure involves the selection of at least three target behaviors of similar complexity that are in need of remediation. It is important to choose a set of targets for which direct transfer of learning is not expected to occur from one behavior to the others. For example, it is inappropriate to include phonemes that differ from each other by only one feature (e.g., voicing). Baseline measures are then obtained to ascertain their pretreatment status. Treatment procedures are then implemented for one of the targets. After criterion has been reached on the trained behavior, the clinician repeats the baseline measures on the untrained targets. If the results show no significant change from the original baseline scores, the clinician can be confident that the treatment, and no other factor, was responsible for the client's improvement on the trained target. One of the remaining targets is then selected for training and the treatment/posttreatment baseline sequence is repeated. This procedure is continued until all therapy targets have been trained.

TROUBLESHOOTING TIPS FOR THERAPY SESSIONS

If your client is not making adequate progress or seems bored and inattentive, ask yourself the following questions:

1. Are the reinforcers that I am using during therapy activities really motivating for this client?
2. Am I delivering the reinforcers fast enough for the client to connect them with the target behavior?
3. Did I shift from a continuous reinforcement schedule to an intermittent schedule too soon?
4. Am I teaching the target behavior in small enough steps?
5. Am I presenting the stimuli when the client is not paying attention or not making eye contact?
6. Is the client bored because the same therapy materials are being used too often?
7. Is the client confused because I tend to phrase instructions in the form of requests rather than directions?

8. Am I programming a sufficient variety of target behaviors during each session to maintain the client's interest and motivation level?
9. Am I providing enough prompts during difficult therapy tasks to ensure that the client is relatively successful?
10. Am I allowing the client to make too many errors in a row without modifying the task?
11. Am I telling the client what he or she does well or giving feedback only about incorrect responses?
12. Am I giving the client enough time to respond before repeating or rephrasing the stimuli?
13. Did I anticipate the unexpected and prepare 50% more material than I thought I needed?

CONCLUSION

This chapter has presented basic information, protocols, and procedures for intervention for communicative disorders at an **introductory** level. This information is intended only as a starting point in the reader's clinical education and training. For in-depth coverage of this area, the following readings are recommended:

Hegde, M. N. (1998). *Treatment procedures in communicative disorders.* Austin, TX: Pro-Ed.

Hegde, M. N., & Davis, D. (2005). *Clinical methods and practicum in speech-language pathology* (4th ed.). Clifton Park, NY: Thomson Delmar Learning.

Paul, R. (2002). *Introduction to clinical methods on communication disorders.* Baltimore: Paul H. Brookes.

ADDITIONAL RESOURCES

Therasimplicity Inc.
832 North Shore Drive
New Richmond, WI 54017
Phone: 800-839-7949
Fax: 715-246-7517
E-mail: info@therasimplicity.com

TSI Software Library
A series of "books" that allow clinicians to access and print therapy materials such as cards, sequences, photographs, and pictures for a wide range of communication disorders. Also includes medical encyclopedia and graphics for creating cards, templates, and certificates. Provides information on products in 23 areas (e.g., feeding, motor development).

APPENDIX 1-A

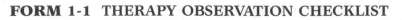

FORM 1-1 THERAPY OBSERVATION CHECKLIST

Date:_____   KEY:

Clinician:_____   4 = Outstanding   1 = Weak

Supervisor: _____   3 = Above average   0 = Unsatisfactory

Client: _____   2 = Average   N/A = Not applicable

Programming

_____ Clear rationale for behavioral objectives/activities

_____ Appropriate written formulation of objectives (do statement, condition, criterion)

_____ Data from previous session used to determine behavioral goals

_____ Skill in revising goals/procedures as necessary during session (branching)

Behavior Modification

_____ Appropriate type of reinforcement

_____ Appropriate schedule of reinforcement

_____ Client behavior managed consistently in a firm yet nonthreatening manner

Key Teaching Strategies

_____ Target behaviors modeled accurately

_____ Target-specific feedback provided consistently

_____ Brief summary of performance given after each activity

_____ Therapy techniques appropriate for client's age/developmental level and disorder

_____ Appropriate home assignments given with written instruction and demonstration

Session Design

_____ Clear preinstruction given for each target behavior

_____ Communication style adapted to needs of the client (vocabulary, language level, nonverbal communication)

(continues)

Appendix 1-A (continued)

_____ Appropriate interpersonal skills; establishing rapport, motivating client

_____ Poised, confident demeanor

_____ Appropriate pace and amount of target productions

_____ Creative and appropriate therapy materials

_____ Appropriate proxemics

_____ Objectives for each client integrated into group sessions

Data Collection

_____ Ability to judge responses accurately

_____ Consistent, accurate data collection

FORM 1-2 WORKSHEET FOR IDENTIFYING BEHAVIORAL OBJECTIVES

Instructions: The objectives listed below are stated incorrectly. Identify the errors in each objective by placing a check mark in the appropriate column(s).

Objective	Do	Condition	Criterion
1. Client will understand the concept of "red" with 90% accuracy when shown 30 cards.			
2. Client will produce /f/ several times given the clinician's model.			
3. Client will produce a complete sentence in four out of five trials.			
4. Client will use the regular past tense with no errors.			
5. Client will improve voice quality while reciting nursery rhymes with less than one parameter break per minute.			
6. To elicit /s/ and /z/ in single words by presenting familiar objects.			
7. Client will produce "is + verb + ing" with 80% accuracy.			
8. Client will comprehend two-stage directions 100% of the time.			
9. Client will use the stuttering modification technique of "pull-out" frequently during a one-minute monologue.			
10. Student will write 10 behavioral objectives that meet the criteria as discussed in this chapter.			

*Answer key is on next page.

(continues)

Appendix 1-B (continued)

ANSWER KEY: WORKSHEET FOR IDENTIFYING BEHAVIORAL OBJECTIVES

Instructions: The objectives listed below are stated incorrectly. Identify the errors in each objective by placing a check mark in the appropriate column(s).

Objective	Do	Condition	Criterion
1. Client will understand the concept of "red" with 90% accuracy when shown 30 cards.	X		
2. Client will produce /f/ several times given the clinician's model.			X
3. Client will produce a complete sentence in four out of five trials.		X	
4. Client will use the regular past tense with no errors.		X	
5. Client will improve voice quality while reciting nursery rhymes with less than one parameter break per minute.	X		
6. To elicit /s/ and /z/ in single words by presenting familiar objects.	X		X
7. Client will produce "is + verb + ing" with 80% accuracy.		X	
8. Client will comprehend two-stage directions 100% of the time.	X	X	
9. Client will use the stuttering modification technique of "pull-out" frequently during a one-minute monologue.			X
10. Student will write 10 behavioral objectives that meet the criteria as discussed in this chapter.		X	X

APPENDIX 1-C

FORM 1-3 WORKSHEET FOR FORMULATING AND WRITING BEHAVIORAL OBJECTIVES

1. Do statement: Maintain phonation of a vowel for an average of 1.8 seconds

   Conditions: Using the inhalation method

   Criterion: 9 correct of 10 trials

   Behavioral Objective: _____

   _____

   _____

2. Do statement: Manipulate objects

   Conditions: Given oral directions containing the concepts up-down, in-out, on-under

   Criterion: With no errors

   Behavioral Objective: _____

   _____

   _____

3. Do statement: Imitate nonspeech vocalizations

   Conditions: Given the clinician's model

                   Given no more than two verbal prompts

   Criterion: 90% accuracy

   Behavioral Objective: _____

   _____

   _____

4. Do statement: Tally instances of disfluency

   Conditions: While watching a videotape of himself speaking

   Criterion: 95% agreement with the clinician's tally

   Behavioral Objective: _____

   _____

   _____

(continues)

Appendix 1-C (continued)

5. Do statement: Produce fricatives /f/, /v/, /s/ in CV syllables

   Conditions: In imitation of the clinician

   In response to pictures

   Criterion: With 90% accuracy over two consecutive sessions

   Behavioral Objective: _____

   _____

   _____

6. Do statement: Use easy onset of phonation

   Conditions: On the telephone

   While reading a written script

   Criterion: With less than two errors

   Behavioral Objective: _____

   _____

   _____

7. Do statement: Sort 20 pictures of common objects

   Conditions: According to categories named by clinician

   Criterion: 18 correct of 20 trials

   Behavioral Objective: _____

   _____

   _____

8. Do statement: Say words with /sw/ in the initial position

   Conditions: While looking in a mirror

   Criterion: 100% accuracy

   Behavioral Objective: _____

   _____

   _____

9. Do statement: Maintain correct production of all forms of the verb "to be"

   Conditions: In spontaneous conversation with the clinician

   Criterion: No more than one error per three-minute segment

   Behavioral Objective:_____

   _____

   _____

APPENDIX 1-D

FORM 1-4 SAMPLE DAILY THERAPY PLAN

Client: __John Adams__   Clinician: __Marie Landers__

Date: __March 8, 2005__   Disorder: __Articulation/Language__

Behavioral Objectives	Data/Results
1. Given 10 pictures for each position and asked to create a sentence for each word, John will produce /f/ in the initial, medial, and final positions (IMF) with 90% accuracy.	/f/ I = 100% /f/ M = 90% /f/ F = 60% He was heard to use /f/ initial correctly in off-task comments. 5/6 errors in final position were ө/f.
2. John will correctly label the position of a block in relation to another object as "on" or "under" with 90% accuracy.	30/40 = 75%. Was only required to say "on" or "under" but on the last six responses, client used a phrase as the answer (i.e., "on the chair").
3. John will follow two-step commands with four linguistic elements in response to clinician's verbal directions for nine out of ten trials.	5/10 – had to be reminded to refrain from responding until entire command was presented.
4. John will imitatively produce CVC words maintaining final consonant with 90% accuracy.	28/50 = 56%

Reinforcement = 1:1 token + verbal praise
20 tokens = 1 puzzle piece

(continues)

Appendix 1-D (continued)

OBSERVATION AND COMMENTS

Client: John has met the criterion for /f/ I and M. Next session we will work only on F position. His spontaneous use of phrases during the preposition activity indicates that he is ready to move beyond the single-word response stage. The data for the two-step command activity suggests that this task needs to be modified. Maybe I will try a tactile prompt by placing my hands over his while presenting each command. I will instruct him that he can start responding as soon as I remove my hands from his. For the final consonant task, John needs some kind of cue to improve his performance. What do you think about using a visual prompt that highlights the concept of "final position" like a train that has three parts: an engine, one car, and a caboose? I gave Mom written instructions for homework for the initial and medial /f/ and for prepositions.

Clinician: The articulation work took up a lot of time today, especially the final consonant activity. I need to design the next session so that an equivalent amount of time is spent on the language and articulation activities. I reviewed the audiotape from today's session and I think my feedback to John was immediate and specific to the targets. I think that my ability to accurately judge correct versus incorrect articulation responses is improving. I need to start fading the continuous reinforcement schedule for the tasks on which John is achieving an accuracy rate of 70% or higher.

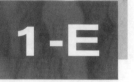

APPENDIX

FORM 1-5 DAILY THERAPY PLAN

Client: _____   Clinician: _____

Date: _____   Disorder: _____

Behavioral Objectives	Data/Results

(continues)

Appendix 1-E (continued)

OBSERVATION AND COMMENTS

FORM 1-6 REPORT OF OBSERVATION HOURS

Name: _____

_____

Semester: _____

KEY:

Age: C = Children   A = Adults

Category: Select from list below
Articulation Language Fluency Voice Other
Hearing Evaluation   Selection/Use of Amplification
& Assistive Listening Devices   Aural Rehabilitation

Date	Client's First Name and Initial	Age	Category	Hours Diag.	Ther.	Supervisor Initials
1						
2						
3						
4						
5						
6						
7						
8						
9						
10						
11						
12						
13						
14						
15						
16						
17						
18						
19						
20						
21						
22						
23						
24						
25						

Total Observed Hours

Number of Speech Hours: _____

Supervisor's Signature: _____

Date: _____

Number of Audiology Hours: _____

Supervisor's Signature: _____

Date: _____

APPENDIX 1-G

INSTRUCTIONS FOR USING DATA RECORDING FORMS

Session Data Log: This is an all-purpose data sheet designed to record an individual client's performance within a single session. Determine the type of notational system that will be used to record client responses (e.g., + or −, o or x, and so on) and enter this information in the box labeled "Key." Write the name or description of tasks in the left column (up to a maximum of eighteen). The numbered boxes indicate the number of trials. Record the accuracy of each response in the appropriate box. If the number of trials on a given task exceeds 20, continue to record on the next line of the grid. Calculate percentage of correct responses and enter this information in the far right column for each task.

Summary Data Log: This form is used to summarize information about an individual client's performance across a maximum of 20 sessions. It is designed to display client progress on specific therapy tasks over time. Enter session numbers or session dates in the boxes indicated at the top of the grid. Write the name or description of tasks in the left column (up to a maximum of 17). Retrieve the percentage of correct responses for each task from previous daily sheets (e.g., Session Data Log) and enter this information under each session date or number.

Summary Data Graph: Like the Summary Data Log, this form is used to summarize information about a client's status across a maximum of 20 sessions. The unique aspect of this form is that it allows the clinician to graph a client's progress on one or more objectives. Select a code for each objective that will be used on the graph to plot client performance. The code can consist of lines of different colors or patterns (e.g., solid, dotted, hatched, and so on). Enter this information along with a brief description of each task in the Key box. Retrieve performance data for each task from daily data sheets. Enter the session dates on the designated line, beginning with the pretreatment baseline session. Plot percentage of performance on the graph for each date (and for each task) and connect the data points to create a visual display of client progress.

Response Data Form: This is an all-purpose data sheet designed to track an individual client's responses on a single task during one session. It allows the clinician to document the specific stimulus items that are presented to a client during a given activity. Write the behavioral objective, therapy materials, and reinforcement type and schedule on the designated lines. Determine the type of notational system that will be used to record client responses (e.g., + or −, o or x, and so on) and enter this information in the Key. Record each stimulus in the left-hand column as it is presented. Note correct versus incorrect responses in column 1. This form can accommodate 20 stimulus items, which can be presented for a maximum of 10 trials each. Count the number of correct and incorrect responses and calculate the percentage of accuracy. Enter this information in the appropriate box at the lower left of the form.

Response Rating Scale: This is a general form that can be used to document an individual client's performance within a single session. This form utilizes a scale that allows the clinician to rate the quality of a client's responses along a **continuum** of accuracy. The continuum is a five-level scale that includes the old error pattern (O), cued responses (C), approximations (A), self-corrections (S), and the new target behavior (T). Enter the task in the left column. The numbered

(continues)

Appendix 1-G (continued)

boxes indicate the number of trials. Record the rating for each response (i.e., O, C, A, S, T) in the appropriate box. If the number of trials on a given task exceeds 20, continue to record on the next line of the grid. Calculate the percentage of each response type, and enter this information in the far right columns for each task.

Articulation Data Sheet: This form is designed to record an individual client's responses during articulation therapy. Determine the type of notational system that will be used to record the client's responses (e.g., + or −, o or x, and so on) and enter this information in the box labeled "Key." This form can be used in at least two ways. It can function as a data sheet for a single session, or it can be used to track a client's progress over time. Enter the session date and the therapy activity in the appropriate boxes. *All* correct and incorrect responses for each activity are recorded in a *single* box under the appropriate level of difficulty (e.g., Isolation, Syllable, Words, and so on). A single box may contain as many as 20 to 30 response notations. The amount of time spent on each activity also can be documented on this form. Count the number of total and correct responses and calculate the percentage of accuracy. Enter this information in the appropriate box.

Individual/Group Quick Tally Sheet: This form is designed for data collection in individual or group therapy sessions. For individual sessions, enter the client's name in the first box on the left. Assign a code or number (e.g., A or #1) for each activity, and enter this information for the first activity in the same box. As the stimuli are presented, record incorrect responses by making a slash mark through the corresponding number. Correct responses are indicated by the lack of a slash mark. Tally the number of correct responses, and calculate the percentage of accuracy. Enter this information on the appropriate lines. Repeat this procedure for each subsequent activity (except for re-writing the client's name). For group sessions, this form can be used in at least two ways depending on the size of the group. For groups of three or fewer, enter the name, activity code, and response data for each individual from left to right across the page in the same row. This orientation permits data to be recorded on a maximum of six activities for each group member. For groups with three to six members, enter the data for each client from top to bottom down the page in the same column. This orientation accommodates a maximum of three activities per group member.

Group Therapy Data Sheet: This form is designed for use in therapy groups that range in size from two to four members. Determine the type of notational system that will be used to record the clients' responses (e.g., + or −, o or x, and so on) and enter this information on the line labeled "Response Key." Enter each group member's name on the indicated line. Assign a code or number (e.g., A or #1) for each activity, and enter this information for each group member in the appropriate box. Record the accuracy of each client's responses in the boxes below the numbers. This data form allows for a maximum of 50 trials (per member) to be recorded for each activity. The amount of time each client spends on a given activity also can be documented on this form. Count the number of correct and total responses and calculate the percentage of accuracy for each client. Enter this information in the appropriate boxes.

Classroom Data Form: This form is an example of a data sheet used in the classroom to track performance of multiple children on eight curriculum-based language goals. Enter one child's name in each block in the first column. Indicate incorrect responses with slash marks through specific stimulus items. This form can be used to calculate percentage of accuracy for individual children on one or more goals. In addition, performance accuracy of the entire group can be monitored for all eight identified goals.

(continues)

Appendix 1-G (continued)

FORM 1-7 SESSION DATA LOG

SESSION DATA LOG

Name of Client: _____

Name of Clinician: _____

Date: _____

KEY:
_____
_____
_____

Trials

Task	1	2	3	4	5	6	7	8	9	10	11	12	13	14	15	16	17	18	19	20	% correct

(continues)

Appendix 1-G (continued)

FORM 1-8 SUMMARY DATA LOG

SUMMARY DATA LOG

Name of Client: _____

Name of Clinician: _____

Date or Session #

Task

(continues)

Appendix 1-G (continued)

FORM 1-9 SUMMARY DATA GRAPH

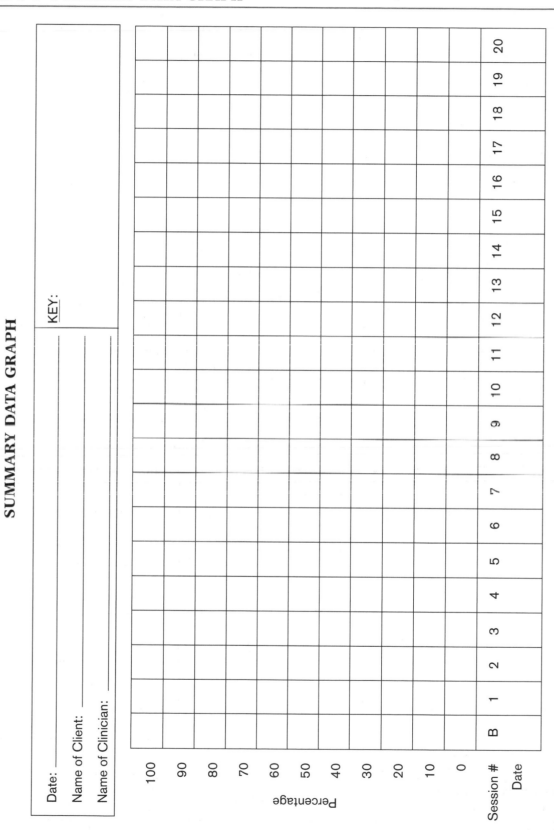

(continues)

Appendix 1-G (continued)

FORM 1-10 RESPONSE DATA FORM

RESPONSE DATA FORM

Name of Client: _____ Date: _____

Name of Clinician: _____

Behavioral Objective: _____

Therapy Materials: _____

Reinforcement Type and Schedule: _____

Trials

Stimulus Presented	1	2	3	4	5	6	7	8	9	10	Comments
1.											
2.											
3.											
4.											
5.											
6.											
7.											
8.											
9.											
10.											
11.											
12.											
13.											
14.											
15.											
16.											
17.											
18.											
19.											
20.											

Total Number of Responses:	<u>KEY</u>:
Total Correct Responses:	
Total Incorrect Responses:	
Percent Correct:	

(continues)

Appendix 1-G (continued)

FORM 1-11 RESPONSE RATING SCALE

RESPONSE RATING SCALE

Name of Client: _____

Name of Clinician: _____

Date: _____

KEY:

O = Old behavior S = Self-correction

C = Cued response T = Target behavior

A = Approximation

Trials

Task	1	2	3	4	5	6	7	8	9	10	11	12	13	14	15	16	17	18	19	20	% O	% C	% A	% S	% T

(continues)

Appendix 1-G (continued)

FORM 1-12 ARTICULATION DATA SHEET

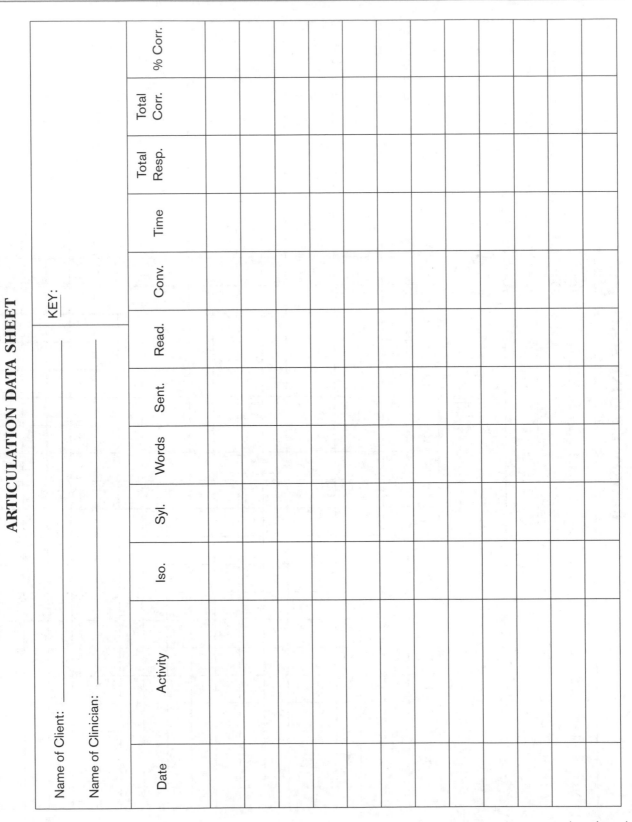

ARTICULATION DATA SHEET

Name of Client: _____

Name of Clinician: _____

KEY: _____

Date	Activity	Iso.	Syl.	Words	Sent.	Read.	Conv.	Time	Total Resp.	Total Corr.	% Corr.

(continues)

Appendix 1-G (continued)

FORM 1-13 INDIVIDUAL/GROUP QUICK TALLY SHEET

INDIVIDUAL/GROUP QUICK TALLY SHEET

Clinician: ______________________ Date: ______________________

Name ______
Activity ______

1	2	3	4	5
6	7	8	9	10
11	12	13	14	15
16	17	18	19	20
21	22	23	24	25
26	27	28	29	30
31	32	33	34	35
36	37	38	39	40
41	42	43	44	45
46	47	48	49	50

Correct ______
% Correct ______

Name ______
Activity ______

1	2	3	4	5
6	7	8	9	10
11	12	13	14	15
16	17	18	19	20
21	22	23	24	25
26	27	28	29	30
31	32	33	34	35
36	37	38	39	40
41	42	43	44	45
46	47	48	49	50

Correct ______
% Correct ______

Name ______
Activity ______

1	2	3	4	5
6	7	8	9	10
11	12	13	14	15
16	17	18	19	20
21	22	23	24	25
26	27	28	29	30
31	32	33	34	35
36	37	38	39	40
41	42	43	44	45
46	47	48	49	50

Correct ______
% Correct ______

Name ______
Activity ______

1	2	3	4	5
6	7	8	9	10
11	12	13	14	15
16	17	18	19	20
21	22	23	24	25
26	27	28	29	30
31	32	33	34	35
36	37	38	39	40
41	42	43	44	45
46	47	48	49	50

Correct ______
% Correct ______

Name ______
Activity ______

1	2	3	4	5
6	7	8	9	10
11	12	13	14	15
16	17	18	19	20
21	22	23	24	25
26	27	28	29	30
31	32	33	34	35
36	37	38	39	40
41	42	43	44	45
46	47	48	49	50

Correct ______
% Correct ______

Name ______
Activity ______

1	2	3	4	5
6	7	8	9	10
11	12	13	14	15
16	17	18	19	20
21	22	23	24	25
26	27	28	29	30
31	32	33	34	35
36	37	38	39	40
41	42	43	44	45
46	47	48	49	50

Correct ______
% Correct ______

Name ______
Activity ______

1	2	3	4	5
6	7	8	9	10
11	12	13	14	15
16	17	18	19	20
21	22	23	24	25
26	27	28	29	30
31	32	33	34	35
36	37	38	39	40
41	42	43	44	45
46	47	48	49	50

Correct ______
% Correct ______

Name ______
Activity ______

1	2	3	4	5
6	7	8	9	10
11	12	13	14	15
16	17	18	19	20
21	22	23	24	25
26	27	28	29	30
31	32	33	34	35
36	37	38	39	40
41	42	43	44	45
46	47	48	49	50

Correct ______
% Correct ______

Name ______
Activity ______

1	2	3	4	5
6	7	8	9	10
11	12	13	14	15
16	17	18	19	20
21	22	23	24	25
26	27	28	29	30
31	32	33	34	35
36	37	38	39	40
41	42	43	44	45
46	47	48	49	50

Correct ______
% Correct ______

Name ______
Activity ______

1	2	3	4	5
6	7	8	9	10
11	12	13	14	15
16	17	18	19	20
21	22	23	24	25
26	27	28	29	30
31	32	33	34	35
36	37	38	39	40
41	42	43	44	45
46	47	48	49	50

Correct ______
% Correct ______

Name ______
Activity ______

1	2	3	4	5
6	7	8	9	10
11	12	13	14	15
16	17	18	19	20
21	22	23	24	25
26	27	28	29	30
31	32	33	34	35
36	37	38	39	40
41	42	43	44	45
46	47	48	49	50

Correct ______
% Correct ______

Name ______
Activity ______

1	2	3	4	5
6	7	8	9	10
11	12	13	14	15
16	17	18	19	20
21	22	23	24	25
26	27	28	29	30
31	32	33	34	35
36	37	38	39	40
41	42	43	44	45
46	47	48	49	50

Correct ______
% Correct ______

Name ______
Activity ______

1	2	3	4	5
6	7	8	9	10
11	12	13	14	15
16	17	18	19	20
21	22	23	24	25
26	27	28	29	30
31	32	33	34	35
36	37	38	39	40
41	42	43	44	45
46	47	48	49	50

Correct ______
% Correct ______

Name ______
Activity ______

1	2	3	4	5
6	7	8	9	10
11	12	13	14	15
16	17	18	19	20
21	22	23	24	25
26	27	28	29	30
31	32	33	34	35
36	37	38	39	40
41	42	43	44	45
46	47	48	49	50

Correct ______
% Correct ______

Name ______
Activity ______

1	2	3	4	5
6	7	8	9	10
11	12	13	14	15
16	17	18	19	20
21	22	23	24	25
26	27	28	29	30
31	32	33	34	35
36	37	38	39	40
41	42	43	44	45
46	47	48	49	50

Correct ______
% Correct ______

Name ______
Activity ______

1	2	3	4	5
6	7	8	9	10
11	12	13	14	15
16	17	18	19	20
21	22	23	24	25
26	27	28	29	30
31	32	33	34	35
36	37	38	39	40
41	42	43	44	45
46	47	48	49	50

Correct ______
% Correct ______

Name ______
Activity ______

1	2	3	4	5
6	7	8	9	10
11	12	13	14	15
16	17	18	19	20
21	22	23	24	25
26	27	28	29	30
31	32	33	34	35
36	37	38	39	40
41	42	43	44	45
46	47	48	49	50

Correct ______
% Correct ______

Name ______
Activity ______

1	2	3	4	5
6	7	8	9	10
11	12	13	14	15
16	17	18	19	20
21	22	23	24	25
26	27	28	29	30
31	32	33	34	35
36	37	38	39	40
41	42	43	44	45
46	47	48	49	50

Correct ______
% Correct ______

(continues)

Appendix 1-G (continued)

FORM 1-14 GROUP THERAPY DATA SHEET

GROUP THERAPY DATA SHEET

Date: _____ Clinician: _____

Name: _____ Response Key: _____

Activity:						Time:				# Correct:					Total Resp.:					% Correct:				
1	2	3	4	5	6	7	8	9	10	11	12	13	14	15	16	17	18	19	20	21	22	23	24	25
26	27	28	29	30	31	32	33	34	35	36	37	38	39	40	41	42	43	44	45	46	47	48	49	50

Name: _____

Activity:						Time:				# Correct:					Total Resp.:					% Correct:				
1	2	3	4	5	6	7	8	9	10	11	12	13	14	15	16	17	18	19	20	21	22	23	24	25
26	27	28	29	30	31	32	33	34	35	36	37	38	39	40	41	42	43	44	45	46	47	48	49	50

Name: _____

Activity:						Time:				# Correct:					Total Resp.:					% Correct:				
1	2	3	4	5	6	7	8	9	10	11	12	13	14	15	16	17	18	19	20	21	22	23	24	25
26	27	28	29	30	31	32	33	34	35	36	37	38	39	40	41	42	43	44	45	46	47	48	49	50

Name: _____

Activity:						Time:				# Correct:					Total Resp.:					% Correct:				
1	2	3	4	5	6	7	8	9	10	11	12	13	14	15	16	17	18	19	20	21	22	23	24	25
26	27	28	29	30	31	32	33	34	35	36	37	38	39	40	41	42	43	44	45	46	47	48	49	50

(continues)

Appendix 1-G (continued)

FORM 1-15 CLASSROOM DATA FORM: BASIC CONCEPTS

CLASSROOM DATA FORM: BASIC CONCEPTS

Date: _____

Child's Name	Names Letter	Names Sound	Names Color	Names Shape	Counts 1–20	Names Number	Names Day	Names Month
	A B C D E F G H I J K L M N O P Q R S T U V W X Y Z	A B C D E F G H I J K L M N O P Q R S T U V W X Y Z	Red Yellow Blue Orange Green White Black	Circle Oval Square Triangle Rectangle	1 2 3 4 5 6 7 8 9 10 11 12 13 14 15 16 17 18 19 20	1 2 3 4 5 6 7 8 9 10 11 12 13 14 15 16 17 18 19 20	Sun Mon Tues Wed Thurs Fri Sat Sun	Jan Feb Mar Apr May June July Aug Sept Oct Nov Dec
	A B C D E F G H I J K L M N O P Q R S T U V W X Y Z	A B C D E F G H I J K L M N O P Q R S T U V W X Y Z	Red Yellow Blue Orange Green White Black	Circle Oval Square Triangle Rectangle	1 2 3 4 5 6 7 8 9 10 11 12 13 14 15 16 17 18 19 20	1 2 3 4 5 6 7 8 9 10 11 12 13 14 15 16 17 18 19 20	Sun Mon Tues Wed Thurs Fri Sat Sun	Jan Feb Mar Apr May June July Aug Sept Oct Nov Dec
	A B C D E F G H I J K L M N O P Q R S T U V W X Y Z	A B C D E F G H I J K L M N O P Q R S T U V W X Y Z	Red Yellow Blue Orange Green White Black	Circle Oval Square Triangle Rectangle	1 2 3 4 5 6 7 8 9 10 11 12 13 14 15 16 17 18 19 20	1 2 3 4 5 6 7 8 9 10 11 12 13 14 15 16 17 18 19 20	Sun Mon Tues Wed Thurs Fri Sat Sun	Jan Feb Mar Apr May June July Aug Sept Oct Nov Dec
	A B C D E F G H I J K L M N O P Q R S T U V W X Y Z	A B C D E F G H I J K L M N O P Q R S T U V W X Y Z	Red Yellow Blue Orange Green White Black	Circle Oval Square Triangle Rectangle	1 2 3 4 5 6 7 8 9 10 11 12 13 14 15 16 17 18 19 20	1 2 3 4 5 6 7 8 9 10 11 12 13 14 15 16 17 18 19 20	Sun Mon Tues Wed Thurs Fri Sat Sun	Jan Feb Mar Apr May June July Aug Sept Oct Nov Dec
	A B C D E F G H I J K L M N O P Q R S T U V W X Y Z	A B C D E F G H I J K L M N O P Q R S T U V W X Y Z	Red Yellow Blue Orange Green White Black	Circle Oval Square Triangle Rectangle	1 2 3 4 5 6 7 8 9 10 11 12 13 14 15 16 17 18 19 20	1 2 3 4 5 6 7 8 9 10 11 12 13 14 15 16 17 18 19 20	Sun Mon Tues Wed Thurs Fri Sat Sun	Jan Feb Mar Apr May June July Aug Sept Oct Nov Dec
	A B C D E F G H I J K L M N O P Q R S T U V W X Y Z	A B C D E F G H I J K L M N O P Q R S T U V W X Y Z	Red Yellow Blue Orange Green White Black	Circle Oval Square Triangle Rectangle	1 2 3 4 5 6 7 8 9 10 11 12 13 14 15 16 17 18 19 20	1 2 3 4 5 6 7 8 9 10 11 12 13 14 15 16 17 18 19 20	Sun Mon Tues Wed Thurs Fri Sat Sun	Jan Feb Mar Apr May June July Aug Sept Oct Nov Dec
	A B C D E F G H I J K L M N O P Q R S T U V W X Y Z	A B C D E F G H I J K L M N O P Q R S T U V W X Y Z	Red Yellow Blue Orange Green White Black	Circle Oval Square Triangle Rectangle	1 2 3 4 5 6 7 8 9 10 11 12 13 14 15 16 17 18 19 20	1 2 3 4 5 6 7 8 9 10 11 12 13 14 15 16 17 18 19 20	Sun Mon Tues Wed Thurs Fri Sat Sun	Jan Feb Mar Apr May June July Aug Sept Oct Nov Dec
	A B C D E F G H I J K L M N O P Q R S T U V W X Y Z	A B C D E F G H I J K L M N O P Q R S T U V W X Y Z	Red Yellow Blue Orange Green White Black	Circle Oval Square Triangle Rectangle	1 2 3 4 5 6 7 8 9 10 11 12 13 14 15 16 17 18 19 20	1 2 3 4 5 6 7 8 9 10 11 12 13 14 15 16 17 18 19 20	Sun Mon Tues Wed Thurs Fri Sat Sun	Jan Feb Mar Apr May June July Aug Sept Oct Nov Dec

CHAPTER 2

Information Reporting Systems and Techniques

PHILOSOPHY

The main purpose of clinical reports is to summarize and interpret information regarding a client's performance or status. In this chapter, the term "report" is used to refer to written records that may vary in length from multiple-page documents to brief notations in client charts. A well-written document does more than report test scores and performance data. It provides an explanation of each data point and specifies its relation to a client's overall communication profile and needs. Numbers alone do not yield this interpretive information. Inferential statements must always be substantiated by supporting data. Adherence to this philosophy of clinical writing promotes clinician accountability by providing justification for the judgments and decisions that occur throughout the treatment process.

Accountability also requires that reports be written with ethical considerations in mind. Prognosis and recommendation statements, in particular, must be written carefully to ensure that they are not misleading or unrealistic. For example, consider the following prognostic statement for a 60-year-old male with moderate aphasia who suffered his stroke 10 years ago:

> Based on Mr. Hanks' high level of enthusiasm, the prognosis for improvement in therapy is good.

This statement is inappropriate for two important reasons. First, a client's degree of enthusiasm is not a reliable indicator of future success. Moreover, the amount of time that has elapsed since Mr. Hanks' stroke (a more meaningful indicator) would warrant a more guarded statement of prognosis. Ethical considerations also significantly influence the development of treatment recommendations. These statements must be based solely on client needs rather than on the type and frequency of service that a particular therapist or facility can provide.

TECHNICAL WRITING STYLE

Clinical reports are formal documents that must be written in an appropriate technical style (Hegde & Davis, 1999; Knepflar & May, 1989). In many cases, written reports may be the first or the only avenue of contact between a speech-language pathologist and other professionals. Poorly written reports can severely compromise a clinician's professional credibility. Imagine the reaction of a physician when reading the following section of a speech-language pathologist's progress report:

> Shirley was initially nervous in the therapy room, particularly when her mother, she thought was going to leave her, she cried. Difficult to illicit spontaneous utterances from her, though she was willing to imitate.

For this reason, the ability to communicate effectively in writing is as important as a clinician's knowledge of communication disorders and their treatment. The following guidelines can assist in the development of professional reports that are clear, concise, and well-organized.

- Avoid writing clinical reports in a conversational style (e.g., "He just didn't get the point" versus "He did not appear to understand the task").

- Use correct spelling, grammar, and punctuation and write in complete sentences.

- Write in the third person (e.g., "The Token Test was administered" rather than "I administered the Token Test").

- Avoid use of contracted verb forms (e.g., isn't, can't, I've).

- Give the full names of tests when first mentioned before using acronyms and other abbreviations in the remainder of the report.

- Express information in behavioral terms (e.g., "followed two-step commands" versus "is able to follow two-step commands").

- Present information (particularly case history) in chronological sequence.

- Differentiate clearly between information reported by others versus information obtained directly through clinician observation.

- List all data such as test scores or baseline measures before providing any interpretative statements. This approach facilitates interpretation of a client's overall profile rather than presenting unrelated descriptions of isolated communication skills.

- Include information about a client's strengths as well as weaknesses in the body of the report.

- Avoid presenting information in the summary section of any report that was not introduced previously in the body of the report.

- Write reports to communicate with colleagues using professional terminology, but include simple explanations and clear examples to make reports meaningful to family members and other nonprofessionals.

- Use language that is specific and unambiguous (e.g., "He demonstrated language skills characteristic of 4-year-old children" versus "He demonstrated poor language skills").

- Avoid exaggeration and overstatement (e.g., "*completely* uncooperative," "*absolutely* intelligible," "*never* produces /s/," "*extremely* motivated").

REPORT FORMATS

In the context of intervention, clinical reports serve three main purposes: (1) to outline the intended intervention plan at the beginning of therapy, (2) to monitor client performance on a session-to-session basis throughout the course of treatment, and (3) to summarize client status periodically and at the end of the treatment program. Report formats for each of these functions can vary greatly among clinicians and service delivery settings. Regardless of the particular format, however, a basic core of information must be included in each of the three types of reports. Following is a framework for each report type.

Initial Therapy Plan

An initial therapy plan (ITP) is developed at the beginning of treatment for each client. It specifies long-term goals and short-term objectives based on diagnostic findings and pretreatment baseline results. Following are the basic content and organization of an ITP.

Identifying Information. List identifying information at the top of the report. This section may include a client's name, age, address, type of disorder, date of report, and so on.

Example

Name:	Jose Rodriguez	Date of Birth:	July 15, 1997
Parents:	Carlos and Maria Rodriguez	Age:	7 years, 3 months
Address:	1800 Knox Street	Date of Report:	October 25, 2004
	College Park, MD 20740	Disorder:	Articulation and Language
		Clinician:	Gary Frost

Background Information. In paragraph form, state the full name and age of the client and the location and date of the initial evaluation, and summarize diagnostic information in one or two sentences. For clients who have received previous therapy, this section should specify the provider, identify the dates of service, and briefly summarize goals and progress.

Example

Jose Rodriguez, a 7-year, 3-month-old male, was evaluated at Children's Hospital on May 23, 2004. While his parents' native language is Spanish, Jose is reported to use English as his primary language in both home and school settings. Results indicated a severe articulation deficit consisting of multiple sound substitutions, final consonant deletion, and cluster reduction. Delayed expressive language skills also were noted and were characterized primarily by the absence of grammatical morphemes. Jose was enrolled at the Edgewater Speech and Language Clinic for twice-weekly therapy sessions from June 10 through August 20, 2004. At the conclusion of this therapy program, Jose demonstrated the ability to:

spontaneously produce final /k/ in single words

imitatively produce initial /bl/ in single words

spontaneously use "is + verb + ing" in sentences

spontaneously use plural marker /s/ in phrases

Present Status. In paragraph form, state the date of client's enrollment in the current therapy program and specify the type, frequency, and duration of therapy sessions to be provided. Describe the client's major speech-language deficits as observed and measured during the first three (approximate) therapy sessions. Report specific baseline data and/or test results in chart form. Make note of any unusual or clinically significant behavior patterns.

Example

Jose began speech-language therapy at this clinic on October 13, 2004 for one-hour sessions on a twice-weekly basis. Baseline results for articulation targets were obtained at the single-word level using the *Clinical Probes of Articulation Consistency* (C-PAC):

Initial	Final
/k/ = 100%	/k/ = 60%
/g/ = 0%	/g/ = 45%
/r/ = 0%	/d/ = 20%

The *Structured Photographic Expressive Language Test* (SPELT II) was administered on October 15, 2004 to assess Jose's expressive language skills:

Raw Score	% Correct	Age Equivalent
28	56	4–6 to 4–11

This score falls below the second standard deviation for Jose's chronological age, indicating a moderate delay. Errors included omission of plural markers, and regular past tense markers, and incorrect use of prepositions.

Baseline measures were obtained for these grammatical morphemes at the phrase level on October 15, 2004:

Plural marker /s/	= 55%
Regular past tense	= 0%
Present progressive	= 90%
Prepositions	= 60%

The data indicate that Jose maintained his previous mastery of final /k/ at the word level and present progressive tense at the sentence level. However, production of the plural /s/ marker at the phrase level dropped significantly to the 55% level of accuracy. Jose cooperated with the tasks presented during the initial therapy sessions. However, it was noted that he frequently initiated a response before the clinician finished presenting task instructions or test items.

Goals and Objectives. In outline form, record pertinent speech-language goals and objectives in a hierarchy of complexity ranging from least to most difficult. (Recall that goals are general statements of what is to be accomplished over the course of the treatment program, whereas objectives specify measurable behaviors that lead to mastery of the long-term goals.) Materials and procedures generally are not included as part of this section.

Example

Articulation

Goal I. To produce final /k/ spontaneously at the sentence level.

    A. Jose will produce final /k/ spontaneously in single words with 90% accuracy over two consecutive sessions while naming picture cards.

    B. Jose will produce final /k/ spontaneously at the carrier phrase level with 90% accuracy over two consecutive sessions in response to clinician questions.

    C. Jose will produce final /k/ spontaneously at the sentence level with 90% accuracy over three consecutive sessions while describing pictures.

    D. Jose will produce final /k/ spontaneously at the carrier phrase level with 90% accuracy over two consecutive sessions in response to clinician questions.

    E. Jose will produce final /k/ spontaneously at the sentence level with 90% accuracy over three consecutive sessions while reading written sentences.

Language

Goal I. To spontaneously use the plural marker /s/ at the sentence level.

    A. Jose will use the plural marker /s/ in single words with 90% accuracy over two consecutive sessions given groups of objects.

    B. Jose will use the plural marker /s/ spontaneously at the phrase level with 90% accuracy over two consecutive sessions while completing oral sentences initiated by the clinician.

    C. Jose will use the plural marker /s/ spontaneously at the sentence level with 90% accuracy over three consecutive sessions during a picture description task.

Reinforcement. In paragraph form, indicate the type and schedule of reinforcers to be used for target productions and behavior management.

Example

A continuous schedule of verbal reinforcement coupled with token reinforcers will be used to shape target behaviors. This will be faded to an intermittent schedule as Jose demonstrates progress. A separate response cost system will be used to reduce Jose's tendency to initiate responses prematurely.

Family Involvement. In paragraph form, discuss how family members will be involved in observation of therapy sessions, conferences/counseling, and homework.

Example

Parent(s) will observe Jose's therapy sessions at least once every two weeks. Formal conferences will be held every three months; brief informal discussions of Jose's progress will take place following every session. Periodic training will be provided to help parents participate in homework assignments.

Generalization Plan. In paragraph form, specify strategies for generalization of target objectives within home, school, or work settings.

> **Example**
>
> Jose will be given weekly homework assignments to facilitate generalization of target behaviors. Parent will be provided with written instructions for these assignments. The clinician will also contact Jose's teacher bimonthly to discuss his status and give suggestions for how therapy objectives can be incorporated into the classroom.

The initial therapy plan can be viewed as the clinician's best prediction of what a client can accomplish in a given amount of time. The client's progress in therapy should be monitored on a periodic basis through the administration of probes to determine whether the plan's original objectives remain appropriate or require modification. (A complete sample ITP is included in Appendix 2-A at the end of this chapter.)

Progress Notes

Once therapy has begun, client performance must be documented on an ongoing basis. Progress notes are short and are written during or after each session. They may be filed in a patient's medical chart or a client's folder or written on the therapy plan itself. Daily notes serve at least three important functions: (1) they enable the clinician to monitor the treatment program on a continual basis and implement any necessary changes immediately; (2) they provide information on a daily basis to other professionals who also may be working with the client (e.g., occupational therapist, social worker); and (3) they facilitate the continuity of treatment by allowing another clinician to provide services in the event of unexpected clinician absence.

One common format of daily progress notes, particularly in medical settings, is known as SOAP notes. SOAP is an acronym that refers to the terms *s*ubjective, *o*bjective, *a*ssessment, and *p*lan.

Subjective: Write your opinion regarding relevant client behavior or status in a brief statement.

Objective: Record data collected for each task during the therapy session.

Assessment: Interpret data for current session and compare to client's previous levels of performance.

Plan: Identify proposed therapy targets for the next session.

> **Example**
>
> S: Jose appeared tired and reluctant to cooperate with the tasks presented.
> O: Final /k/ in single words = 85% (17/20); plural /s/ in spontaneous phrases = 50% (20/40).
> A: Fading of clinician model to a 5:1 ratio on plural task may have been premature. Today's score of 50% constitutes a decrease in accuracy compared to Jose's performance of the same task over the two previous sessions (70% and 75%).
> P: Continue work on both tasks at the same levels but decrease clinician modeling for the plural task to a 2:1 ratio.

Progress and Final Reports

A report is written for each client at specific intervals throughout treatment and when intervention services are terminated. These reports also may be referred to as interim summaries, annual reviews, discharge reports, or final summaries, depending on the clinical setting. Progress and final reports document a client's mastery of the goals and objectives outlined in the ITP and implemented over the course of treatment. Following are the basic content and organization of these reports.

Identifying Information. List identifying information at the top of the report. This section may include a client's name, age, address, type of disorder, dates of service and date of report, and so on.

Example

Name:	Jose Rodriguez	Date of Birth:	July 15, 1997
Parents:	Carlos and Maria Rodriguez	Age:	8 years, 4 months
Address:	1800 Knox Street	Date of Report:	November 25, 2005
	College Park, MD 20740	Disorder:	Articulation and
Service Dates: October 13, 2004 to			Language
	November 21, 2005	Clinician:	Gary Frost

Background Information. In paragraph form, state the full name and age of the client and include the following information: (1) date of first therapy session, (2) client's speech and language status at that time, and (3) session frequency and duration.

Example

Jose Rodriguez, an 8-year, 4-month-old male, began speech and language therapy at this clinic on October 13, 2004. At that time, he presented with a severe articulation deficit characterized by multiple sound substitutions, final consonant deletion, and cluster reduction. He also demonstrated an expressive language delay consisting primarily of grammatical morpheme deletions. Jose received therapy twice weekly for 1-hour sessions.

Therapy Objectives and Progress. In outline form, restate all the short-term objectives listed for each goal in the ITP, indicate the highest level at which the client met criterion, and cite supporting data for mastery of that objective. Compare the client's current performance levels to the pretreatment baseline data for that target area. Comment on the degree of improvement represented by this comparison (e.g., significant, moderate, minimal). Note any special procedures, strategies, tasks, or cues that facilitated the client's performance.

Example

Articulation

Goal I. To produce final /k/ spontaneously at the sentence level.

    A. Jose will produce final /k/ spontaneously in single words with 90% accuracy over two consecutive sessions while naming picture cards.

    B. Jose will produce final /k/ spontaneously at the carrier phrase level with 90% accuracy over two consecutive sessions in response to clinician questions.

    C. Jose will produce final /k/ spontaneously at the sentence level with 90% accuracy over three consecutive sessions while describing pictures.

    D. Jose will produce final /k/ spontaneously at the carrier phrase level with 90% accuracy over two consecutive sessions in response to clinician questions.

    E. Jose will produce final /k/ spontaneously at the sentence level with 90% accuracy over three consecutive sessions while reading written sentences.

Criterion met at the level of objective E: Jose used final /k/ spontaneously at the sentence level with 90% accuracy on September 12, 2005 and 100% accuracy on September 14, 2005 and September 18, 2005. This represents significant improvement over the pretreatment baseline measure of 60% accuracy at the carrier phrase level. Moreover, Jose was observed to spontaneously generalize correct production of this velar consonant to its voiced cognate /g/ in both initial and final word positions. In the initial stages of therapy, it was noted that Jose's performance was greatly enhanced by use of a mirror to monitor and maintain correct tongue placement.

Language

Goal I. To spontaneously use the plural marker /s/ at the sentence level.

    A. Jose will use the plural marker /s/ spontaneously in single words with 90% accuracy over two consecutive sessions given groups of objects.

    B. Jose will use the plural marker /s/ spontaneously at the phrase level with 90% accuracy over two consecutive sessions while completing oral sentences initiated by the clinician.

    C. Jose will use the plural marker /s/ spontaneously at the sentence level with 90% accuracy over three consecutive sessions during a picture description task.

Criterion met at objective B: Jose demonstrated mastery of the plural marker /s/ at the spontaneous phrase level with 95% accuracy on October 30, 2005 and 100% on November 2, 2005. This represents minimal progress over pretreatment baseline measures of 55% accuracy at the phrase level. Jose benefited from visual cues in the form of written numbers that signaled the need for him to use the plural marker in his response.

Summary and Additional Information. Summarize all the preceding "criterion met" statements. This summary should provide an overall profile of the client's progress over time rather than a simple reiteration of previously stated information. In separate paragraphs, include information about the following:

- Reinforcement (for both targets and attending behaviors)
- Completion of homework assignments
- Family participation/observation
- Parent/client conferences
- Other pertinent issues such as results of additional testing; significant medical information (e.g., changes in medication); change in educational placement, and so on

---

Example

Overall, Jose's communicative skills have shown uneven improvement this semester. Jose has mastered production of final /k/ at the spontaneous sentence level and has demonstrated generalization to /g/, an untreated target sound. Use of plural tense marker /s/ remains an area of difficulty for Jose. From a functional perspective, Jose's parents report that his general intelligibility seems to have improved based on the increasing number of verbal messages he is able to convey without adult and peer requests for clarification or repetition.

A continuous verbal reinforcement schedule was used to establish target behaviors. As accuracy improved, an intermittent schedule was introduced. A behavior management system was implemented in which Jose was given 10 tokens at the beginning of each session. He was told that these could be traded in at the end of the session for a small prize that "costs" 10 tokens. However, one token would be subtracted from his pile for each instance of noncompliant behavior (e.g., off-task talking) during therapy activities.

Homework practice was assigned weekly. Mrs. Rodriguez reported working with Jose on homework assignments on a daily basis. Mrs. Rodriguez observed therapy at least once every two weeks. Jose's progress was discussed with her informally after each session and formally during parent conferences held every three months.

It was noted that Jose's educational placement changed in September 2005 to a private school with a higher teacher-student ratio.

Recommendations. State whether continued speech-language intervention is warranted. If so, give suggestions for specific goals and objectives. Make any other pertinent recommendations (e.g., psychological testing).

Example

Jose's parents are withdrawing him from therapy at this facility because his new educational placement will include on-site intervention. Therapy goals should continue to focus on stabilization of final /k/ and plural marker /s/ at the conversational level. New goals for past tense markers and prepositions should be initiated.

(A complete sample Progress Report is included in Appendix 2-B at the end of this chapter.)

TIPS FOR PROOFREADING CLINICAL REPORTS

Students, beginning clinicians, and supervisors can use the following set of proof-reading questions to edit and monitor the quality of clinical reports.

- Are spelling, grammar, and punctuation correct?

- Are professional terms used accurately?

- Is there redundancy of word usage or sentence type?

- Are any sentences too lengthy, rambling, or unfocused?

- Is all the important client information included in the report?

- Is information presented only in the germane sections of the report (e.g., recommendation statements should not be included in the background information section)?

- Does the report follow a logical sequence from one section to the next (i.e., from background, to data and interpretation, to summary and recommendations)?

- Are raw data interpreted and not merely reported?

- Are all conclusions and assumptions supported by sufficient data?

- Are speculative statements explicitly identified as such?

- Does the report contain seemingly contradictory statements without adequate explanation?

- Is the wording clear or are some statements vague and ambiguous?

- Is content presented with appropriate emphasis (e.g., Has any critical information been overlooked? Has any minor point been overemphasized?)?

- Is the report written with ethical/legal considerations in mind?

INDIVIDUALIZED EDUCATION PLAN (IEP)

The Education of All Handicapped Children Act (PL 94-142) was passed in 1975 to ensure that all children, ages 3 to 21 years with special needs, receive a free, appropriate public education. Speech-language pathology is a designated special education service under this law. This legislation was updated in 1997 through authorization of PL 105–17, the Individuals with Disabilities Education Act (IDEA). Final regulations for Part B of the amendment were released in 1999. These regulations pertain to services in school settings. At the time of this writing, IDEA is currently undergoing reauthorization by Congress. Interested readers are encouraged to visit ASHA's Web site at www.asha.org for updated information.

Each eligible child must have an annual written Individualized Education Plan (IEP) that documents the need for the provision of special education services. The purpose of this plan is to identify specific areas for remediation. Unlike other clinical reports, the IEP generally does not include a description of the actual intervention procedures that will be used to accomplish the specified annual goals.

The IEP is generated as part of a process that begins with a referral. A comprehensive assessment is then conducted by an appointed team and the findings are reviewed at a meeting of all involved parties (including therapists, teachers, parents). The participants develop and approve a written IEP, which is implemented over the subsequent school year and reviewed annually. When speech-language therapy is the sole or primary special education service to be provided, the SLP may assume principal responsibility for writing the IEP. (For an overview, summary, and questions and answers about the IDEA and the IEP process, see the American Speech-Language-Hearing Association's Web site at www.asha.org.

IEP Content

To ensure a measure of uniformity and accountability nationwide, federal law requires that all IEPs contain the following basic information:

- *Present levels of performance:* This section of the document includes information regarding a child's current status in all pertinent developmental and educational domains. For speech-language pathology, test scores and clinical analysis of observed performance are presented. The team must also consider a list of other factors, including the child's strengths, parents' concerns, need for assistive technology, and specific needs of children with limited English proficiency. This section must also state how the disability affects the child's educational performance and progress in the general curriculum. This information should be discussed in sufficient detail to provide a basis for development of intervention goals and objectives.

- *Annual goals:* The goals are long-term projections of what a child is expected to accomplish over the entire school year. These goals must be linked to the general curriculum. Statements about needed supplementary aids and services must be included as well as any modifications necessary for participation in state or districtwide assessments. There is no mandate concerning the number of goals and objectives that must be included in an IEP. Finally, the IEP must include a statement regarding the mechanism by which parents will be informed about their child's progress and how often these updates will occur.

- *Special education and related services:* This section identifies the special services needed by a child to achieve the stated goals. The type and frequency of services must be specified. A typical example for speech-language pathology might be: "Articulation therapy will be delivered two times per week in 30-minute group sessions." Assistive technology devices and services may be identified as necessary for some children. The IEP team determines whether use of school-purchased devices in the child's home or other settings is necessary for a free and appropriate education.

- *Placement recommendation and justification:* This section indicates the specific educational setting into which preschool or school-aged children will be placed. By law, this setting must be the **least restrictive environment** (LRE) that provides an appropriate education to meet a child's individualized needs. LRE means that, to the maximum extent possible, children with disabilities are educated with children who have no disabilities.

Recommendations for placements other than a regular classroom in the child's home school must be accompanied by a written rationale. (Eligibility requirements vary among local educational agencies.) The percentage of time that a child will spend in regular versus special education is documented in this section. Parents must be participating members of teams that make placement decisions.

- *Initiation and duration of services:* The IEP must state the dates that services will begin and the projected duration of the services. The duration of services typically is one year because IEPs are reviewed on an annual basis. Reevaluation of the child's performance is conducted as conditions warrant but must occur at least every three years.

These five categories comprise the basic structure of an IEP. Individual states or local educational agencies may impose additional requirements pertaining to format or content information.

Due Process

The IDEA (1997) provides legal and procedural safeguards throughout the educational placement process, including time lines for completion of each step, parental notification and consent, and an appeal system to ensure due process for all parties involved. The parent or guardian must be notified prior to any changes in a child's educational program. The due process system provides a formal mechanism for parents to protest decisions they consider inappropriate or unfair to their child.

INDIVIDUALIZED FAMILY SERVICE PLAN (IFSP)

In 1986, the federal mandate for a free and appropriate education was extended by enactment of PL 99-457 (Part H) to include infants and toddlers with special needs between birth and 3 years of age. This legislation is notable not only for its emphasis on the importance of early intervention but also the stipulation that all services be provided by qualified personnel (i.e., professionals who meet the highest requirement in the state for a given discipline).

This legislation requires the development of an Individualized Family Service Plan (IFSP), which is similar to an IEP. Both documents require specification of (1) a child's present level of performance, (2) long-term goals and short-term objectives, (3) recommended special services, and (4) dates of initiation and duration of services.

The IFSP differs from the IEP in that its main focus is on the family as a unit rather than solely on the child. The written document must include the following types of information that are not part of an IEP:

- *Family strengths and needs:* This section provides a description of the family's strengths and weaknesses as they relate to enhancing the development of the child. It also includes a statement of the impact that the child's disability has on family functioning. In addition, individual families can specify their desired levels of involvement in the intervention plan.

- *Case manager:* The IFSP specifically identifies the individual from the profession most relevant to the needs of the infant and family. The case manager is responsible for the development of the IFSP and for implementation, coordination, and monitoring of all services. The SLP is frequently named as case manager for infants and toddlers whose primary handicapping condition consists of communication or oral-motor disabilities.

- *Transition:* This section outlines the procedures that will be employed to facilitate the transition to services provided under PL 94-142 if the child continues to need special services beyond age 2 years, 11 months.

In addition to the differences outlined above, this legislation extends eligibility to "at-risk" youngsters rather than restricting services to children with recognized disabilities. Moreover, these services can be provided through agencies outside the public school system (e.g., social welfare, respite care, and so on). PL 99-457 also contains provisions for home-based instruction as well as family education and counseling. The IFSP is reviewed every six months rather than annually.

PROFESSIONAL CORRESPONDENCE

In addition to clinical treatment reports, speech-language pathologists often interact with other professionals and agencies through written correspondence. These documents may vary with respect to length, content, and format, but all professional correspondence should be written in a clear, concise manner with correct spelling, grammar, and punctuation. Typically, written correspondence involves authorizing the release of information, making referrals to other professionals, and acknowledging referrals from colleagues.

HIPAA is the acronym for the Health Insurance Portability and Accountability Act of 1996. It is designed to regulate the storage and/or electronic transmission of health care data and ensures confidentiality for all personal patient information. This federal law includes protection of all forms of identifiable client information generated and transmitted by speech-language pathologists in settings such as private practice, schools, nursing homes, hospitals, clinics, and other institutional settings. For more detailed information on HIPAA, refer to Centers for Medicare and Medicaid Services Web site at www.cms.hhs.gov/hipaa.

It is essential that clients authorize the release of confidential evaluation or treatment information, whether it is to be written or verbally communicated. It is the sole prerogative of the client to determine the type and amount of information to be shared with teachers, physicians, or other therapists. Correspondence related to referral issues provides documentation for record-keeping purposes and is an important aspect of professional courtesy.

Pages 69 through 74 contain reproducible release of information authorization forms and sample referral letter and acknowledgment formats.

FORM 2-1 AUTHORIZATION FOR RELEASE OF INFORMATION FROM ANOTHER AGENCY OR PHYSICIAN

The person named below has requested the services of our facility _____

_____. We understand that this individual has been

seen by you. Kindly forward any hearing, speech, language, medical, psychological,

educational, or social records regarding this individual. Below is written authorization for the

release of these records. Please send this information to the attention of _____

_____ at the following address:

_____

_____

_____

Thank you for your cooperation.

This will certify that you have my permission to release information concerning

_____

(Client Name)

to the following facility: _____

Signature: _____ Date: _____

FORM 2-2 AUTHORIZATION FOR RELEASE OF INFORMATION TO ANOTHER AGENCY OR PHYSICIAN

Name: _____ Date of Birth: _____

I hereby consent to the release of any and all hearing, speech, and language records concerning the above-named individual to:

Name/Agency: _____

Address: _____

_____

_____

Signature: _____ Date: _____

FORM 2-3 REFERRAL LETTER FORMAT

Date: _____

Name of Recipient: _____

Address: _____

Dear _____,

_____ is being referred to you for _____

_____.

He/she was seen at our facility for _____

_____ on/from _____.

His/her communication status is characterized by _____.

I am making this referral because _____

_____. Enclosed please find a copy of _____

_____, along with the client's written authorization for

the release of this information. If you have any questions, please contact me at

_____.

Sincerely,

_____
Signature and Title

FORM 2-4 SAMPLE REFERRAL LETTER

April 25, 2004

Timothy Anderson, M.D.

866 Manor Drive

College Park, MD 20742

Dear Dr. Anderson,

Franklin Pearl is being referred to you for a laryngoscopic examination. He was seen at our facility for a voice evaluation on April 24, 2004. His communication status is characterized by harsh voice quality, intermittent aphonia, and accompanying throat pain.

I am making this referral to verify Mr. Pearl's medical status prior to the initiation of therapy services. Enclosed please find a copy of the diagnostic report, along with the client's written authorization for the release of this information. If you have any questions, please contact me at 301-555-1212.

Sincerely,

Mary Ann Schilling, M.S., CCC-SLP

Speech-Language Pathologist

FORM 2-5 ACKNOWLEDGMENT OF REFERRAL FORMAT

Date: _____

Name of Recipient: _____

Address: _____

Dear _____ ,

    Thank you for referring _____ to our clinic.

He/she was seen for _____

on/from _____ .

    I have enclosed a copy of my full report, including recommendations regarding future

services. If you have any questions, please do not hesitate to contact me at _____

_____ .

    We appreciate your referral and look forward to continued collaboration with you.

Sincerely,

_____

Signature and Title

FORM 2-6 SAMPLE REFERRAL ACKNOWLEDGMENT

April 27, 2004

Kim Davidson, M.D.

31 Azalea Lane

Kendall, FL 02113

Dear Dr. Davidson,

Thank you for referring Barbara Hawley to our clinic. She was seen for an initial speech and language evaluation on April 18, 2004.

I have enclosed a copy of my full report, including recommendations regarding future services. If you have any questions, please do not hesitate to contact me at 305-555-1846.

We appreciate your referral and look forward to continued collaboration with you.

Sincerely,

Marian Kirley, M.A., CCC-SLP
Speech-Language Pathologist

ADDITIONAL RESOURCES

Allyn & Bacon
160 Gould Street
Needham Heights, MA 02494
Phone: 800-852-8024
Fax: 781-455-7024
Web site: www.ablongman.com

What's Best for Matthew?
Uses a case study of a boy with autism, named Matthew, to help clinicians and teachers develop and write IEPs for disabled students. Provides assistance in writing an IEP for Matthew using a step-by-step approach, which can then be used to write IEPs for individual clients. Also includes a special notepad feature that allows the clinician to sort relevant IEP information into categories, such as communication and written language, which can be saved and accessed when needed during the writing process.

American Speech-Language-Hearing Association
10801 Rockville Pike
Rockville, MD 20852-3279
Phone: 888-498-6699
E-mail: productsales@asha.org
Web site: www.ideapractices.org

Discover IDEA Supporting Achievement for Children with Disabilities: An IDEA Practices Resource Guide (by ASPIRE)
The package is organized around the key topics in special education in an accurate, easy-to-use format. This resource package brings you immediate access (through the Discover CD 2002) to hundreds of books, handouts, transparencies and Web links. It provides connections to the centers and programs addressing topical areas in special education, and in addition, it infuses the IDEA regulations within each area in a strategic and easy-to-follow format.

LinguiSystems
3100 Fourth Avenue
East Moline, IL 61244
Phone: 800-776-4332
Fax: 800-577-4555
Web site: www.linguisystems.com

The SLP's IDEA Companion
A resource for goals and objectives that match the guidelines outlined in the Individuals with Disabilities Education Act (IDEA). Therapy goals link to the classroom curriculum, and appropriate benchmarks for students are determined as well as levels of performance using the baseline measures provided in the book. Classroom expectations are provided for grades K–12 in the areas of fluency, semantics, syntax, voice, word finding, pragmatics, phonological awareness, oral-motor, articulation, and narrative/expository writing.

Parrot Software

P.O. Box 250755
West Bloomfield, MI 48325
Phone: 800-727-7681
Fax: 248-788-3224
E-mail: parrot@mcs.net
Web site: www.parrotsoftware.com

Instant IEP and Report Writing Demo
Designed to help SLPs create personalized and detailed IEPs. Clinicians specify a clinical area, such as voice, and a list of goals is presented for that area. After a goal is chosen, three lists are displayed: Objectives, Methods, and Evaluation Procedures. Select specific items appropriate for the client from these lists and the program then automatically generates a personalized IEP. Contains more than 1,000 entries in the database; additional items can be entered for recall within the report.

Pro-Ed

8700 Shoal Creek Boulevard
Austin, TX 78757-6897
Phone: 800-897-3202
Fax: 800-397-7633
Web site: www.proedinc.com

Report Writing for Speech-Language Pathologists and Audiologists, Second Edition
This is a resource that includes all necessary information to be included in reports of various types. There is information about referral acknowledgements, diagnostic evaluation reports, integrated diagnostic reports, treatment plans and reports, IEPs, and progress reports.

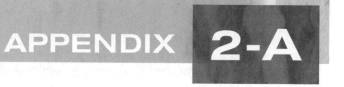

APPENDIX 2-A

SAMPLE INITIAL THERAPY PLAN

University of Maryland Speech and Hearing Clinic
COLLEGE PARK, MD 20742
(301) 555-4218

Name:	Jamie Rose	Date of Birth:	April 24, 1998
Parents:	Jim and Kathy Rose	Age:	5 years, 10 months
Address:	2635 Drake Court	Date of Report:	February 14, 2004
	Fairfax, VA 20901	Category:	Articulation and Language
Phone:	(703) 555-9587	Clinician:	Ilana Anderson, M.S., CCC-SLP

Background Information

Jamie Rose, a 5-year, 10-month-old female, was evaluated at the University of Maryland Speech and Hearing Clinic on April 28, 2003. At that time, she exhibited a severe phonological disorder characterized by initial consonant devoicing, stridency deletion, velar fronting, stopping of fricatives and affricates, cluster simplification, and liquid simplification. She also presented with an idiosyncratic process of gliding fricatives and affricates. In addition, results from the Structured Photographic Expressive Language Test-II (SPELT-II) indicated that Jamie was moderately to severely impaired on measures of syntax and morphology. Her speech was reported to be unintelligible when the context was unknown.

Jamie began speech and language therapy at the University of Maryland Speech and Hearing Clinic in June 2003 and continued therapy through the fall 2003 semester. By the end of the fall semester, Jamie's production of /f/, /g/, and /k/ improved significantly. She produced each of these sounds in the initial and final position of words at the carrier phrase level with 100% accuracy. It was noted that Jamie also was producing these sounds correctly in conversational speech. In addition, she reached 100% accuracy in her production of /s/ and /l/ in the initial and final position of single words and appropriately used the pronouns "he" and "she" with 100% accuracy while telling a story. However, Jamie continued to have some difficulty with her production of /θ/ IF.

Present Status

Jamie began speech and language therapy for the spring 2004 semester at the University of Maryland on January 31, 2004, on a twice-weekly basis. The Goldman-Fristoe Test of Articulation-2 was administered to assess her current articulation status.

Jamie's errors on the Goldman-Fristoe were as follows (error/target):

Initial: ʒ/dʒ, t/θ, w/v

Medial: ʒ/dʒ, j/z, v/ð

Blends: fr/dr

(continues)

Appendix 2-A (continued)

Jamie's performance indicates significant improvement in articulation when compared with her performance on this test in April 2003.

The Khan-Lewis Phonological Analysis was used to analyze the errors from the Goldman-Fristoe. Jamie's raw score on the Khan-Lewis was 18, which placed her below the 15th percentile with an age equivalent of 3 years, 11 months. The following phonological processes and their indices of severity were indicated:

Deletion of final consonants	Average
Initial voicing	Moderate
Deaffrication	Moderate
Velar fronting	Average
Consonant harmony	Average
Stopping of fricatives/affricates	Minimal
Cluster simplification	Average
Final devoicing	Minimal
Liquid simplification	Average

This represents a less severe phonological profile when compared with Jamie's performance in April 2003, despite persistence of initial voicing and deaffrication. Thus, a phonetic rather than phonological process approach will be used in remediation.

The following baseline measures for articulatory targets were obtained at the single-word level on January 31, 2004, and February 2, 2004:

Initial	Medial	Blends
/dʒ/ = 10%	/l/ = 60%	/sn/ = 100%
/tʃ/ = 0%		/sk/ = 25%
		/sl/ = 100%
		/sw/ = 87%
		/sp/ = 87%
		/st/ = 87%

The Structured Photographic Expressive Language Test-II (SPELT-II) also was administered to assess Jamie's current language status. She achieved a raw score of 25/40 with a percentile rank of 9, thus placing her performance more than one standard deviation (SD) below the mean for her age group. Her most consistent errors involved omission of the auxiliary "is" in present progressive and future progressive constructions (e.g., "She is climbing" and "She is going to jump," respectively).

A sample of Jamie's spontaneous conversational speech was analyzed for errors in articulation and morphology. Articulation errors in conversation were consistent with those indicated by the standardized assessment measures. In addition, the copula "is" was omitted 17% of the time in obligatory contexts, while the auxiliary verb forms "is" and "are" were omitted 24% of the time in obligatory contexts. These errors are consistent with those on the SPELT-II. There was some evidence of overregularization of irregular past tense verbs (e.g.,"goed" and "falled"), as well as errors in subject-verb agreement (e.g., "he were").

The following baseline measures for language targets were obtained at the spontaneous sentence level with picture prompts on February 7, 2004:

(continues)

Appendix 2-A (continued)

Auxiliary "is" = 55%
Auxiliary "are" = 55%
Copula "is" = 60%
Copula "are" = 50%

Goals and Objectives

Articulation

Goal I. To produce medial /l/ spontaneously in sentences.
    A. Jamie will produce medial /l/ imitatively in single words when prompted with picture stimuli with 90% accuracy over two consecutive sessions.
    B. Jamie will produce medial /l/ spontaneously in single words when prompted with picture stimuli with 90% accuracy over two consecutive sessions.
    C. Jamie will produce medial /l/ in carrier phrases when prompted with picture stimuli with 90% accuracy over two consecutive sessions.
    D. Jamie will produce medial /l/ in spontaneous sentences when prompted with picture stimuli with 90% accuracy over two consecutive sessions.

Goal II. To produce the following /s/ blends in spontaneous sentences: /sw/, /sp/, and /st/.
    A. Jamie will produce /s/ blends in carrier phrases when prompted with picture stimuli with 90% accuracy over two consecutive sessions.
    B. Jamie will produce /s/ blends in spontaneous sentences when prompted with picture stimuli with 90% accuracy over two consecutive sessions.

Goal III. To produce initial /dʒ, tʃ/ in carrier phrases.
    A. Jamie will produce /dʒ, tʃ/ in isolation with clinician modeling with 90% accuracy over two consecutive sessions.
    B. Jamie will produce initial /dʒ, tʃ/ imitatively in single words when prompted with picture stimuli with 90% accuracy over two consecutive sessions.
    C. Jamie will produce initial /dʒ, tʃ/ spontaneously in single words when prompted with picture stimuli with 90% accuracy over two consecutive sessions.
    D. Jamie will produce initial /dʒ, tʃ/ in carrier phrases when prompted with picture stimuli with 90% accuracy over two consecutive sessions.

Language

Goal I. To produce the appropriate auxiliary verb "is" or "are" in spontaneous speech.
    A. Jamie will produce the appropriate auxiliary verb imitatively to describe action picture stimuli with 90% accuracy over two consecutive sessions.
    B. Jamie will fill in the appropriate auxiliary verb in carrier phrases to describe action picture stimuli with 90% accuracy over two consecutive sessions.
    C. Jamie will produce the appropriate auxiliary verb in spontaneous sentences to describe action picture stimuli with 90% accuracy over two consecutive sessions.

Goal II. To use the appropriate copula "is" or "are" in spontaneous sentences.
    A. Jamie will produce the appropriate copula imitatively to describe picture stimuli with 90% accuracy over two consecutive sessions.
    B. Jamie will fill in the appropriate copula in carrier phrases to describe picture stimuli with 90% accuracy over two consecutive sessions.

(continues)

C. Jamie will produce the appropriate copula in spontaneous sentences to describe picture stimuli with 90% accuracy over two consecutive sessions.

Although irregular verb past tense will not be targeted this semester, several of these verbs will be used in carrier phrases to stimulate correct use through incidental learning. For example: "I *went* to the store to buy _____," "My book *fell* right on the _____."

Reinforcement

A continuous verbal reinforcement system coupled with tangible reinforcement will be used when shaping target behaviors, fading to an intermittent schedule as Jamie demonstrates progress. Jamie will receive turns at a game, pieces of puzzles, or art projects to assemble when predetermined criterion levels of responses have been achieved.

Family Involvement

Parent conferences will be held formally twice during the semester and informally after each therapy session. In addition, the parent will observe periodically and will be asked to participate in Jamie's homework assignments.

Generalization Plan

Jamie will be given regular homework assignments to facilitate generalization of specific goals. The clinician will review the home program with the parent, explain the instructions, and provide demonstrations as needed. Mrs. Rose will also monitor Jamie's production of error sounds in normal conversation and during homework assignments.

(continues)

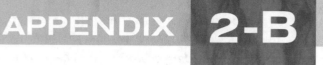

APPENDIX 2-B

SAMPLE PROGRESS REPORT

University of Maryland Speech and Hearing Clinic
COLLEGE PARK, MD 20742
(301) 555-4218

Name:	Jamie Rose	Date of Birth:	April 24, 1998
Parents:	Jim and Kathy Rose	Date of Report:	May 2, 2004
Address:	2635 Drake Court	Age:	6:0
	Fairfax, VA 20901	Category:	Articulation and Language
Phone:	(703) 555-9587	Service Dates:	January 31, 2004
Clinician:	Ilana Anderson,		to May 2, 2004
	MS, CCC-SLP		

Background Information

Jamie Rose, a 6-year-old female, began speech and language therapy at the University of Maryland Speech and Hearing Clinic in June 2003. At that time, she presented with a severe phonological disorder and was moderately to severely impaired on measures of syntax and morphology. At the beginning of the current semester, Jamie's performance on the Goldman-Fristoe Test of Articulation-2 indicated significant improvement in articulation. A Khan-Lewis Phonological Analysis showed an improved phonological profile, although some deaffrication and initial voicing persisted. Her performance on the Structured Photographic Expressive Language Test-II (SPELT-II) and baseline measures indicated errors involving auxiliary and copula verb forms. There was also some evidence of overregularization of irregular past tense verbs, as well as errors in subject-verb agreement in her spontaneous speech.

Therapy Objectives and Progress

Articulation

I. Jamie will produce medial /l/ in spontaneous sentences when prompted with picture stimuli with 90% accuracy over two consecutive sessions.

Criterion met: Jamie produced medial /l/ with 100% accuracy in spontaneous sentences when prompted with picture stimuli on April 18, 2004 and on April 20, 2004 (baseline: 60% accurate in single words on January 31, 2004). This represents significant progress over baseline performance.

II. Jamie will produce /s/ blends in spontaneous sentences when prompted with picture stimuli with 90% accuracy over two consecutive sessions.

Criterion not met: Jamie produced /sw/, /sp/, and /st/ in carrier phrases when prompted with picture stimuli with 85% accuracy on April 20, 2004 (baseline: 87% for /sw/, /st/, and /sp/ in single words on February 2, 2004). Although criterion was not met for these blends, this performance represents significant progress over baseline behavior.

(continues)

Appendix 2-B (continued)

III. Jamie will produce initial /dʒ/ and /tʃ/ in carrier phrases when prompted with picture stimuli with 90% accuracy over two consecutive sessions.

Criterion not met: Jamie produced initial /dʒ/ in single words when prompted with picture stimuli with 96% accuracy on April 9, 2004 and 99% accuracy on April 14, 2004 (baseline: 10% accurate in single words on January 31, 2004). Jamie produced initial /tʃ/ imitatively in single words with 90% and 95% accuracy on April 14, 2004 and April 18, 2004, respectively. This represents substantial improvement over her baseline performance of 0% in single words on February 2, 2004. Although terminal criterion was not met during therapy, Jamie's mother reports that /dʒ/ and /tʃ/ are accurately and consistently produced in conversation.

Language

I. Jamie will produce the appropriate auxiliary verb in spontaneous sentences to describe action picture stimuli with 90% accuracy over two consecutive sessions.

Criterion not met: Jamie produced the auxiliary verbs "is" and "are" in carrier phrases to describe action pictures with 80% accuracy on April 23, 2004 and with 80% accuracy on April 30, 2004 (baseline: 55% accurate in sentences describing action pictures on February 7, 2004); however, production in spontaneous speech was noted to be inconsistent. This performance represents improvement over baseline performance.

II. Jamie will produce the appropriate copula in spontaneous sentences to describe picture stimuli with 90% accuracy over two consecutive sessions.

Goal was not addressed due to time constraints.

Additional Information

The clinician used continuous verbal reinforcement and corrective feedback to shape target behaviors, fading to an intermittent schedule as Jamie's performance improved. During therapy, Jamie received turns at a game, stickers, or token reinforcement, which were then traded for a reward at the end of the task or session.

Jamie made steady and significant progress on articulation targets throughout the semester. The observance of target sounds in her spontaneous conversation indicates that she has begun to generalize to situations outside the clinic environment. Jamie's progress was discussed with her mother informally after each session and formally during two parent conferences. Mrs. Rose observed all therapy sessions and facilitated the achievement of target behaviors by helping Jamie complete homework assignments and by monitoring her conversational speech.

It was noted, however, that Jamie continued to demonstrate some language errors in her spontaneous speech, including overregularization of regular past tense verbs, subject-verb disagreement, and omission of auxiliary and copula verbs. On April 27, 2004, Jamie was given the following standardized tests to assess her current expressive and receptive language skills (RS = Raw score, SS = Standard score, %ile = Percentile, AE = Age equivalent, SD = Standard deviation):

Test	RS	SS	%ile	AE
Analysis of the Language of Learning (ALL)				
(Mean SS = 100, SD = 15)				
Generating Words	8	120	86	6.11
Segmenting Words	2	96	43	5.4

(continues)

Appendix 2-B (continued)

Test	RS	SS	%ile	AE
Test of Word Knowledge (TOWK)				
(Mean SS = 10, SD = 3)				
Expressive Vocabulary	7	7	16	–
Receptive Vocabulary	18	13	84	–
Clinical Evaluation of				
Language Fundamentals-3 (CELF-3)				
(Mean SS = 10/100, SD = 3/15)				
Linguistic Concepts	16	9	37	–
Sentence Structure	23	10	50	–
Oral Directions	9	9	37	–
Receptive Language Score	–	95	–	–
Word Structure	22	7	16	–
Formulated Sentences	42	12	75	–
Recalling Sentences	62	13	84	–
Expressive Language Score	–	104	–	–
Total Language Score	–	99	37	6.5

The Generating Words subtest of the Analysis of the Language of Learning (ALL) assesses a child's awareness that phonemes (sounds) serve to begin and end words. By 6 years of age, children have little difficulty producing words given initial phonemes; however, it is not unusual for children 8 or 9 years of age to continue to have difficulty producing words given final phonemes. Jamie's performance on this subtest was above average. It also reflects the differential production ability given initial versus final phonemes that is typical of a child her age. The Segmenting Words subtest assesses a child's ability to divide words into component sounds. Jamie had some difficulty with this task, although her performance indicated an awareness that words are composed of multiple, separate sounds.

The Expressive Vocabulary subtest of the Test of Word Knowledge (TOWK) assesses the ability to name pictures that represent nouns and verbs. Jamie's score on this test places her performance one SD below the mean (16th percentile). The Receptive Vocabulary subtest assesses the ability to select appropriate pictures that represent nouns, verbs, or modifiers. Jamie's score on this test places her one SD above the mean (84th percentile). Based on these subtests, Jamie's receptive vocabulary skills exceed her expressive vocabulary skills.

The Clinical Evaluation of Language Fundamentals-3 (CELF-3) assesses both receptive and expressive language skills. Linguistic Concepts is a receptive subtest that assesses comprehension of concepts related to inclusion, exclusion, coordination, time, condition, and quantity. Jamie's score on this test places her at the 37th percentile. Sentence Structure assesses comprehension of structural rules at the sentence level. Jamie's score on this test places her at the 50th percentile. Oral Directions assesses comprehension, recall, and execution of oral commands of increasing complexity. Jamie's score places her at the 37th percentile. Together, these subtests provide an **overall receptive language score** of 95 (23rd percentile) for Jamie.

The Word Structure subtest of the CELF-3 is an expressive subtest that assesses knowledge of morphological rules. Jamie's score on this subtest places her at the 16th percentile.

(continues)

Appendix 2-B (continued)

Although errors in production of regular and irregular past tense on this subtest may have been due to Jamie's failure to understand the directions, similar errors have been noted in analyses of her spontaneous language samples. Formulating Sentences assesses formulation of simple, compound, and complex sentences. Jamie performed at the 75th percentile on this subtest. Recalling Sentences assesses recall and reproduction of surface structure as a function of syntactic complexity. Jamie performed at the 84th percentile on this test.

Together, the subtests of the CELF-3 provide an overall **expressive language score** of 104 for Jamie. A comparison of the overall receptive and expressive scores on the CELF-3 suggests, unlike the TOWK, that Jamie's expressive skills and receptive skills both fall in the average range. A **total language score** of 99 indicates that Jamie's performance is appropriate for her age (age equivalent score = 6:5). However, analyses of her spontaneous language sample indicate that Jamie demonstrates continuing difficulty with the correct use of regular and irregular tense and number markers.

Recommendations

It is recommended that Jamie continue speech-language therapy on a twice-weekly basis. The following goals are recommended: (1) monitor Jamie's use of auxiliary verbs and copulas, (2) improve Jamie's productive control of regular and irregular plural forms, and (3) improve her use of regular and irregular past tense markers.

Jamie has made significant progress on articulation targets since beginning speech-language therapy, and Mrs. Rose has been an active facilitator in Jamie's therapy. Thus, it is recommended that one-third (rather than one-half) of each session be devoted to articulation programming. It is also recommended that an intense home program for articulation be established and monitored.

PART TWO

PROVIDING TREATMENT FOR COMMUNICATION DISORDERS

CHAPTER 3

Intervention for Articulation and Phonology in Children

This chapter focuses on the management of articulation and phonological disorders demonstrated by children. An articulation model emphasizes the motor component of speech, whereas a phonologic orientation stresses the linguistic aspect of speech production. Most articulation approaches focus on the incorrect production of individual phonemes, traditionally classified as substitution, omission, and distortion errors. In contrast, phonological approaches concentrate on rule-governed errors that affect multiple speech sounds that follow a predictable pattern.

Articulation disorders can be classified as functional or organic in nature. Articulation disorders are considered functional when no known pathology is causing the errors. Organic disorders result from known physical causes, such as cleft palate, neurological dysfunction, or hearing impairment. Some children may demonstrate both functional and organic deficits.

The information provided in this chapter is based on Standard American English. (See Appendix D at the end of this book for International Phonetic Alphabet symbols.) It is imperative that clinicians take a child's cultural and linguistic background into account in determining whether the production of a given speech sound represents an error or a dialectal difference. (See Appendix C: Multicultural Tables, at the end of the book.)

TREATMENT EFFICACY/EVIDENCE-BASED PRACTICE

Gierut (1998) reviewed 64 publications whose subject matter includes intervention effectiveness for functional articulatory/phonological disorders in children. The summary includes mainly small n studies that focused on the treatment of consonant sounds. The overall conclusion is that intervention is effective in improving correct sound production and increasing speech intelligibility. Additional conclusions include the following:

- Minimal pair treatment and cycles approach treatment generally result in phonological gains.

- Computerized instruction is an effective supplement to direct clinical intervention.

- Efficacy data are needed to determine the relative effectiveness of specific treatment procedures as well as their efficiency (i.e., time needed for completion of the therapy programs).

GENERAL CONSIDERATIONS FOR INTERVENTION PROGRAMMING

There are two primary approaches for choosing initial therapy targets for children with articulation/phonological disorders: developmental and nondevelopmental.

Developmental: In this approach, therapy targets are identified based on the order of acquisition in normally developing children. Table 3-1 provides a list of English consonants in the order of their emergence. Table 3-4 outlines the most common phonological processes exhibited by young children.

TABLE 3-1
Age of Acquisition of English Consonants

Consonant	Poole (1934)	Templin (1957)	Prather et al. (1975)	Smit et al. (1990)	
				Females	Males
m	3½	3	2	3	3
n	4½	3	2	3½	3
h	3½	3	2	3	3
p	3½	3	2	3	3
f	5½	3	2–4	3½	3½
w	3½	3	2–8	3	3
b	3½	4	2–8	3	3
ŋ	4½	3	2	7–9	7–9
j	4½	3½	2–4	4	5
k	4½	4	2–4	3½	3½
g	4½	4	2–4	3½	4
l	6½	6	3–4	6	6
d	4½	4	2–4	3	3½
t	4½	6	2–8	4	3½
s	7½	4½	3	7–9	7–9
r	7½	4	3–4	8	8
tʃ	—	4½	3–8	6	7
v	6½	6	4	5½	5½
z	7½	7	4	7–9	7–9
ʒ	6½	7	4	—	—
θ	7½	6	4	6	8
dʒ	—	7	4	6	7
ʃ	6½	4½	3–8	6	7
ð	6½	7	4	4½	7

Note: Variability in reported ages of acquisition is partly due to the different criterion levels used across studies to determine mastery of each sound. Poole (1934) = 100%, Templin (1957) = 75%, Prather et al. (1975) = 75%, Smit et al. (1990) = 90%.

Nondevelopmental: In this approach, developmental norms are not used in the selection of target behaviors. Instead, the determining factors fall into two groups. One strategy is client-specific and bases the selection of therapy objectives on several factors:

1. Target(s) that are most relevant to a child or parent (e.g., a sound in the child's name)
2. Target(s) that are most stimulable in a given child's error repertoire regardless of developmental sequence
3. Target(s) that are most visible when produced (e.g., /θ/ versus /g/)

The second strategy is based on the degree of perceived deviance associated with a child's errors.

Articulatory

1. Omission errors contribute most to unintelligibility, followed by substitutions, and then distortions.
2. Errors in the initial position of words contribute most to unintelligibility, followed by medial, and then final.
3. Errors that occur on the most frequent sounds in a language contribute significantly to unintelligibility.

Phonological

1. Patterns of initial consonant deletion and glottal replacement of medial consonants tend to contribute significantly to listener perception of unintelligibility.

In addition to choosing therapy targets, clinicians must determine the most appropriate "goal attack strategy" for each client (Fey, 1986). Several strategies/ options can be utilized in the design of a client's therapy program: vertical, horizontal, and cyclical. The basic assumption of **vertical** training is that the best route to target mastery is through intense practice on a limited number of targets. The clinician focuses on one or two targets until the client achieves some predetermined level of mastery, usually at the level of conversation. Therapy then moves on to the next target(s) identified in a hierarchical level of difficulty. This "deep" approach to intervention tends to be most appropriate for clients with relatively few articulatory/phonological errors.

In contrast to training deeply, a **horizontal** strategy attacks goals broadly. It assumes that simultaneous exposure to a wide variety of targets will facilitate a client's ability to produce phonemes or sound patterns. The clinician provides less intense practice on a larger number of targets, even within the same session. This strategy focuses on efficient generalization of target behaviors across the speech sound system and tends to be most appropriate for clients with multiple errors.

Clinicians may choose to combine aspects of the vertical and horizontal strategies into a **cyclical** approach. Instead of attacking therapy targets deeply or broadly, this strategy provides a client with practice on a given target for a predetermined amount of time, and then moves on to another target (Hodson & Paden, 1991). This approach gives the client an opportunity to internalize the original sound/pattern while the clinician introduces the new target. Focus on the original target resumes later in the therapy program. This cycle is repeated until the target(s) emerges in spontaneous speech.

ORAL-MOTOR CONSIDERATIONS

Some children with speech impairments (particularly those with organically-based disorders) may exhibit deficits in oral-motor function that affect the neuromuscular control and organization needed for the production of intelligible speech. These deficits may manifest themselves as hyposensitivity (reduced reactions to sensation); hypersensitivity (overly strong reactions to sensation); or weakness or incoordination of oral structures, including the jaw, tongue, lips, or palate. It is important to realize that speech is not an isolated act but the product of a highly complex and synchronized oral-motor system. Further, oral-motor treatment must be conducted with regard for a child's overall neuromuscular profile.

Oral-motor therapy for children with functional articulation disorders generally consists of a variety of tongue, lip, and jaw exercises. Most proponents of this approach subscribe to one or more of the following basic rationales: a) speech is founded on earlier-developing nonspeech motor patterns such as sucking and chewing (Marshalla, 1985; Ruark & Moore, 1997); b) reduced muscle tone in the oral-facial area results in limited strength of speech articulators (Robin, Somodi, & Luschei, 1991); c) the Piagetian construct that normal movement and sensation significantly influence motor learning (Piaget, 1951; Thelen & Smith, 1994); and d) speech is a highly complex behavior that is more easily learned when broken into smaller components (Magill, 1998). However, controversy exists regarding this approach to intervention. The few controlled studies present correlational rather than causal findings and report no significant connection between oral-motor exercises and speech sound production (Love, 2000; Moore & Ruark, 1996; Nittrouer, 1993). (See Forrest, 2002 and Lof, 2003 for a comprehensive discussion of the efficacy of oral-motor intervention for functional articulation errors.)

Given the scarcity of research-based evidence on this topic, clinicians are encouraged to combine available information with "professional wisdom" (Whitehurst, 2002). Accordingly, the decision to use oral-motor intervention requires careful consideration and a sound theoretical rationale. We suggest that this rationale serve as the basis for a set of systematic implementation guidelines which can be developed by individual practitioners, specific facilities, or regional school districts. These guidelines necessarily include (but are not limited to) the following factors: age, type of disorder, severity of impairment, number and type of speech errors, and individual responsiveness to this treatment approach.

The authors of this book do not specifically endorse the use of oral-motor techniques for any specific clients or groups of clients. The remaining coverage of this topic is included for general informational and educational purposes.

Proponents of an oral-motor approach to treatment (Alexander, Boehme, & Cupps, 1993; Mackie, 1996; Morris & Klein, 1987) suggest that children who exhibit the following speech characteristics are potential candidates for such therapy:

- Weak production of bilabials (/p,b,m/) resulting from decreased lip strength and control

- Poor production of sounds requiring tongue elevation (/t,d,n,l/) as a result of decreased tongue strength and coordination

- Poor differential production of midrange vowels (/ɚ,ʌ,ɝ/) as a result of inadequate jaw stabilization

- Weak production of plosives, fricatives, and affricates (/p,b,s,z,ʃ/) in the presence of hypernasality as a result of inadequate velar movement

The basic goals of an oral-motor therapy program for improving speech intelligibility are as follows:

- To heighten conscious awareness of the oral mechanism

- To normalize (increase or decrease) sensitivity to stimulation of the oral area
- To inhibit primitive or abnormal reflex patterns in the oral mechanism, while enhancing normal movement patterns
- To increase differentiation and stabilization of the oral structures
- To refine articulation movements by increasing the strength and range of motion of oral mechanism components

Following is a basic introductory hierarchy of oral-motor treatment steps along with sample intervention activities.

Hierarchy of Oral-Motor Treatment Steps

1. *Address postural and positioning issues to ensure adequate balance and alignment of the hip, shoulder, neck, and head.*

   Sample activity: Consult with occupational therapist (OT) or physical therapist (PT) to determine optimal positioning for conducting effective oral-motor therapy.

2. *Normalize oral sensitivity (both hypo- and hypersensitivity).*

   Sample activity: Gradually introduce firm, graded pressure along the child's gums from front to back using fingertips or textured implement. If child reacts negatively, modify the activity by applying the pressure to an area where touch has been tolerated previously.

3. *Increase jaw control to provide a stable base for finely graded movements of the lips and tongue.*

   Sample activity: Place fingers on the child's jaw. Use thumb to quickly pull the jaw down in a firm, gentle manner. Tell child to try to close mouth while clinician guides upward movement with index finger.

4. *Strengthen lip movement/increase muscle tone.*

   Sample activity: Use pads of fingers to stroke diagonally from cheekbones to lips. Tell child to hold a straw horizontally with lips for at least five seconds. Release and repeat.

5. *Improve tongue control for elevation and lateralization.*

   Sample activity: Place finger or tongue depressor flat against tongue tip. Instruct child to try to push tongue tip up against pressure.

Certain general guidelines should be kept in mind when implementing oral-motor therapy:

- Apply stimulation systematically and follow the same sequence of steps each time.
- Begin stimulation with outer body parts and move in toward midline (e.g., work from the cheeks to the lips to the tongue).
- Use firm, slow touch rather than light, quick strokes.

- Use visual feedback (e.g., mirror) to facilitate child's ability to categorize new perceptions and improve tolerance of stimulation.

- Explain procedures as each is being implemented (e.g., "Okay, now I'm stroking from your cheek down to your mouth. Good, you let me touch your face.")

FUNCTIONAL ARTICULATION DISORDERS

Children with functional articulation disorders demonstrate speech production errors in the absence of any identifiable etiology. These children present with adequate hearing acuity and intellectual abilities and with no signs of significant structural abnormalities or neurological dysfunction. The specific errors displayed vary greatly from one child to the next and are not as readily predictable as those found in organically based disorders. The selection of initial therapy targets for functional articulation disorders can be approached from either a developmental or nondevelopmental perspective.

Example Profiles

Below are three commonly seen profiles of childhood articulation problems. These examples have been designed to illustrate the selection of intervention targets as well as specific therapy activities and materials. Most of the chosen activities are easily implemented in either individual or group therapy settings.

For many children, it may be necessary to teach the phonetic placement of target sounds prior to the introduction of actual activities. Appendix 3-A provides specific instructions for establishing the correct placement for consonants that are typically considered difficult to elicit.

The first profile describes a *young child with multiple errors*.

PROFILE 1

Jill is 3 years old and demonstrates the following articulation errors (error sound/ intended target):

Initial	Medial	Final
d/g	d/g	ʃ/tʃ
j/l	w/r	-/s
b/v	f/θ	-/k
-/s	j/l	-/d
p/f	ʔ/t	s/ʃ
b/m	j/n	-/ŋ
	-/s	

Blends: b/bl, f/fl, w/kl, t/sl, t/skw, fw/kr, b/br, d/dr, w/pr

Selection of therapy targets using a developmental approach. Based on this child's chronological age, the errors to be targeted first are d/g, b/m, p/f, j/n,-/ŋ because these are the earliest emerging sounds as can be seen in Table 3-1. The second set of target sounds consists of -/k,-/d, and ʔ/t. The remaining errors would not be considered appropriate targets for intervention because they emerge well beyond 3 years of age.

Selection of therapy targets using a nondevelopmental approach. The errors to be targeted are /θ/, /v/, /m/, /f/, /g/, and /s/. The /θ/ and /v/ sounds were chosen despite developmental considerations because Jill was highly stimulable for these sounds in isolation during the diagnostic session. The /m/ and /f/ sounds were selected because they are visible when produced, which facilitates learning of correct articulatory placement. The /f/ and /g/ sounds were included as beginning targets because their status as initial-position errors makes them significant contributors to Jill's overall unintelligibility.

Sample Activities

1. Modify a board game, such as Candy Land, by requiring a child to produce a target sound in isolation following the clinician's model in order to move a game piece. Close approximations, rather than accurate productions, of the target phoneme may be acceptable in the very early stages of therapy. Once the child improves her performance by 30% to 50% over baseline measures, clinician models should be faded. Three consecutive spontaneous productions can then be required for the child to take a turn in the game.

2. Create a game with construction paper fish. Each fish has a picture on it designed to elicit a target sound in the desired position. Attach paper clips to the back of each fish and give the child a "fishing pole" with a magnet on the end of its string. Have the child dangle the magnet over the fish. Instruct the child to respond by producing the stimulus item three times as she "lands" each fish. The difficulty level of the response can be programmed to vary from single words to lengthy sentences.

3. Assemble 25 4-by-4-inch squares of colored construction paper with one stimulus picture on each. One of the squares should be marked in a special way (e.g., with a star or a sticker). Cover one wall with the squares so that the stimulus pictures are facing the wall. Tell the child that she is going to pretend to be a detective who has to find the "magic square" in the dark. Hand the child a penlight, turn out the lights, and instruct her to aim the beam at the square that she thinks is the magic one. As each square is lit up, the child is asked to produce the target item at the appropriate level of complexity.

4. Assemble the following materials to make two puppets: two glue sticks, two brown paper bags, yarn, two sets of construction paper cutouts of facial features, and other accessories such as earrings, mustaches, and eyeglasses. Collect 25 pictures containing the targeted therapy sounds and place them in a pile on the table. Explain that the clinician and child will construct puppets using the paper bags and other materials. The clinician selects one picture from the pile, models correct production of the word, and then glues one feature/accessory to one of the bags. Instruct the child to select the next picture from

the pile, produce the word correctly three times, and glue a feature/accessory on the other bag. Alternate turns until both puppets are completed.

The second profile describes a school-age child with *multiple articulation errors.*

PROFILE 2

Joe is 6 years old and demonstrates the following errors:

Initial	*Medial*	*Final*
j/l	j/l	j/l
	s/θ	s/θ
ʃ/tʃ	ʃ/tʃ	ʃ/tʃ
		-/d
ʃ/f	ʃ/f	s/f
b/v	b/v	
w/r	w/r	

Blends: s/sl, b/bl, k/kl, fw/fl, fw/fr, tw/tr, k/skw, fw/kr, t/st

Selection of therapy targets using a developmental approach. Based on this child's chronological age, the errors to be targeted first are -/d, ʃ/f, b/v, j/l because these are the earliest emerging sounds as can be seen in Table 3-1. The second set of targets consists of the remaining sound and blend errors because all these are typically acquired by 6 years of age.

Selection of therapy targets using a nondevelopmental approach. The errors to be targeted are /r/, /fr/, /fl/, and /θ/. The /r/ was chosen because it is one of the most frequently occurring sounds in English (see Table 3-2, Frequency of Consonant Occurrence in English). The /fr/ and /fl/ blends were selected because these are the only phonetic contexts in which Joe can correctly produce his otherwise misarticulated /f/ sound. The blends can provide a starting point for facilitating the correct production of /f/ as a singleton. Finally, the /θ/ was chosen because its articulatory placement is highly visible and is therefore relatively easy to approximate.

Sample Activities

1. Draw 10 pictures on a blackboard, each containing one instance of a target sound. Give the child a squirt gun and tell him to hit one of the pictures. Instruct the child to produce the stimulus item at the appropriate level of complexity (e.g., single word, carrier phrase, sentence, narrative).

2. For a group activity, gather at least 20 pictures/objects that contain the target sound(s) and place them around the room. Give each child a "suitcase" (box) and tell them that the group is going on a trip. Say, "I'm going to Disney World. I'll take you too if you bring the right things in your suitcase." Have

TABLE 3-2
Frequency of Consonant Occurrence in English

Sound	Percentage of Occurrence	Cumulative Percentage
n	12.0	12.0
t	11.9	23.9
s	6.9	30.8
r	6.7	37.5
d	6.4	43.9
m	5.9	49.8
z	5.4	55.2
ð	5.3	60.5
l	5.3	65.8
k	5.1	70.9
w	4.9	75.8
h	4.4	80.2
b	3.3	83.5
p	3.1	86.6
g	3.1	89.7
f	2.1	91.8
ŋ	1.6	93.4
j	1.6	95.0
v	1.5	96.5
ʃ	0.9	97.4
θ	0.9	98.3
dʒ	0.6	98.9
tʃ	0.6	99.5
ʒ	<0.1	99.6

Source: From "Computer-Assisted Natural Process Analysis (NPA): Recent Issues and Data," by L. D. Shriberg and J. Kwiatkowski, 1983, p. 11, in *Seminars in Speech and Language, 4*(4). Adapted by permission.

the children take turns retrieving stimulus items from around the room. They may place them in their suitcases upon correct production of the appropriate target sounds.

3. Assemble at least 20 pictures/objects that contain target sound(s) and place them on the table. Introduce a "shopping game" by presenting a carrier phrase such as "I went to the food store and bought _____, _____, and _____." Have the child remove the corresponding pictures from the table. Then instruct the child to take a turn at making a shopping list by producing the same carrier phrase with three new food items chosen from the remaining picture stimuli. The type of store named in the carrier phrase can be varied to expose/reinforce the child's ability to organize lexical items into semantic categories (e.g., clothing, toys, pets). Each list can also be written on a blackboard or chart paper to emphasize the connection between writing, reading, and speaking. The activity can be easily adapted for small group sessions.

4. Write each verse of the following song on a sheet of paper. Place clip art or other icons above words containing a targeted sound (e.g., /θ/). Provide a

microphone and arrange a spotlight using a flashlight in a darkened room. Explain that in this activity the child will pretend to be on stage. Teach the child to sing the song using the melody from Simon and Garfunkel's "I'd Rather Be a Hammer Than a Nail" or another suitable tune.

> I'd rather use a bathtub than a booth
> I'd rather have a toothache than no tooth
> I'd rather have a birthday than a wreath
> I'd rather be an athlete than a thief
>
> *Refrain*
> Yes I would
> If I only could
> I surely would
>
> I'd rather use a thumbtack than a thorn
> I'd rather have a thick one than a thin
> I'd rather have some mouthwash than a bath
> I'd rather be a Matthew than a Keith
>
> *Repeat refrain*

The third profile describes an *older school-age child with persistent /r/ and /s/ substitution errors.*

PROFILE 3

Sammy is 8 years old and demonstrates the following errors:

Initial	Medial	Final
w/r	w/r	w/r
θ/s	θ/s	θ/s

Blends: Sammy has the same substitution pattern for all /r/ and /s/ blends.

Selection of therapy targets using a developmental approach. A developmental approach for therapy target selection is not relevant in this case. The /r/ and /s/ sounds are typically acquired by 8 years of age, and, therefore, both would be considered appropriate therapy objectives.

Selection of therapy targets using a nondevelopmental approach. The /s/ phoneme is selected as the primary therapy target because Sammy was stimulable for this sound in isolation. It is also considered a particularly relevant objective for Sammy because /s/ is the first sound in his name.

Sample Activities

1. Draw a football field on a chalkboard with the yard lines (e.g., 10-yard line, 20-yard line, and so on) and end zones clearly delineated. Make a football from construction paper/cardboard and affix masking tape or other adhesive

to the back. The therapist and child select team names. The child takes control of the ball at the 50-yard line because he represents the home team. Model stimulus items containing the target sound and instruct the child to repeat the stimulus item five times. He can move the football five yards toward his end zone for every correct response. If the child produces no correct responses, the clinician gets to move the ball five yards toward the other end zone. The difficulty level of this game can be modified in various ways: fading the therapist model, increasing the number of required responses, and increasing the length and complexity of the target response from isolation to complex sentences. This activity also works well in small group sessions.

2. Design a game sheet with at least six or eight drawings of blank TV screens. Instruct the child to name television shows containing the target sound. A correct production allows the child to draw or write something related to that show on one of the TV sets on the game sheet. For example, for the target sound /r/, the child may name shows such as R*oad* R*unner*, P*ower* R*angers*, R*ocky and Bullwinkle*, and *Mister* R*oger's Neighborhood*. Once all the TV sets are filled in, begin a guessing game in which the child is instructed to describe one of the TV shows without using the title, and the therapist has to guess the name of the show. All correct spontaneous productions of the target sound during this conversational task should be reinforced. If the child meets a predetermined criterion for accuracy of sound production, a paper "Emmy" can be awarded. Task difficulty can be increased to more complex levels by requiring the child to summarize an episode of a show or describe one of its characters in order to fill in a blank TV set on the game sheet. This activity is easily adapted for group sessions.

3. On slips of paper, write 25 single words containing the target sound /s/ in initial, final, or medial position. Fold slips of paper and place them in a container or pile them on the table. Affix a Nerf basketball hoop (or equivalent) to a therapy room wall at least three feet higher than the child's standing height. Explain that this game requires the child to select a slip of paper from the pile and produce a sentence using the word written on the slip. If the target sound is produced correctly, the child is allowed to crumple the paper slip and shoot it at the basketball hoop. If target sound /s/ is incorrectly produced, the slip of paper is returned to the pile or container. The game continues until the pile is depleted and all paper slips have been crumpled and shot.

4. Gather materials to play "detective," including a badge and a small notebook with pencil. Design several simple crime scenarios that contain multiple instances of the target sound. One example of a possible scenario follows:

> *S*ue is lying dead on the floor beside a window*s*ill in a *s*ealed room. *S*cattered on the floor, there is water and broken gla*ss*. *S*imon is a*s*leep on the *s*ofa acro*ss* the room. Mr. *S*oaps, a window washer, *s*pots *S*ue and calls the police to report his *s*uspicions.

Tell the child to play a detective and ask questions of the witness, Mr. Soaps (played by therapist), to solve the crime. The child should be encouraged to ask questions that contain as many instances of the target sound as possible.

To facilitate this, all questions could begin with, "Well, Mr. Soaps . . . " Appropriate questions for this scenario include "What sort of clothes was Sue wearing when you saw her?"; "How old is Simon?"; "Where do you suppose the broken glass came from?"

(Solution: Sue is a goldfish and Simon is a cat.)

Helpful Hints

1. Do not include more than one error sound in a stimulus word, phrase, or sentence during the initial stages of therapy.

2. Pay attention to the phonetic context of words that contain a child's target sounds. Certain consonant-vowel sequences may facilitate or impede correct production.

3. In some ways, the production of speech sounds is a motor skill like that of playing a piano. Therapy sessions that elicit the greatest number of sound productions will be the most effective in establishing correct production as an automatic behavior.

4. Children with persistent errors that appear to be functional should be evaluated for the presence of oral-motor difficulties.

5. Use books that contain target sounds as immersion activities. The books can be given to parents to use at reading time with their child. For our example child Sammy, good choices include *Rotten Ralph* by J. Gantos, *Rain Makes Applesauce* by J. Scheer, *Miss Nelson Is Missing* by H. Allard and J. Marshall, and *My Mama Says* by J. Viorst. For further suggestions, see *Books Are for Talking Too!* by J. Gebers (1990).

6. It is important to counsel parents to respond consistently to the content of their child's utterances before pointing out speech errors or modeling correct productions. This is particularly relevant in the early stages of therapy to avoid frustration and other negative feelings.

ORGANIC ARTICULATION DISORDERS

Three pathologies associated with severe articulation problems in children are cleft palate, hearing impairment, and developmental verbal dyspraxia. The selection of initial therapy targets for organic disorders is based on a nondevelopmental approach because the accompanying articulation deficits are the direct result of structural/neurologic anomalies and are not developmental in nature.

Cleft Palate

This is a congenital malformation of the palate and/or lip that results from the failure of oral structures to fuse at midline during the first trimester of pregnancy (4 to 12 weeks gestation). A cleft can be unilateral (one-sided) or bilateral. Clefts of the palate have substantially more severe effects on speech intelligibility than do isolated clefts of the lip. Management of children with clefts generally is carried out by an interdisciplinary team that includes a speech-language pathologist. Surgical repair of labial clefts is completed at approximately 3 months of age or earlier; palatal repairs generally occur before the child's second birthday (Osborn & Kelleher, 1983; Peterson-Falzone, Hardin-Jones, & Karnell, 2001; Shprintzen & Bardach, 1995). Pharyngeal flap procedures are considered secondary surgical interventions and involve joining a flap of soft tissue from the posterior pharyngeal wall to the palate, creating a bridge that partially occludes the velopharyngeal space. This procedure is performed primarily for the purpose of facilitating velopharyngeal closure during speech. Speech therapy may begin before surgical repairs are completed but is primarily provided following surgical intervention. McWilliams, Morris, and Shelton (1990) recommend a three-month postsurgical recovery period before therapy is initiated or resumed.

The most significant speech problem associated with cleft palate is velopharyngeal incompetence (VPI). VPI is the inability to close off the oral cavity from the nasal cavity during speech due to inadequate velar movement. This results in audible nasal emission of air, hypernasal resonance, and articulation errors. Audible nasal emission occurs when air flows at an excessive rate through the nasal passages, creating turbulence and generating distracting noise during speech. This leakage of air results in reduced oral breath pressure for the production of pressure consonants (i.e., fricatives, affricates, and plosives). Hypernasal resonance, or hypernasality, occurs when the balance between oral and nasal resonance shifts to such a degree that speech is perceived by listeners to be "nasal." This phenomenon is particularly noticeable during the production of vowels, especially when the degree of mouth opening is restricted.

In misarticulations related to VPI, the most frequent errors occur on fricatives, affricates, and plosives. The most common types of errors demonstrated by cleft palate speakers are distortions and omissions, with occasional substitutions in the form of glottal stops and pharyngeal fricatives. In general, the provision of therapy is appropriate only for children who have VP competence or questionable/marginal incompetence, as determined by the cleft palate team (Kuehn & Moller, 2000; McWilliams, et al., 1990). Therapy focusing on oral direction of the breath stream is not usually recommended for children who demonstrate clear evidence of VPI. It may lead to elevation of the larynx and result in voice disorders.

The most common patterns of speech errors of children with cleft palates are as follows:

- The most frequent errors occur on fricatives and affricates, followed by plosives.

- Distortions and omissions are the most common error types, followed by substitutions.

- Singleton fricatives and affricates are most likely to be distorted.

- Consonants in blends are most likely to be omitted.

- Glottal stops tend to be substituted for plosives.

- More misarticulations occur on voiceless consonants than their voiced cognates, especially in young children.

- Most errors occur in the final position, followed by medial and initial positions, respectively.

Example Profile

Following is a typical profile for cleft palate. This example has been designed to illustrate the selection of intervention targets as well as specific therapy activities and materials. The chosen activities are easily implemented in either individual or group therapy settings.

PROFILE

Eddie is 4 years old, has undergone successful palatal repair, and demonstrates adequate VP closure in nonspeech activities. His speech is characterized by audible nasal emission of air, hypernasality, and the following articulation errors:

	Initial	Medial	Final
Distortions	s,z,ʃ	s,z,ʃ	s,z,ʃ
	k,g,p,b	f,θ,k,g	f,θ,k,g
	t		
Omissions	-r/pr*	-l/pl*-	s/st*
Substitutions	n/d	ʔ/p, ʔ/b	ʔ/p, ʔ/b
		ʔ/d, ʔ/t	ʔ/d, ʔ/d

*Consonant blends are consistently reduced to singletons in all positions and, therefore, are too numerous to list individually.

Selection of therapy targets. The five main goals of speech therapy with children with cleft palate are (1) correct articulatory placement, (2) light articulatory contacts, (3) greater mouth opening, (4) decrease hypernasal resonance quality, and (5) promote more anterior placement of articulatory production (Hall & Golding-Kushner, 1989; Shelton, Hahn, & Morris, 1968; Witzel, 1995). Given these goals, the errors to be targeted for intervention are /p/, /b/, /s/, /θ/, /k/, /g/, /t/, /d/, and vowels. The first four sounds were chosen to decrease Eddie's tendency to move frontal articulatory placements to the back of the vocal tract. The /k/, /g/, /t/, and /d/, as well as /p/ and /b/, were selected because pressure consonants are the most effective vehicles for demonstrating light articulatory contact (less forceful movements of oral muscles). Vowels were included because they are the most appropriate targets for encouraging increased or exaggerated mouth opening as a means of improving the balance between oral and nasal resonance.

Sample Activities

1. Compile a set of 20 pictures that are clear demonstrations of the concept of front versus back (e.g., train, dog, car, house, horse, truck) and cut them in half. (In addition, decorate a blank sheet of paper with 25 drawings or stickers of balloons without strings for later use.) Shuffle the pictures and place them facedown on the table. Tell the child that this is a memory game in

which he and the clinician will take turns selecting pictures, one at a time, to try to match the pairs that represent the front and back of each object. The child is instructed to identify each picture piece as it is uncovered (e.g., "This is the front of a train"). Each correctly matched pair is given to the player who found both pieces. The player with the most pairs at the end of the game is the winner.

Once it is established that the child understands "front/back" in relation to everyday objects, explain that this concept also applies to his mouth. Tell him that some sounds are made at the front of the mouth, like /p/ and /t/, and others are made at the back like /k/ and /g/. Sit with the child in front of a mirror and model the anterior placement of simple syllables (i.e., /pa/, /bæ/, /so/, /θi/). Engage the child in a "Simon Says" game in which he has to imitate sounds made by the clinician. For each correct production, the child may draw a string under one balloon on the prepared sheet. The object of the game is to fill the sheet with strings on all of the balloons.

2. Obtain two puppets with easily manipulable mouths (e.g., Lamb Chop). Introduce the puppets to the child. Explain that one uses very hard (forceful) movements of his mouth when he talks, while the other uses soft (light) movements. The clinician's speech and hand movements should demonstrate forceful versus light contacts as the explanations are given. To ensure the child's understanding of the basic concept, model several exaggerated examples of both articulatory contact types, and have the child point to the puppet that uses that speech pattern. Once the child can reliably discriminate between "hard" and "gentle," hide both puppets in a bag or box, and instruct the child to close his eyes and pull one out and place it on his hand. The clinician provides a model of the type of contact used by the chosen puppet at the syllable level. Models should focus on pressure consonants in the initial position (e.g., /ka/, /gu/, /ti/, do/, /pa/, and /bæ/). The child is then required to imitate the clinician's stimulus and should be encouraged to use appropriate hand and mouth movements simultaneously. Return the puppet to its hiding place and repeat the activity for 20 or more trials. The level of response complexity can be increased from imitative to spontaneous and also can be programmed to vary from syllables to lengthy sentences.

3. Draw or attach two pictures of frogs to a blackboard. One should be depicted as having an exaggerated open-mouth posture, while the other frog's mouth is only slightly opened. Instruct the child to throw a beanbag at either of the frogs. The clinician should model a vowel production with the degree of mouth opening that corresponds to the frog that is struck by the beanbag. The child is required to imitate the clinician's model five times for another turn at the game. The vowels /a/, /æ/, /o/, and /e/ are good candidates for the initial phase of training.

4. Cut out a 12-inch circle from poster board to use as a "pizza." Use a marker to draw lines dividing the pizza into eight equal slices. Affix three to five small pieces of Velcro to each slice. Gather 24 to 40 small pictures containing targeted therapy sound(s) and attach Velcro strips to each. Explain that the child will decorate the pizza with picture "toppings." Instruct the child to

name a picture with emphasis on the target sound. If production is correct, the child can place the topping on the pizza. Repeat this sequence until all toppings have been used.

Helpful Hints

1. Children who show only glottal and pharyngeal place of articulation should have therapy to assess adequacy of fricative and plosive production before any pharyngeal flap surgery is considered.

2. If the child has questionable VPI, delay training of /k/ and /g/ to avoid the tendency to adopt compensatory movements.

3. Children with cleft palates often have persistent dental anomalies that may result in lateralization of fricatives and affricates which are not amenable to articulation therapy.

4. In general, speech therapy should be initiated at the earliest possible age to take advantage of sensitive periods in speech development.

5. Self-monitoring skills in children with nasality problems may be strengthened with the use of biofeedback devices such as the See-Scape (The Speech Bin, 2003) and the Nasometer II (Kay Elemetrics Corporation, 2003). These devices detect nasal emission/resonance and display this information visually or auditorily. The child uses the displayed information to monitor and eventually control velopharyngeal function.

6. The therapeutic process for children with oral-facial anomalies frequently must address the emotional well-being of the child and the family as well as the symptoms of the physical defect.

7. Parents of infants with clefts may require gentle but firm encouragement to engage in natural smiling and vocal interactions with their babies. Parents may need guidance to see beyond the obvious craniofacial defect to bond successfully with their child.

8. Clinicians treating children with cleft palates should be prepared to make referrals to parent support groups or to counseling professionals who have expertise in the area of birth defects.

Hearing Impairment

Hearing impairment refers to a significant loss in auditory acuity. There are two major types of hearing impairments: conductive and sensorineural. A conductive, or peripheral, hearing loss refers to a disruption in the mechanical transmission of sounds from the external auditory canal to the cochlea (inner ear) (Northern & Downs, 2002). Conductive losses do not exceed 60 dB HL and generally are amenable to medical treatment. A common cause of conductive hearing loss in young children is otitis media, an inflammation in the middle ear. A sensorineural loss involves a deficit in the neural transmission of sound impulses through the cochlea hair cells or the auditory nerve. Losses of this type usually do not respond to medical treatment and are generally irreversible. A disruption that occurs simultaneously in both pathways is termed a mixed hearing loss.

The degree of loss can range in severity from mild to profound. The majority of children with hearing losses are typically labeled hard of hearing (loss of < 80 dB HL) and can derive significant benefit from articulation therapy. Children who are profoundly hearing impaired or deaf (loss of > 80 dB HL) experience great difficulty acquiring intelligible speech even with intervention. In general, greater degrees of hearing loss result in more severe disruptions of speech development. It is important to note, however, that a loss as mild as 10 to 15 dB HL may be handicapping in the classroom setting with an ambient noise level of 25 to 35 dB. Deficits in speech production may not be marked if the hearing loss is unilateral rather than bilateral. Table 3-3 outlines the effects of different degrees of hearing loss on children's speech production abilities.

Speech intelligibility also is significantly affected by several other factors, including age of onset, configuration of hearing loss, age of identification, and degree of linguistic complexity (Martin & Clark, 1996; Radziewicz & Antonellis, 2002). With regard to amplification, important factors include the age at which appropriate amplification is fitted, the type and amount of habilitation, and the consistency of device use. Age of onset is a particularly critical factor. Children who are born with or sustain significant hearing losses prior to the critical language learning period (before age 3 years) will have more severe articulation deficits than children whose losses occurred later in life.

Following is a list of the most common types of speech errors exhibited by children with hearing impairment. The first four are characteristic of children whose hearing losses fall in the moderate range. Children who are profoundly hearing-impaired or deaf will likely display all these behaviors.

- Omission of final consonants
- Substitution of voiced consonants for voiceless
- Substitution of stops for nasals, fricatives, and affricates
- Omission of consonants in blends
- Omission of initial consonants
- Substitution of schwa for other vowels (neutralization)
- Insertion of schwa into words or added to the ends of words
- Substitution of vowels for other vowels
- Nasalization of vowels

Treatment approaches. There are three basic approaches to intervention for children with hearing impairment: oral, manual, and total communication. **Oral** programs emphasize spoken language as the primary mode of communication through the use of strategies such speechreading, amplification, auditory training, and explicit speech-language instruction. **Manual** programs focus on the earliest possible acquisition of a linguistic system, generally via American Sign Language (ASL), fingerspelling, and/or manually coded English systems. **Total communication** is a philosophy that encourages any combination of modalities (e.g., speech, writing, signing, gestures, and facial expression) which is most effective in facilitating an individual child's acquisition of language. Recently, a **bilingual/bicultural** model of education has been implemented for children

TABLE 3-3	
Effects of Hearing Loss on Articulation Development	
Degree of Loss	**Characteristics**
Slight (16–25 dB HL)	No noticeable difficulty in relatively quiet listening environments
Mild (26–40 dB HL)	Occasional difficulty with voiceless consonants; vowels and voiced consonants generally intact
Moderate (41–70 dB HL)	Some difficulty with sounds characterized by low intensity, high frequency, or short duration (e.g., final consonant omission, distortion of fricatives and affricates)
Severe (71–90 dB HL)	Significant difficulty in consonant production with additional confusion of voiced/voiceless consonants and omission of consonants in blends
Profound (91 dB HL or greater)	Global speech production impairment with the addition of neutralization (schwa), substitution, addition, and nasalization of vowels as well as the omission of initial consonants

Sources: Adapted from Oller & Kelly (1974), Hudgins & Numbers (1942), Nober (1967), and Clark (1981).

with significant hearing loss. In this approach, children are exposed to ASL as their first language for communication and learn English in the school setting to develop reading and writing skills. Lively debate continues regarding the educational, social, and cultural impact of these different approaches. (See Lieberth, 1990 and Winefield, 1987 for comprehensive discussion of the topic.)

The most recent advance in rehabilitation for children with deafness is the use of **cochlear implants**. The following discussion represents the most current data available at the time of this edition. Since state-of-the-art knowledge in this area is evolving rapidly, clinicians are encouraged to seek out additional, updated information.

Unlike a traditional hearing aid, a cochlear implant directly stimulates surviving auditory nerve fibers. One component of the device is a body-worn processor that highlights speech signals and minimizes background noise. These signals are routed first to a receiver implanted in the mastoid bone. Then the signals travel to an array of electrodes implanted in the cochlea which transfers the sound to the auditory nerve (Wilson, 2000). The cochlear implant devices currently approved by the U.S. Food and Drug Administration (FDA) for implantation in children provide multichannel stimulation and continue to evolve technologically. Thus far, the cochlear implant literature suggests that four important factors are associated with improved speech production skills: years of device use, nonverbal intelligence, oral communication as primary mode post-implant, and number of active electrodes with a wide dynamic range (Geers, 2002; and Tobey, Geers, Brenner, Altuna & Gabbert, 2003).

Example Profile

Following is a typical profile for pediatric hearing loss. This example has been designed to illustrate the selection of therapy targets as well as specific therapy activities and materials. The chosen activities are easily implemented in either individual or group therapy settings.

| PROFILE |

Sherry is 7 years old with a congenital moderate-severe bilateral sensorineural hearing loss, is fitted with binaural hearing aids, and demonstrates the following errors. These errors are illustrative of the misarticulations of children with this degree of hearing impairment.

1. Omission of final consonants
   -/s
   -/z
   -/t
   -/d
   -/k
   -/g
   -/tʃ

2. Substitution of voiced for voiceless consonants
   v/f
   b/p
   d/t
   g/k
   ð/θ

3. Substitutions of stops for nasals, fricatives, and affricates
   d/n
   g/ŋ
   t/s
   d/z
   d/tʃ
   t/ʃ

4. Substitution of schwa for other vowels*
   ə/æ (hat)
   ə/ɛ (bet)
   ə/ʊ (boot)

*Errors of this type may not be found in all children with this degree of hearing loss.

Selection of therapy targets. The errors to be targeted are -/s,-/z,-/t,-/d, ə/æ, ə/ɛ, ə/ʊ, v/f, b/p, and ð/θ. Final consonant omissions and schwa substitutions were identified as priorities because these error types have a significant negative impact on perceived speech intelligibility. The four deletion errors listed (-/s,-/z,-/t,-/d) were chosen because, in the word final position, these sounds also function as plural and tense markers. The ə/æ, ə/ɛ, and ə/ʊ were included because these three substitutions have highly contrastive lip configurations that facilitate differential production. The voiced/voiceless confusion is an appropriate initial target because two of the three critical characteristics of these phonemes (i.e., place and manner) are already present in the child's repertoire, thus increasing the likelihood of early success in therapy. The v/f, b/p, and ð/θ confusions were selected because they are highly visible, which eliminates the need for placement cues and allows training to focus solely on voicing. Production of /ʃ/ also was included as a therapy target because it is the initial sound of Sherry's name. This sound will be programmed at the sentence level since Sherry demonstrates relatively consistent production at the level of isolated words.

Sample Activities

1. Draw three "speech flowers" on large pieces of paper, each with a distinct rounded center and ten petals (similar to daisies). From construction paper, cut 30 loose flower petals that are the same size as the drawn petals and place them in a pile on the table. Write a different consonant-vowel (CV) syllable on every petal and a different final consonant in the three flower centers. The combination of each CV syllable with the final consonant should constitute a real word (e.g., fa + t = fat; be + t = bet, and so on). Explain to the child that the activity will focus on the production of final sounds in words. Provide a glue stick or other adhesive. Instruct the child to pick a petal from the pile and fit it in an empty petal on the drawing. The clinician then glides a finger from the top of the petal to the flower center as the child produces the syllable plus final sound and forms a real word. After five correct productions of the target word, the child may glue the petal to the flower. Repeat this sequence until all the CV petals have been attached. The completed flowers can be used for home practice. (This activity can also be used to facilitate language awareness by using rhyming stimuli.)

2. Draw three Charlie Brown (or another character) faces on separate pieces of paper or poster board, each depicting distinctly different mouth configurations corresponding to the target vowels. The mouth posture representing /æ/ should be drawn with an exaggerated lowering of the mandible. The /ɛ/ should depict clear lip retraction (similar to a smile), and the /ʊ/ drawing should display a pursed, rounded lip position that is slightly opened. For each vowel sound, gather or prepare 10 picture cards representing common monosyllabic words for a total of 30 cards (e.g., cat, bag, pen, bed, boot, shoe, and so on). Draw a gallows on the blackboard in preparation for a "hangman" game. Place the three Charlie Brown cue cards on the table and put the shuffled card deck face side down in front of the child. Explain the rules of hangman and emphasize that the game will focus on correct vowel production. Begin the game by having the child turn over the top card of the deck and place it next to the corresponding Charlie Brown cue card. Instruct the child to produce the correct vowel in isolation, making sure to match mouth configuration to that of Charlie Brown's, and then name the card five times. Each incorrect production allows the clinician to fill in one part of the hangman drawing. The object of the game is to deplete the picture deck before the hangman is completed.

3. With masking tape, create an outline on the floor of a mountain range with at least six peaks. Provide a small toy train or other vehicle and tell the child that the train is going on a long journey up and down the mountain peaks.

The clinician introduces a voiced/voiceless cognate pair (e.g., v/f) and instructs the child to produce the voiced sound while moving the train *up* the mountain and to produce the voiceless sound as the train is moved *down* the mountain. Instruct the child to monitor voice onset and offset by placing her free hand on her throat (tactile cue) throughout the journey. Repeat this activity with each target cognate pair.

4. Engage the child in a hand-clapping or jump rope activity using the following chant. Explain that the chant emphasizes correct production of the /ʃ/ in lots of different words. Teach one verse at a time to control task difficulty level. Use pictures and/or written words as needed.

> *Sh*eila the fi*sh*, fi*sh*, fi*sh*
> *Sh*e had one wi*sh*, wi*sh*, wi*sh*
> To have a bowl, bowl, bowl
> Without a hole, hole, hole.

> *Sh*e called up Jo*sh*, Jo*sh*, Jo*sh*
> Who said, Oh go*sh*, go*sh*, go*sh*
> Do you have a ga*sh*, ga*sh*, ga*sh*
> Or a red ra*sh*, ra*sh*, ra*sh*?

> *Sh*e said, Oh *s*ure, *s*ure, *s*ure
> Quite an eyesore, sore, sore
> My bowl was sma*sh*ed, sma*sh*ed, sma*sh*ed
> When the table cra*sh*ed, cra*sh*ed, cra*sh*ed.

> Jo*sh* said, let's ru*sh*, ru*sh*, ru*sh*
> Or the water will gu*sh*, gu*sh*, gu*sh*
> Get the me*sh* net, net, net
> So you stay wet, wet, wet.

> *Sh*eila the fi*sh*, fi*sh*, fi*sh*
> Was plopped in a di*sh*, di*sh*, di*sh*
> And said, Oh *sh*eesh, *sh*eesh, *sh*eesh
> I thought I'd be qui*ch*e, qui*ch*e, qui*ch*e.

> After a while, while, while
> *Sh*e began to smile, smile, smile
> At first sluggi*sh*, i*sh*, i*sh*
> *Sh*e now goes swi*sh*, swi*sh*, swi*sh*.

Helpful Hints

1. Cued speech can be a helpful tool for teaching place, manner, and voicing in the initial stages of therapy for children with hearing losses greater than 85 dB HL. (See Cornett, 1967; Paul, 2000; and Scheetz, 2001, for more information and specific techniques.)

2. Try to incorporate alternative sensory modalities (i.e., visual, tactile, and so on) in the early stages of each therapy task. These cues can be faded out as soon as they are no longer required to elicit a target sound.

3. For school-age children whose hearing losses also result in language impairments, select stimulus words that are related to the classroom curriculum (e.g., spelling words, science vocabulary).

4. Always ensure that the child's amplification system is in working order during therapy sessions to maximize residual hearing capabilities. Good sources for tips regarding troubleshooting hearing aids are Hull, 2001; Bentler, 2000; and Schow, 2001.

5. Auditory trainers are often used in the classrooom environment to facilitate the child's ability to monitor his or her own speech production as well as that of the teacher. Auditory trainers are high-fidelity systems in which the speaker's voice is fed into a microphone, amplified, and then directed to the child through a receiver. These devices make it possible for the child to receive speech input with minimum background noise (a high signal-to-noise ratio). One widely used system consists of a microphone/transmitter worn by the teacher, which broadcasts directly to an FM receiver worn by the child.

6. As counselors, clinicians may be asked to provide information regarding a child's academic aptitude and recommendations for appropriate educational placement.

7. Clinicians should anticipate that some children may demonstrate confusion or fear when experiencing sound input for the first time (via devices such as hearing aids and cochlear implants). Comfort with sound stimulation and auditory awareness develops gradually.

Developmental Verbal Dyspraxia

Developmental verbal dyspraxia (DVD), sometimes called developmental apraxia of speech, is a speech-motor planning disorder characterized by a reduced ability to volitionally sequence movements of the articulators for speech in the absence of paralysis, incoordination, or weakness of the oral musculature (dysarthria). (See Appendix 3-B for normative data on diadochokinetic rates for children.) DVD is thought to result from neurologic dysfunction, although currently no definitive evidence of specific brain pathology exists. There is much controversy in the literature as to whether DVD constitutes a discrete clinical entity (e.g., Rosenbek & Wertz, 1972; Shriberg, Aram, & Kwiatkowski, 1997a,b,c; Waldron, 1998; Williams, Ingham, & Rosenthal, 1981; Yoss & Darley, 1974). However, several behavioral features have been identified across studies as characteristic of children who are described as exhibiting DVD. In general, these children demonstrate receptive language abilities that are significantly superior to their speech production skills and frequently exhibit an accompanying oral apraxia. Children with severe DVD are highly unintelligible; at the most severe levels, these children may be categorized as nonverbal (i.e., the virtual absence of oral expressive output). They frequently demonstrate awareness of and frustration with their reduced ability to communicate.

Following is a list of the speech production characteristics most frequently associated with DVD:

- Repertoire of phonemes is extremely restricted.
- There is reduced ability to imitate sounds modeled by others, especially at the multisyllabic level.

- Speech production errors are highly inconsistent.
- Omission errors predominate; substitution, distortion, addition, prolongation, and metathetic errors (transposition of sounds) also occur.
- Vowel distortions may be present.
- There is a higher percentage of errors in sounds requiring complex oral movements (e.g., fricatives, affricates, consonant clusters).
- Prosodic disturbances are evident, particularly in the appropriate use of stress patterns.
- Struggling or groping movements of the oral musculature are present.
- Number of errors increase as the length and complexity of utterances increase.
- The ability to sequence phonemes in words/phrases and diadochokinetic tasks is reduced.

DVD is noted for its resistance to remediation. That is, DVD does not respond easily to traditional articulation techniques. A set of basic factors to be considered in developing treatment programs for this population includes:

- Progress in therapy is slow and marked by poor retention and generalization of therapy targets across treatment sessions.
- Although repeated practice is an integral component of therapy for all types of articulation disorders, it is important to provide intensive, systematic drill for children with DVD in order for them to master the necessary speech-motor patterns.
- Based on the first two factors, sessions which are shorter and more frequent may be helpful in facilitating generalization and avoiding speech system fatigue.
- Children with DVD have great difficulty learning articulatory patterns through auditory input alone. For this reason, the use of visual and tactile cues is essential for establishing these sensory/motor patterns.
- Remediation should include an early emphasis on improving children's ability to monitor their own speech production, particularly through tactile and/or kinesthetic modalities (e.g., concentrate on how sounds "feel" and where the tongue is during movement sequences).
- Intervention should incorporate a focus on the melody and rhythm patterns of connected speech.
- For children with extremely unintelligible speech, it may be necessary to introduce an augmentative/alternative system to provide the child with a functional means of communication. This option may be temporary in nature or serve as the child's long-term communication mode.

Example Profile

Following is a typical profile of developmental verbal apraxia. This example has been designed to illustrate the selection of intervention targets as well as specific therapy activities and materials. The chosen activities are easily implemented in either individual or group therapy settings.

PROFILE

Billy is almost 3 years old and presents with unintelligible speech. His phoneme repertoire is limited to four consonant sounds /b, m, t, d/, which he substitutes for several other sounds. He sometimes produces the same CV syllables for many different words (e.g., /ba/ for *ball*, *table*, *telephone*, *door*, and *paper*). In addition, Billy demonstrates a significant number of omission errors (sounds and syllables), which occur in all word positions (e.g., /tɔ/ for truck, /ət/ for *dog*, /oh/ for *open*). Billy also demonstrates occasional vowel errors characterized by the substitution of schwa for other vowels, especially diphthongs.

Selection of therapy targets. The primary areas to be targeted are poor oral-motor skills, restricted phoneme repertoire, and limited speech-sound sequencing abilities. The oral-motor skills selected for remediation were tongue-tip elevation, tongue lateralization, tongue protrusion/retraction, lip pursing, and lip retraction because these movements are highly visible. (Children who demonstrate an accompanying oral apraxia may find these tasks very frustrating.) The phonemes /p/ and /f/ were chosen as targets to be added to Billy's consonant repertoire for several reasons. These sounds appear early developmentally, are highly visible, and are sufficiently different from one another to avoid confusion during training. In addition, these consonants are voiceless and therefore require the mastery of one less feature for correct production than do voiced sounds. The complexity level selected for work on sequencing skills was reduplicative CV and VC syllables in which the consonant and vowel remain constant across syllables. The phonemes identified for use in the sequencing tasks were /b,m,t,d/ because these sounds are already present in Billy's consonant repertoire at the single-syllable level.

Sample Activities

1. Gather two sets of five to ten items of varying texture, size, shape, and temperature (e.g., ice, tongue depressor, straw, warm liquid, rubber toy). Encourage the child to use each of the objects in a set to engage in oral-exploratory play. Imitate each of the child's play behaviors using the objects in the second set. Establish the child's conscious awareness of oral-motor sensations by commenting on what the child is doing and how it makes the mouth feel. Promote expansion of the number and variety of oral-motor play movements demonstrated by the child. This task is most effective when used as a warm-up activity at the beginning of a therapy session.

2. Sit next to the child in front of a large mirror. Tell the child that he is going to play a "clown" game and show him a clown hat/wig made from construction paper/yarn. Instruct the child that this game involves taking turns making funny faces in the mirror. The clinician takes the first turn by putting on the clown hat and modeling a target tongue or lip movement. Have the child imitate the target movement a minimum of five times to earn a chance to be the clown. (In the early stages of therapy, it may be necessary to reinforce any voluntary oral-motor movement that occurs in response to the clinician's stimulus.) Explain that it is now the child's turn to wear the hat and make a

funny face for the clinician to imitate. Repeat this sequence with other oral-motor movements that are absent from the child's repertoire. This activity also works well as a warm-up procedure at the beginning of a session (5 to 10 minutes) and may be repeated at intervals throughout the session to reinforce targeted motor patterns. (Refer to the Oral-Motor Treatment section at the beginning of this chapter for additional information.)

3. Gather four large sacks (pillowcases, trash bags, grocery bags, and so on), fill each one with at least five objects whose names begin with a target sound (avoid blends), and attach the sacks to the wall. For example, objects for the target sound /p/ might include pencil, puzzle, paint, puppet, pot. Give the child a beanbag and tell him to throw it at one of the sacks. The clinician removes the sack that was hit from the wall and tells the child to close his eyes and pick one object at a time from the sack. The clinician holds the object next to his or her mouth and models the target phoneme in isolation for the child to imitate three successive times. When the sack is empty, give the child the beanbag and start the game again.

4. Cut an egg carton in half lengthwise, turn it upside down, and color or paint each of the six protruding sections a different color. Hide the last three sections from the child's view by covering them with a piece of aluminum foil or other material. Obtain a large plastic dinosaur or other animal with a large mouth opening and collect at least 25 marbles. Explain to the child he is going to play a game in which he has to sing silly sounds in exactly the same way as the clinician to earn a chance to feed marbles to the very hungry dinosaur. The clinician then "sings" a string of three reduplicative CV syllables that are constructed from the identified consonant targets /b, m, t, d/. The clinician produces these strings with a distinctive intonational contour pattern, while simultaneously tapping the egg carton protrusions to pace each CV syllable as it is "sung." Intonational contour patterns might include rising/falling intonation, primary stress on a particular syllable, and increased/decreased loudness on initial/medial/final syllables. Instruct the child to imitate the clinician's syllable sequence using the same intonational pattern and pacing cues as the clinician. Following the successful imitation of at least three different sequences, the child is allowed to feed a marble to the dinosaur. Continue this activity using varied combinations of phonemes and intonation patterns until the dinosaur has eaten all the marbles. The level of difficulty can be modified by increasing the number of syllables in the reduplicative CV/VC strings or by introducing nonreduplicative syllable strings.

Note: This activity represents a simplified adaptation of Melodic Intonation Therapy (Sparks, Helm, & Albert, 1974) in which rhythm and intonation patterns are used to facilitate speech output.

Helpful Hints

1. Oral-motor movements can be used to facilitate articulatory placement for the acquisition of new consonants. For example, after work on tongue-tip elevation, you can add voice to it to produce /l/.

2. Capitalize on an acceptable speech-motor pattern at the moment of its production when the experience is most recent and vivid in the child's mind. Have the child repeat the utterance immediately for multiple trials to reduce probability that the articulatory gesture will fade (Chappell, 1973; Hall, Jordan, & Robin, 1993).

3. Early therapy should focus on a child's ability to produce *accurate* responses. As the child improves, the focus can be shifted to *speed* of response by requiring rapid automatic production of the accurate articulatory movements.

4. Rhymes and songs can be used as stimulus materials to facilitate oral-motor sequencing abilities for children who can produce sentence-length utterances.

5. For children at the single-word level, it may be helpful to introduce words that contain reduplicative syllables (e.g., mama, bye-bye, night-night, dada). Such utterances highlight the rhythm of speech and can provide a transition to other bisyllabic words (e.g., cookie, allgone, open).

6. Given that children with DVD frequently demonstrate intact language comprehension skills and normal intelligence, there are two commonly occurring counseling issues: (a) the child may be significantly frustrated by the inability to intelligibly convey his/her ideas and thoughts, and (b) parents may inaccurately perceive the inconsistent nature of their child's poor speech production as an indicator of laziness or lack of motivation.

7. Clinicians should make every effort to ensure that therapy remains a positive experience for the child because intervention with this disorder consists largely of repetitive drill.

8. Clinicians interested in facilitating parent/family understanding of this disorder are encouraged to consult the series of "Letters to the parent of . . . " by Hall (2000) which explains the nature, causes, and treatment of DVD in clear, simple language.

PHONOLOGICAL DISORDERS

The phonological system governs the ways in which sounds in a language can be combined to form words. Children with phonologically based problems demonstrate difficulty in acquiring a phonological system, not necessarily in production of the sounds. These children do not simply possess an incomplete system of speech sounds; rather, their errors have logical and coherent principles underlying their use. Therefore, the philosophy of intervention with these children differs markedly from traditional approaches to either functional or organic articulation problems.

Two of the main approaches to the remediation of phonological rule disorders focus on phonological processes and distinctive features. A phonological process is a strategy used by young, typically developing children between 1½ and 4 years of age to simplify the production of an entire class of adult speech sounds (Hodson & Paden, 1981; Khan & Lewis, 2002; Oller, 1975). For example, young children frequently omit weakly stressed syllables in multisyllabic words (e.g., ephant/elephant, jamas/pajamas); reduce consonant clusters (e.g., bue/blue, dek/desk); assimilate consonants in words (e.g., goggie/doggie, chichen/chicken); and delete final consonants (e.g., ba/ball, hou/house). Children who persist in using these processes beyond the age of 4 are frequently referred for speech-language services because their speech is now perceived as difficult to understand. Some children exhibit phonological processes that are not typical of normally developing children. These nondevelopmental processes include (1) backing: substitution of sounds that are more posterior than the usual place of production (e.g., koe/toe, mackiz/matches, gipper/zipper); (2) initial consonant deletion: omission of the first sound in a word (e.g., ouse/house, amp/lamp, ellow/yellow); and (3) glottal replacement: substitution of a glottal stop for a consonant (e.g., boʔle/bottle, chiʔen/chicken, miʔey/mickey). Table 3-4 describes the most common phonological processes exhibited by normally developing children.

TABLE 3-4
Selected Developmental Phonological Processes

Process	Definition	Examples
Dropped by 3 years		
Assimilation (harmony)	A sound becomes similar to or is influenced by another sound in the same word	guck/duck toat/coat doddie/doggie
Final consonant deletion	Omission of the last sound in word	be/bed fi/fish so/soap
Syllable deletion	Omission of weak or unstressed syllable(s)	nana/banana agator/alligator zert/dessert
Dropped after 3 years		
Cluster reduction	Omission of at least one consonant from a cluster	top/stop mall/small net/nest
Epenthesis	Addition of sounds in a word	bulack/black sthoap/soap pulay/play
Fronting	Substitutions are produced anterior to their usual place of production	tome/come cats/catch dum/gum
Metathesis	The order of sound segments is reversed	aminal/animal flutterby/butterfly bakset/basket
Stopping	Fricatives/affricates are replaced by stops	tun/sun dat/that dump/jump
Voicing/devoicing	Voiced consonants replace voiceless sounds in the initial position; in the final position voiced consonants become voiceless	gup/cup doe/toe bet/bed

Source: Based on the work of Bauman-Waengler (2004); Bernthal & Bankson (2004); Hodson (1986); and Shriberg & Kwiatkowski (1980).

Distinctive features are defined in terms of articulatory patterns and acoustic properties. Each phoneme in a language consists of a bundle of binary features, in which the presence or absence of these features is specified (e.g., +voicing/-voicing, +nasal/-nasal, +continuancy/-continuancy) (Jakobson, 1968). Some phonemes, such as /t/ and /d/, differ by only one feature contrast, in this case, voicing. Other phonemes, such as /s/ and /g/, differ by many feature contrasts, including voicing, continuancy, placement, and stridency. Table 3-5 presents a complete list of the eleven distinctive features originally identified by Chomsky and Halle (1968). For the purposes of clinical application, however, sounds are usually analyzed according to three basic feature categories: place, manner, and voicing. This breakdown is illustrated in Table 3-6.

TABLE 3-5
Distinctive Feature Analysis Chart

Features	Consonants																								
	k	g	t	d	p	b	f	v	θ	ð	s	z	ʃ	ʒ	tʃ	dʒ	m	n	ŋ	l	r	h	w	j	?
Vocalic	-	-	-	-	-	-	-	-	-	-	-	-	-	-	-	-	-	-	-	+	+	-	-	-	-
Consonantal	+	+	+	+	+	+	+	+	+	+	+	+	+	+	+	+	+	+	+	+	+	-	-	-	-
High	+	+	-	-	-	-	-	-	-	-	-	-	+	+	+	+	-	-	+	-	-	-	+	+	-
Back	+	+	-	-	-	-	-	-	-	-	-	-	-	-	-	-	-	-	+	-	-	-	+	-	-
Low	-	-	-	-	-	-	-	-	-	-	-	-	-	-	-	-	-	-	-	-	ı	-	-	-	+
Anterior	-	-	+	+	+	+	+	+	+	+	+	+	-	-	-	-	+	+	-	+	-	-	-	-	-
Coronal	-	-	+	+	-	-	-	-	+	+	+	+	+	+	+	+	-	+	+	+	+	-	-	-	-
Voice	-	+	-	+	-	+	-	+	-	+	-	+	-	+	-	+	+	+	+	+	+	-	+	+	-
Continuant	-	-	-	-	-	-	+	+	+	+	+	+	+	+	-	-	-	-	-	+	+	+	+	+	+
Nasal	-	-	-	-	-	-	-	-	-	-	-	-	-	-	-	-	+	+	+	-	-	-	-	-	-
Strident	-	-	-	-	-	-	+	+	-	-	+	+	+	+	+	+	-	-	-	-	-	-	-	-	-

– = Absence of feature
+ = Presence of feature

Vocalic = Oral cavity constriction is less than required for the high vowels /i/ and /u/
Consonantal = Marked constriction in the midline region of the vocal tract
High = Body of the tongue is raised above the neutral or resting position
Back = Body of the tongue is retracted from the neutral or resting position
Low = Body of the tongue is lowered below the neutral or resting position
Anterior = Point of constriction is farther forward than required for /ʃ/
Coronal = Tongue blade is elevated toward alveolar ridge/palate from the neutral position
Voice = Vocal folds vibrate during sound production
Continuant = Partial constriction of oral cavity; sound can be sustained in a steady state
Nasal = Velum is lowered to allow sound stream to escape through the nose
Strident = Turbulent noise is created by rapid airflow released through a small opening

TABLE 3-6
Place, Manner, and Voicing Chart for English Consonants

Manner	Place	Voiced	Voiceless
Stop	Bilabial	b	p
	Alveolar	d	t
	Velar	g	k
	Glottal	—	ʔ
Fricative	Labiodental	v	f
	Linguadental	ð	θ
	Alveolar	z	s
	Palatal	ʒ	ʃ
	Glottal	—	h
Affricate	Palatal	dʒ	tʃ
Glide	Bilabial	w	—
	Palatal	j	—
Liquid	Alveolar	l	—
	Palatal	r	—
Nasal	Bilabial	m	—
	Alveolar	n	—
	Velar	ŋ	—

Example Profiles

Following are two profiles commonly seen in children with phonological rule problems. The first case depicts a process approach to intervention; the second case illustrates a modified distinctive feature strategy. These examples have been designed to illustrate the selection of intervention targets as well as specific therapy activities and materials. Most of the chosen activities are easily implemented in either individual or group therapy settings. Following are examples of the types of errors that a child might demonstrate; some children may produce additional errors within each of these categories.

PROFILE 1

Gerry is 5 years old and demonstrates the following phonological processes:

1. Final consonant deletion
   -/s
   -/v
   -/p
   -/d
   -/k

2. Unstressed syllable deletion
   tephone/telephone
   way/away

tato/potato
amance/ambulance

3. Cluster reduction
-t/st
-m/sm
p-/pl
-t/sk
n-/nd

4. Fronting
t/k
d/g

5. Voicing
b/p
d/t
z/s
v/f

6. Initial consonant deletion
-/k
-/l
-/h
-/p
-/t

7. Glottal replacement
ʔ/t
ʔ/k
ʔ/g

Selection of therapy targets. The processes to be targeted are final consonant deletion, fronting, voicing, and initial consonant deletion. The first five
processes in the preceding list are exhibited by typically developing children and
are therefore considered developmental in nature. Final consonant deletion and
fronting were targeted because these developmental processes drop out of children's speech production repertoires earlier than the other two (by 3 years of age).
The last two processes occur much less frequently among typically developing
children. Initial consonant deletion was selected as a therapy target because of its
severe impact on intelligibility (Khan & Lewis, 2002; Leinonen-Davies, 1988;
Yavas & Lamprecht, 1988).

Sample Activities

1. Cut out a large dinosaur (about 3 feet in length) with a very long detachable
tail (e.g., tyrannosaurus rex) from poster board or construction paper and
obtain a small paint bottle with a sponge top (bingo marker). Collect a pile of
25 pictures for the child to name. The names should be monosyllabic and
contain a variety of singleton final consonants, including examples of his

deletion errors as well as any that he might be able to produce spontaneously. Remove the tail from the dinosaur and explain to the child that words have sounds at the ends just like dinosaurs have tails. Instruct the child to select a picture from the pile and name it, making sure to put the ending sound on the word. Following each correct response, illustrate the parallel between the dinosaur's tail and the final sound of the word by allowing the child to reattach the dinosaur's tail and decorate it with one dot of sponge paint. The ultimate goal of this activity is to decorate the dinosaur's tail completely and attach it permanently for the child to take home. This activity can be used effectively up through the level of conversation and narration.

2. Create or collect a deck of picture cards for the game "Go Fish" depicting pairs of identical words and minimal contrast words that incorporate the child's fronting errors. Minimal pairs consist of two words that are identical except for a single distinctive feature or phoneme (Elbert & Gierut, 1991). This approach is designed to emphasize the concept that even small sound contrasts can signal differences in word meanings. Examples include *tap* and *cap*, *top* and *cop*, *date* and *gate*, *pit* and *pick*, *bed* and *beg*. Begin the game by dealing three cards to each player and placing the remainder in a pile in the middle of the table. Explain to the child that the object of the game is to make pairs for all the cards in his hand with *identical* pictures by asking other players, "Do you have any _____?" A correct production allows the child to continue requesting cards. If the child uses a fronting error during a turn at requesting a card, he should be given the picture that corresponds to his actual, not intended, production. For example, if the child says *date* when attempting to match his picture of *gate*, he will receive the card depicting a date on a calendar and therefore not obtain the match. The clinician should model the intended production for the child to imitate. A correct imitation is rewarded with the desired picture match, but the turn passes to the next player. The player who has the most pairs at the end of the game is the winner.

3. Gather pictures for the parenthesized words in the following sentences and arrange them on a table. Explain that the clinician will say a sentence with a word missing at the end. Instruct the child to finish the sentence by selecting the picture that sounds almost the same as a word in the sentence, except for using "voice on" or "voice off." The clinician reads one sentence at a time with particular emphasis on the italicized word. (Note: The clinician provides the child with a hint that the target word rhymes with one of the words in the sentence.)

> The *pig* is ____ (big).
>
> Put the *coat* on the ____ (goat).
>
> The *fan* is in the ____ (van).
>
> I *see* the letter ____ (Z).
>
> Put the *pin* in the ____ (bin).
>
> Don't *tip* over the ____ (dip).
>
> The *girl* has a ____ (curl).
>
> *Sue* likes the ____ (zoo).

Dan is very ____(tan).

Go *down* to the ____(town).

He *came* to play the ____(game).

Put the *pack* on your ____(back).

4. Cut out a minimum of 30 construction paper turtles that are approximately eight inches in length. Two-thirds of the turtles should have their heads protruding out from their shells, while the heads of the remaining third should not be visible. Place the turtles in an obstacle course-like path around the room so that a child can hop easily from one turtle "stepping-stone" to another. Gather a deck of 20 pictures whose names begin with the child's initial consonant deletion errors. Prepare numerous slips of paper that instruct the child to perform one of the following: (a) hop forward one turtle, (b) hop forward two turtles, (c) hop backward one turtle, and (d) hop backward two turtles. Fold these paper slips and place them in a paper bag. Tell the child that to play the "turtle stepping-stone" game, he has to hop on the turtles and say some words. For each turn, he has to choose a slip of paper from the bag without looking and follow its instruction. As he lands on a turtle, the clinician holds up one card from the picture deck. If the child is on a turtle that has no head, he should name the picture three times without producing its initial consonant sound. If the turtle has a head, the word must be produced five times with its initial consonant sound present. The object of the game is to reach the final turtle on the obstacle course.

Note: It is important to remember that the focus of these three activities is on phonological processes rather than the production of particular sounds. For this reason, in the early stages of therapy, the clinician should reinforce any responses that demonstrate a child's use of the targeted phonological process, regardless of the actual phoneme(s) produced. For example, during work on the final consonant deletion process, a child may be reinforced for producing "bat" or "bam" instead of his habitual "ba" when naming a picture of "bag."

PROFILE 2

Grace is 5 years old and demonstrates the following feature errors:

Manner Errors	*Examples*
Stops for fricatives:	zoo → /doo/; soap → /toap/
Fricatives for affricates:	porch → /porsh/
Glides for liquids:	right → /yight/
Place Errors	
Alveolars for velars:	tuptake/cupcake; det/get
Alveolars for palatals:	sue/shoe; trezure/treasure
Voicing Errors	
Voiced for voiceless:	gow/cow; doe/toe
Voiceless for voiced:	loose/lose; stofe/stove

For clarity, the examples in the preceding list reflect a single feature contrast between the error sound and the intended target. However, children frequently produce errors that differ from the target by two or more feature contrasts (e.g., late → /jet/ differ in both place and manner; sip → /gip/ differ in all three features).

Selection of therapy targets. The first set of therapy targets includes one error contrast from each of the three feature categories. The manner contrast of stop/fricative was selected because fricatives emerge earlier developmentally than the other two sound classes listed under this category (i.e., affricates and liquids). In addition, fricatives have a higher frequency of occurrence in English than affricates. The place contrast of alveolar/velar was chosen because palatals are acquired much later in the developmental sequence than velars. The voiced/voiceless contrast was included because this feature error generally occurs in word-initial position, which contributes heavily to perceived unintelligibility.

Sample Activities

1. Using masking tape, create a hopscotch grid with eight squares on the floor. Draw a long slide on a blackboard or piece of paper, and obtain a spinner with numbers. Provide a doll or stuffed animal figure and tell the child that "Harry" uses different types of sounds when playing these two different activities. Demonstrate that Harry produces "short hopping" sounds (stops) such as /b, p, d/ as he jumps on the hopscotch grid. Then demonstrate that Harry produces "long sliding" sounds (fricatives) such as /s, z, v, f/ as he goes down the slide. Check the child's grasp of the concepts involved by modeling alternating examples of each manner of sound production and asking the child to place Harry on the corresponding activity.

   Start with the hopscotch game and explain that the child will jump from the beginning to the end of the grid while holding Harry. The clinician models examples of stops (such as /t/ or /k/) when the child lands on each square. The child must produce three imitations of the stop before jumping to the next square. After completing the hopscotch grid, move on to the slide activity. Emphasize the feature contrast between stops and fricatives by reminding the child that Harry uses "long sliding" sounds with this activity. Have the child use the spinner to determine the number of times Harry can go down the slide. The clinician models an example of a fricative sound with exaggerated duration (such as /fffff/ or /sssss/). Tell the child to place Harry at the top of the slide and move him down slowly while imitating the clinician's exaggerated production. Repeat as many times as indicated by the spinner and then have the child spin again for another turn. The clinician should model different fricatives for each turn. Allow the child four more turns with the spinner and then return to the hopscotch game to reinforce the targeted feature contrast.

   Once the child demonstrates mastery at this level, the clinician can introduce more complex stimulus items such as syllables and words.

2. Create a race track game board with starting and finishing lines that are connected by 20 squares. Provide a small race car game piece. Make a spinner with numbers, half colored green and half red. Tell the child that the race car

moves forward when the spinner indicates a green number and backward with a red number. Explain that, whenever the spinner points to a green number, the child will imitate the clinician's model of a "forward" sound (alveolar such as /d/ or /t/), while moving the game piece. If the spinner points to a red number, a contrasting "backward" sound (velar such as /g/ or /k/) will be modeled for imitation. A variety of sounds that highlight the alveolar/velar place contrast should be modeled throughout the game. The object of the game is to cross the finish line.

3. Make a 24-square bingo card (six rows of four squares) and place pictures/ stickers of butterflies and bumblebees in alternating columns on the card. Collect a deck of 24 pictures for the child to name. One-third of the names should have voiced consonants in the initial word position (e.g., *boy, girl, duck, zipper, jump*) and the other two-thirds should have voiceless initial consonants (e.g., *soup, table, chair, cat, piano*). Provide 24 game tokens. Explain to the child that bumblebees and butterflies "make" two different kinds of sounds. The bumblebee uses sounds that buzz, like /zzzzz/, and the butterfly uses sounds that do not buzz, like /sssss/. The clinician then selects a picture card from the deck and holds it up. Instruct the child to name the picture and then to categorize the initial phoneme as a bumblebee or butterfly sound. If the child responds correctly to both parts, she is able to place a game token on one of the picture squares that corresponds to the sound category of the target word (i.e., bumblebee versus butterfly). The object of the game is to fill an entire column of squares with tokens.

4. Gather a plastic tablecloth and napkins for a pretend tea party and arrange them on a table in the therapy room. Collect 20 pictures of objects/animals that have easily identifiable front portions and back portions, and cut them in half (e.g., train, horse, car, dog, snake, airplane, pencil, bus, giraffe, fish). Separate the front and back pieces into two piles. Briefly review that certain sounds are made in the front of the mouth (e.g., /p/, /t/) while others are made in the back (e.g., /k/, /g/). Practice a few examples of each with the child.

   Explain that the tablecloth and napkins need to be decorated in a special way for the tea party. Model a front or back sound in a CV syllable and instruct the child to identify it as "front" or "back" and imitate three times. If identification and production responses are correct, the child picks a picture from the appropriate pile and pastes/tapes it to the tablecloth or napkins. Alternate CV models between front and back sounds until all picture pieces have been used as decorations.

Helpful Hints

1. When using a phonological processes approach, it is sometimes useful to teach the underlying concepts in nonspeech activities before moving to speech production tasks.

2. One consideration in the selection of phonological processes for therapy is the relative consistency of their use. Processes that a child demonstrates only occasionally may be more easily modified than those used on a consistent basis.

3. In the initial stages of distinctive feature therapy, selection of target sounds that differ by only a single feature contrast may increase the likelihood of early success.

4. Distinctive feature theory predicts that generalization will most likely occur from trained phonemes to phonemes that share the same feature. Thus, it is important to regularly probe these untrained sounds to determine whether any have been acquired spontaneously and will not require subsequent intervention.

5. Clinicians may need to explain to parents that therapy for phonological disorders focuses on appropriate use of linguistic rules rather than acquisition of correct motor movements. This may eliminate a parent's confusion in the early stages of therapy when the clinician reinforces a seemingly incorrect response (e.g., toat/boat when targeting initial consonant deletion) when, in fact, the child is now using the correct rule.

CONCLUSION

This chapter has presented basic information, protocols, and procedures for intervention for articulation and phonology at an **introductory** level. This information is intended only as a starting point in the reader's clinical education and training. For in-depth coverage of this area, the following readings are recommended:

Bauman-Waengler, J. (2004). *Articulatory and phonological impairments: A clinical focus.* Needham Heights, MA: Allyn & Bacon.

Bernthal, J. E., & Bankson, N. W. (2004). *Articulation and phonological disorders.* Needham Heights, MA: Allyn & Bacon.

Creaghead, N. A., Newman, P. W., & Secord, W. A. (1989). *Assessment and remediation of articulatory and phonological disorders.* Columbus, OH: Charles E. Merrill.

Oral-Motor Dysfunction

Alexander, R., Boehme, R., & Cupps, B. (1998). *Normal development of functional motor skills: The first year of life.* Tucson, AZ: Therapy Skill Builders.

Bahr, D. C. (2001). *Oral motor assessment and treatment: Ages and stages.* Boston: Allyn & Bacon.

Mackie, E. (1996). *Oral-motor activities for young children.* East Moline, IL: Lingui-Systems.

Morris, S. E. & Klein, M. D. (1987). *Pre-feeding skills: A comprehensive resource for feeding development.* Tucson, AZ: Therapy Skill Builders.

ADDITIONAL RESOURCES

Articulation

The Psychological Corporation
19500 Bulverde
San Antonio, TX 78259
Phone: 800-872-1726
Fax: 800-232-1223
Web site: www.psychcorp.com — Go to Speech and Language section

Pictures, Please: Picture Gallery Articulation, Language, and Adult Language
More than 1,000 black-and-white illustrations on CDs, for clients from 3 years
through adult. Drawings of common objects, actions, and situations covering
24 consonants and 19 vowels/diphthongs. Search by the vocabulary level, word
length, and various clinical features and select whether you want the picture, the
word, or both to appear.

Speechviewer III for Windows (CD-ROM)
Computer software presents speech stimuli for clients to practice and analyze
their speech.

Super Duper Publications
P.O. Box 24997
Greenville, SC 29616
Phone: 800-277-8737
FAX: 800-978-7379
Web site: www.superduperinc.com

Webber Articulation Cards (Sets I, II, and III)
Decks of cards with colored pictures designed to elicit 15 target phonemes in all
word positions; duplicate cards are included to make the decks suitable for many
children's card games.

The Big Book of Sounds
246-page book of drill-based activities with sections for initial, medial, and final
position. Includes syllable drills, syllable rhymes, word lists, word rhymes, short
sentences, and word list enhancements for each sound.

Month by Month Artic Carry-Over Fun
Open-ended pages that can be customized for any sound. Each month contains
two types of activity pages: four-part pages with separate topics (which can be
completed in different ways) and full-page sheets with word scenes, fill-in blanks,
etc. Parent letter included.

Artic Chipper Chat
Sixty different game boards each filled with sound loaded pictures. Students pick
a question card and search their boards for the correct picture answer. As they
answer questions, they fill up their boards with magnetic chips. It focuses on 12 different sounds targeting the initial, medial, and final position and/or combination.

The Speech Bin
1965 Twenty-Fifth Avenue
Vero Beach, FL 32960
Phone: 800-4-SPEECH
Fax: 888-FAX-2BIN
Web site: www.speechbin.com

Sound Therapy Lite
Displays lists of words containing specified phonemes and encourages clients to
practice speech sounds and words in a game format.

Photo Articulation Library

1,085 real-life photos arranged by sounds and word positions—350 cards in each set, suitable for all ages. Twenty-seven categories include events, communication, actions, games and toys, occupations, transportation, and more organized by consonants, vowels, and word position.

LinguiSystems

3100 Fourth Avenue
East Moline, IL 61244
Phone: 800-776-4332
Fax: 800-577-4555
Web site: www.linguisystems.com

50 Quick-Play Articulation Games

More than 50 creative, fun, interactive games on reproducible sheets for ages 5–10. Games target these sounds in all positions: *p, b, m, k, g, t, d, f, v, sh, ch, j, s, z, r, l, l* blends, *r* blends, *s* blends, and voiced and voiceless *th*. There are 50 path games, 15 card games, 11 noncompetitive games, plus a *Make Your Own Game* path and a *Target the Stars* motivational sheet.

Artic Shuffle

Fifty-two different pictures per deck to give student tons of articulation practice by playing Go Fish, Crazy Eights, or Memory. Students match suits, numbers, and face cards so there is no need for picture pairs. Ten card decks cover 12 sounds plus sounds in blends.

Sally's Circus: An Articulation Game

For ages 4–9. The stimulus items provide articulation practice in a variety of speaking contexts. Students practice using their target sounds in three levels of production: short phrases, sentence completion tasks, and silly rhymes or tongue twisters. Contains 300 game cards to target these sounds in all positions: *k, g, l, s, z, r, ch, sh, j,* and voiced and voiceless *th*.

Phonology

Parrot Software

P.O. Box 250755
West Bloomfield, MI 48325-0755
Phone: 800-PARROT-1
Fax: 248-788-3224
Web site: www.parrotsoftware.com

Minimal Contrast Stories Plus

Provides 40 minimal contrast stories and accompanying pictures representing several patterns of misarticulations: final consonant deletion, denasalization, gliding, stopping, and fronting.

Pro-Ed

8700 Shoal Creek Boulevard
Austin, TX 78758-9965
Phone: 800-897-3202

Fax: 800-FXPROED
Web site: www.proedinc.com

Remediation of Common Phonological Processes
A semantically based approach that uses minimal word pair contrasts to remediate phonological process errors; includes decks of stimulus cards for nine different phonological processes.

More Picture Pairs: Games and Activities for Remediating Phonological Processes
Colorful pictures of minimal pairs allow you to use minimal pairs in conversational practice. The manual provides nearly 50 picture card activities, 17 poster activities, 32 reproducible worksheets (4 worksheets for each of the 8 processes), complete instructions for the games, recordkeeping forms for tracking your clients' progress, and 60 additional pairs you can form using the picture cards in the kit. Processes targeted include final consonant deletion, cluster reduction, devoicing of final consonants, prevocalic voicing, velar fronting, fronting of palatals, and stopping and gliding of liquids.

Phonology for Groups: Thematic Activities for Everyday Settings
Assist students in targeting phonology while working in a natural setting. Focuses on the repetitive cyclical approach to teaching phonology. Forty-eight lesson plans, each with a topic of the day, provide structured sessions of Circle Time Activities, Art Card Activity, Small-Group Production, Movement/Music, Snack Time, Play Centers, Review of Target Patterns/Good-bye, and Probing. Includes a variety of games and coloring and cutting activities.

The Speech Bin
1965 Twenty-Fifth Avenue
Vero Beach, FL 32960
Phone: 800-4-SPEECH
Fax: 888-FAX-2BIN
Web site: www.speechbin.com

Minimal Pair Cards
Four decks of illustrated three-by-five-inch cards remediate five common phonological processes—stopping, fronting, gliding, cluster reduction, final consonant deletion—and develop vocabulary, language, and game playing skills in K–3 children.

Oral-Motor

LinguiSystems
3100 Fourth Avenue
P.O. Box 747
East Moline, IL 61244
Phone: 800-776-4332
Fax: 800-577-4555
Web site: www.linguisystems.com

Oral-Motor Activities for School-Aged Children
For older children to improve oral-motor function for better speech production.

Oral-Motor Activities for Young Children
Uses simple snack foods to achieve oral-motor function and stimulate accurate speech production.

Easy Does It for Articulation
Includes specific techniques to develop better oral-motor control, precision, strength, and coordination for accurate speech sound placement.

The Speech Bin
1965 Twenty-Fifth Avenue
Vero Beach, FL 32960
Phone: 800-4-SPEECH
Fax: 888-FAX-2BIN
Web site: www.speechbin.com

Whistle Kit & Blow Toy Kit
The Whistle Kit is a nine-piece collection of motivating whistles featuring moving parts. The Blow Toy Kit gives you colorful toys to encourage prolonged blowing without sound and ocular tracking.

Super Duper Publications
P.O. Box 24997
Greenville, NC 29616
Phone: 800-277-8737
Fax: 800-978-7379
Web site: www.superduperinc.com

Oral-Motor Fun and Games
For preschool and school-aged children. Includes drill exercises for tongue and lip strengthening and movement with game boards, cut-and-paste activities, and manipulatives. Can be used as therapy materials or homework assignments.

Visual Health Information
P.O. Box 44646
11003 A Street South
Takoma, WA 98444
Phone: 800-356-0709
Fax: 253-536-4944
Web site: http://www.vhikits.com

Oral Sensory and Motor Treatment Kit
For older school-aged children and up. Provides a comprehensive program of oral exercises for lips, cheeks, jaw, tongue, and palate. Small cards describing exercises are categorized by motor versus sensory and are indexed by anatomical area. Illustrations of target behaviors are provided along with an index of corresponding phonemes.

Miscellaneous

Smit, A.B. (2004). *Articulation and phonology resource guide for school-age children and adults.* Clifton Park, NY: Thomson Delmar Learning.

APPENDIX 3-A

PHONETIC PLACEMENT INSTRUCTIONS FOR DIFFICULT-TO-TEACH SOUNDS

/ɚ/

1. Open your mouth and put your tongue up like this (model tongue tip in center of mouth almost touching hard palate, using mirror). Close your mouth until teeth are almost clenched and say /ɚ/.
2. Open your mouth and get ready to say /k/ (or /g/). Put your tongue tip up and say /ɚ/.
3. Say /u/ while raising your tongue tip to produce /ɚ/.
4. Raise the tip of your tongue toward the roof of your mouth just as you do for /l/. While making the /l/ sound, curl your tongue tip back toward your throat to make the /ɚ/ sound.
5. Stick out your tongue. (Touch edges of client's tongue with tongue blade to show him where the tongue should be touching the teeth.) Bring your tongue back into your mouth, touching its edges to the teeth. Raise the tongue tip slightly and say /ɚ/.
6. Pretend you are a puppet. I am going to pull an imaginary string attached to the back of your head. You should raise the back of your tongue slightly and say /ɚ/ as I pull the string.
7. (Spread the sides of the child's mouth with your fingers.) Make a really long /n/ sound, while curling the tip of your tongue toward your throat to produce /ɚ/.
8. Make a long /i/ sound with your lips really tight, like a big smile. While continuing to make the sound, relax your lips and move your tongue back gradually to produce /ɚ/.

/s, z/

1. Make a long /th/ sound and slowly draw the tip of your tongue back behind your teeth to produce /s/.
2. Position your tongue for the /t/ sound. Hold the /t/ sound and drop your tongue tip slightly to produce /s/.
3. (Move a tongue depressor or straw down the midline of child's tongue to indicate the appropriate pathway of airflow.) Hold the sides of your tongue against the edges of your upper side teeth. Point your tongue tip toward the exact center of your upper front teeth and blow airstream straight out the middle of your tongue to make the /s/.
4. (Draw a picture of the two upper and two lower central incisors in contact with one another. Make a circle on the picture to show the small center opening where the four teeth meet to indicate the correct direction of the airstream.) Make your top and bottom teeth touch the same way as in the picture. Use your tongue to seal off all the way around your mouth except the very small center opening between your middle front teeth like the circle in the picture. Let the /s/ sound come out only from that small opening in a very fine stream just as if you poked a tiny little hole in a water hose.
5. Make a little smile with your teeth nearly closed. Hide your tongue behind your teeth. You can keep the tip of your tongue up or down. Rest the sides of your tongue against the inside of your top teeth. Let the airstream come out the front to make the /s/ sound.

(continues)

/θ, ð/

1. Put your tongue between your top and bottom teeth so that it peeks out a little bit. Rest the sides of your tongue against the sides of your top teeth. Blow air out the front of your mouth to make the /θ, ð/ sound.
2. Make a long /s/ sound and slowly stick out your tongue tip slightly to make the /θ, ð/ sound.
3. (Use a mirror to contrast the articulatory placements for /θ, ð/ with the child's sound substitution. For example, show the child that the /θ, ð/ are made with the tongue placed slightly between the front teeth, while /f/ requires the upper teeth to touch the lower lip.)

/ʃ, ʒ/

1. Hold your index finger straight up and touch it to your lips as if to make a hushing sound and say /ʃ, ʒ/.
2. Make a long /s/ sound and gradually round your lips, letting a little extra air rush out the front of your mouth.
3. Elevate tongue tip toward hard palate and allow the lateral edge of the tongue to touch the side teeth and blow air out centrally.

/tʃ, dʒ/

1. Produce /t/ and then /ʃ/. Repeat these two sounds more and more rapidly until they blend into one /tʃ/ sound.
2. Make the sound of a train coming down the tracks by saying "choo-choo." (This takes advantage of children's tendency to produce nonspeech sounds without the errors evidenced in their real word productions.)
3. Make a long /n/ sound and add /sh/. Repeat this combination stronger, louder, and faster until it blends into /tʃ/.

/l/

1 Put the tip of your tongue on the bumpy part behind your upper front teeth and drop it while saying /a/.
2. (For w/l substitutions, contrasting the lip postures using a mirror is particularly helpful. For /w/, explain and show the child that the lips are visibly rounded and protruded, whereas /l/ is made with the lips separated at the corners and somewhat lax.)
3. Close your mouth, put your tongue behind your top teeth, open your mouth while keeping your tongue up. Now let your tongue down as you say /la/.

/k, g/

1. Put the back of your tongue up against the roof of your mouth and hold your breath for a second. Drop your tongue quickly and release your breath with a coughing sound to produce /k/.
2. Pretend you are a puppet with an imaginary string attached to the back of your head. As I pull the string, raise the back of your tongue against the roof of your mouth. Drop your tongue quickly to allow a sudden escape of air to say /k/ as I let go of the string.

(continues)

3. (Use a tongue depressor to hold down the tongue tip while at the same time pushing the tongue backward and upward until it comes into contact with the soft palate.) When I remove the tongue depressor, quickly lower the back of your tongue to say /k/.

Note: All these instructions can be adapted for the voiced cognates by directing the child to "turn his/her voice on" or "make his/her throat buzz." In addition, a mirror can be used to highlight sounds whose articulatory placements are visible (e.g., /θ/, /p/, /l/).

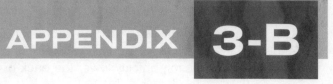

APPENDIX 3-B

DIADOCHOKINETIC RATES FOR CHILDREN

Age/Years	pʌ*	tʌ	kʌ	pʌtəkə**
6	4.0–5.6	3.9–5.9	4.6–6.4	7.2–13.4
7	3.8–5.8	4.0–5.8	4.3–6.3	7.4–12.6
8	3.5–4.9	3.7–5.1	4.1–5.5	6.2–10.4
9	3.4–4.6	3.5–4.7	3.9–5.3	5.8–9.6
10	3.3–4.1	3.4–4.2	3.8–4.8	5.6–8.6
11	3.0–4.2	2.9–4.3	3.4–4.6	5.1–7.9
12	3.0–3.8	3.0–4.0	3.3–4.5	4.8–8.0
13	2.7–3.9	2.8–3.8	3.1–4.3	4.3–7.1

Source: Adapted from Fletcher, 1972; Kent, Kent & Rosenbek, 1987.

*Scores represent time range (in seconds) required for 20 repetitions of single syllables (i.e., pʌ, tʌ, kʌ).

**Scores represent time range (in seconds) required for 10 repetitions of trisyllables (i.e., pʌtəkə).

CHAPTER 4

Intervention for Language in Infants and Preschool Children

This chapter focuses on the treatment of childhood language disorders. A **language disorder** can be defined as the abnormal acquisition, comprehension, or use of spoken or written language. This includes all receptive and expressive language skills. The disorder may involve any aspect of the form, content, or use components of the linguistic system. Children with language disorders are not a homogeneous population in several respects, including the following:

- *Primary versus secondary disorder:* For some children, the reduced ability to acquire language is their primary deficit in the relative absence of impairment in other developmental areas. For other children, the language deficit occurs in association with other impairments (e.g., mental retardation).

- *Developmental versus acquired:* Developmental language disorders are present from birth or occur prior to the onset of normal language acquisition. Acquired disorders involve the loss or interruption of language function due to illness or trauma.

- *Delayed versus deviant acquisition:* Children with delayed language proceed through the same sequence of acquisition as typically developing children but at a substantially slower rate. In contrast, children with deviant language demonstrate acquisition patterns that differ significantly from the normal developmental sequence.

- *Range of severity:* The severity of language deficits can range along a continuum of mild to profound impairment.

CLASSIFICATION OF LANGUAGE DISORDERS

A disorder can involve both the comprehension and production of language. Language **comprehension** (receptive language) refers to the ability to derive meaning from incoming auditory or visual messages. Language **production** (expressive language) involves the combination of linguistic symbols to form meaningful messages. Language disorders are generally classified according to the major components of the linguistic system.

Semantics involves the meaning of individual words and the rules that govern the combinations of word meanings to form meaningful phrases and sentences. Impairments in this subsystem can take the form of reduced vocabulary; restricted semantic categories; word retrieval deficits; poor word association skills; and difficulty with figurative (nonliteral) language forms such as idioms, metaphors, and humor.

Morphology involves the structure of words and the construction of individual word forms from the basic elements of meaning (i.e., morphemes). Deficits in this component are manifested as difficulties with inflectional markers such as plurals, past tense, auxiliary verbs, possessives, and so on.

Syntax involves the rules governing the order and combination of words in the construction of well-formed sentences. Syntactic deficits are characterized by problems with simple and complex sentence types such as negatives, interrogatives, passives, and relative clauses as well as occasional word-order difficulties.

Pragmatics involves the rules governing the use of language in a social context. Pragmatic impairments can include a reduced repertoire of communicative

TABLE 4-1
Behavioral Characteristics Associated with Language Disorders

Behavior	Definition
Inattention	Impairment of concentration characterized by difficulty with completing tasks, attending to details, following through on instructions, and tuning out distracting stimuli
Impulsivity	The abrupt performance of actions without sufficient deliberation or consideration of the consequences
Hyperactivity	An excessively high level of activity accompanied by a reduced ability to inhibit the activity volitionally
Attention deficit disorder (ADD)	Disorder characterized by one or more of the above features: inattention, impulsivity, or hyperactivity
Perseveration	Inappropriate and often involuntary continuation of a motor or verbal response when it is no longer relevant
Echolalia	Excessive and developmentally inappropriate repetition of the speech of others, generally with the same intonation; may be immediate or delayed

intentions, turn-taking difficulties in conversation, an inability to repair messages that are not understood by the listener, and difficulty with narrative discourse such as storytelling.

Phonology involves the particular sounds (i.e., phonemes) that comprise the sound system of a language and the rules that govern permissible sound combinations. (For a discussion of phonological impairments, see Chapter 3.)

In addition to language deficits, children may demonstrate certain associated behavioral characteristics, the most common of which are defined in Table 4-1.

Childhood language disorders affect a diverse group of children who present with differing profiles of language impairment. Intervention with this population is the subject of an enormous literature that covers an age span from infancy through adolescence. To organize this body of information in a manner that is clinically useful for the reader, the remainder of this chapter presents an overview of basic treatment principles and specific intervention information for children from birth through the preschool years. Intervention information for school-age students and adolescents will be the subject of Chapter 5. The information in this chapter is provided as a general guideline regarding language acquisition and treatment. The relative applicability of this material will depend on a host of factors, including the sociocultural background of any particular client.

RELATIONSHIP BETWEEN ORAL LANGUAGE AND LITERACY

It is now recognized that speech-language pathologists play a significant role in the development of literacy. Literacy involves the development of reading and writing skills. From a basic perspective, reading consists of two component processes:

decoding and comprehension. Decoding is the ability to assign sound-letter correspondences to printed symbols (the alphabetic principle), while comprehension involves the ability to derive meaning from printed text. Writing involves the acquisition of spelling and the ability to compose text at the sentence level and beyond. Spelling is the ability to construct words using the conventional orthography (i.e., written symbols) of a given language, while composition is the formulation of coherent units of connected language including narrative and expository texts.

Oral language serves as the basis for the development of reading and writing skills, beginning with the period known as "emergent literacy," which extends from birth through the preschool years. Emergent literacy is a child's increasing awareness of the world of print and an understanding of the functions of literacy. During the preschool period, children develop foundational knowledge about print through everyday, naturally occurring experiences in their home and preschool/daycare environments. These experiences prepare them for the formal literacy instruction that begins in the early elementary school grades.

Of the oral language skills studied thus far, metalinguistic awareness is the area that has been most closely linked to literacy acquisition. Metalinguistic awareness is the explicit knowledge of and ability to manipulate aspects of the linguistic system independently of the meaning conveyed by the message. Phonological awareness is a metalinguistic skill that involves manipulation of the sound structure of language through tasks such as rhyming, blending, and segmenting of words, syllables, or phonemes. In particular, a child's control of sounds at the phoneme level (i.e., phonemic awareness) is highly predictive of decoding and spelling skills. A common example of a phonemic awareness task is asking a child to say a word such as "fat" and then to say it again without the /f/. In turn, acquisition of decoding skill leads to subsequent improvement of phonemic awareness ability. (Note: Phonics is the written language counterpart to this ability and focuses on sound-letter correspondences.) Children and adolescents with language and learning impairments demonstrate considerable difficulty with phonemic awareness tasks. There is evidence that these children can benefit from direct phonological awareness instruction (Torgesen, Wagner, & Rashotte, 1994). Intervention in this skill area is most effective when delivered in conjunction with training on the alphabetic principle and results in measurable gains in reading and spelling (Torgesen & Davis, 1996).

Other aspects of oral language that are associated with literacy development are vocabulary knowledge and word retrieval. Vocabulary size during the toddler years appears to be related to a child's ability to accurately decode single words in first and second grades (Scarborough, 1998; Scarborough & Dobrich, 1990). Once a child reaches middle elementary school years, the focus of reading shifts away from decoding, and vocabulary size becomes predictive of reading comprehension skill (Stanovich, 1986; Baker, Simmons, & Kameenui, 1998). With regard to word retrieval, naming accuracy is predictive of current and future decoding skill, while naming speed has been found to be strongly related to reading comprehension (Scarborough, 1998; Wolf, 1984, 1991). Importantly, deficits in vocabulary and word retrieval are among the most common characteristics of language impairment throughout childhood and adolescence.

Role of the Speech-Language Pathologist in Literacy

The traditional scope of practice for speech-language pathologists (SLPs) has evolved over the past several years to incorporate more emphasis on literacy-related issues. Accordingly, in 2000, ASHA developed a position statement, guidelines, and several other documents to address the roles and responsibilities of SLPs in serving children with reading and writing difficulties. These documents clearly indicate that " . . . SLPs play a critical and direct role in the development of literacy for children and adolescents with communication disorders . . . " and are based on the following premises:

- Oral language is the basis for the acquisition of reading and writing.

- There is a reciprocal relationship between oral and written language in that each builds on the other.

- Children and adolescents with oral language deficits often have difficulty acquiring the ability to read and write (and vice versa).

- Reading and writing deficits can involve any of the subsystems of language: phonology, morpho-syntax, semantics, and pragmatics.

- SLPs have knowledge of typical and atypical patterns of language development as well as experience in assessment and intervention for children and adolescents.

- Literacy development requires an interdisciplinary approach in which SLPs participate collaboratively with other professionals, families, and students.

The ASHA guidelines also identify the various roles and responsibilities that SLPs may undertake to foster literacy development. These include, but are not limited to:

- Prevention: Promote opportunities to participate in oral and written language experiences that facilitate literacy (e.g., shared bookreading, alphabet/letter exposure, adult modeling of reading and writing)

- Identification: Provide screening/early detection of children with or at risk for reading and writing problems as a result of oral language difficulties

- Assessment: Evaluate reading and writing abilities in relation to oral language skills using a comprehensive battery of norm-referenced and descriptive measures

- Intervention: Implement evidence-based instruction for reading and writing problems that emphasizes the reciprocal relationships between oral language and literacy

- Other roles: Collaborate/advocate for effective literacy practices in general and special education settings; advance the knowledge base regarding the relationship between oral language and literacy

TREATMENT

There are different theoretical orientations to language intervention. These arise, in part, from different philosophies about the nature of normal language acquisition and differing viewpoints regarding the application of normal language acquisition to children with language disorders. Theoretical models differentially stress the primacy of cognitive, linguistic, or behavioral variables (e.g., Bates & MacWhinney, 1987; Chomsky, 1965; Piaget, 1954; Pinker, 1989, 1996; Skinner, 1957; Vygotsky, 1962). Other models propose an integrative approach and incorporate elements of several philosophies (Bruner, 1974; Snow, 1978, 1981). Regardless of theoretical perspective, intervention practices should be evidence-based. Clinicians implement effective strategies and procedures in conjunction with their own judgment and knowledge acquired through professional experience.

These models lead to different strategies of language intervention. In general, a behavioral orientation results in a nondevelopmental approach to therapy. Language targets are selected without consideration of prerequisite skills, and behaviors are taught solely through the use of stimulus-response-consequence procedures. In contrast, other models are associated with developmental strategies in which target selection is determined by known sequences of acquisition, whether cognitively, linguistically, or pragmatically based. (See Appendix 4-A for major developmental language milestones.) For most children who present with a profile of delayed language, a developmental treatment strategy is generally utilized. A nondevelopmental approach may be adopted for atypical patterns of language acquisition (e.g., children with severe-profound mental retardation).

Intervention with Infants (Birth to 2 Years)

During this early developmental period, the infant masters the cognitive, social, and communicative behaviors that underlie the acquisition of the linguistic system. It is generally agreed that early intervention is crucial for infants who do not demonstrate these prerequisite skills within the typically expected time frame. Early intervention also is critical for children who are considered at risk for developing language difficulties due to factors such as prematurity, low birth weight, family history, medical complications, and so on. For at risk children, intervention can be provided indirectly through monitoring of developmental progress or directly through infant stimulation programs. Some programs extend this focus to the concept of prevention in which attempts are made to reduce or eliminate the risks and conditions that ultimately may result in communication disorders. Intervention provided during the first 2 years of life is thought to be extremely productive because it capitalizes on the rapid neural growth and learning potential of the young brain.

Early intervention is characterized by a primary emphasis on family involvement and education. A family-centered approach addresses the child's needs within the sole relevant context for the child—the family unit. This model also acknowledges the cultural, social, and economic factors that may affect family dynamics. Early intervention services can be implemented in home- or center-based settings. With infants, more than with any other single age group, the clinician will likely work in an interdisciplinary or transdisciplinary model of service delivery. In an interdisciplinary model, each team member functions within his or her specific discipline and shares information with other team members through established channels such as team meetings. In contrast, members of a transdisciplinary team cross traditional professional boundaries. They receive training in other disciplines and interchangeably provide services as needed by the child and family.

The goal of early intervention is the development of basic skills thought to be critical to successful language learning. **Repeated exposure** and **stimulation** are the primary therapy strategies for infants. The prelinguistic and early language skills that comprise the main therapy targets for infant intervention programs are presented as follows.

Localization. Infants demonstrate awareness of sounds in their environment by turning toward and visually searching for the source of a sound. This auditory-visual association marks the beginning an infant's conceptual grasp of cause-effect relations.

A clinician can enhance the localization behaviors of an infant by presenting a sound stimulus (e.g., rattle or other noisy object) outside the baby's visual field. This will require an observable head turn for the baby to locate the sound source. If this response is not observed, the clinician can gently turn the infant's head toward the sound to reinforce the auditory-visual association. The following developmental sequence can be used as a guideline for choosing the appropriate response level for a given infant.

3 to 4 months:	Primitive attempt to turn head
4 to 7 months:	Localization to side only
7 to 13 months:	Localization to side or below
13 to 21 months:	Localization to side, below, or above
21 to 24 months:	Direct localization to any angle

Joint Attention (Joint Reference). A shared focus underlies successful communication. Joint attention between an adult and infant highlights the relationship between the adult's utterances and the concepts/objects they represent. According to Bruner (1977), joint visual attention is the prerequisite for all subsequent communication. One effective method for facilitating joint attention or shared reference is to place an attractive or noisy object in front of the infant, look at it, and comment on it. The adult may point to the object, shake it, or gently turn the infant's head to encourage eye contact with the object. Sometimes it may be necessary to follow the infant's gaze to a particular object and then point to and label it to promote joint visual regard.

Mutual Gaze. This eye gaze pattern is a characteristic of early communicative development in which the infant and caregiver look at each other during social interactions. It is thought to form the basis for attachment/bonding between infant and caregiver (Rossetti, 2001) and serves as a basic building block for later development of the important skill of turn-taking in conversation (Owens, 2001). Immediate parental response to the infant's initiation of eye contact increases the baby's motivation to communicate and ultimately results in more frequent and varied interactions (Brockman, Morgan, & Harmon, 1988). Establishment and maintenance of mutual gaze with infants can be enhanced when adult eye contact is accompanied by smiling and other facial expressions, touching, and novel/entertaining vocalizations.

Joint Action and Routines. Joint action between an adult and infant occurs in play sequences known as sound-gesture games or routines such as peekaboo, patty-cake, or "I'm gonna get you." A routine is a prepackaged or ritualized exchange between an adult and infant. It has a definite structure with a clearly marked beginning, middle, and end with clearly specified positions for appropriate vocalization or verbalization. This structure allows for the anticipation of events and increases the potential for successful adult-child interaction. It ensures that each partner knows what to expect from the other, thus making the order of events highly predictable. Ratner and Bruner (1978) point out that the semantic content of the mutual play is highly restricted and within the conceptual repertoire of the child. It is generally believed that the regularity and invariance of these routines allow the infant to make his or her first attempts at "cracking the linguistic code" and acquiring the first words (Ferrier, 1978; Newson, 1979). Many investigators also believe that these routines facilitate turn-taking behavior and role shifting in dialogue, both important building blocks of conversational exchanges.

Clinicians can initiate these playful routines in therapy and select the target response for an infant based on the typical acquisition sequence noted for young children.

- At approximately 6 months, infants show enjoyment and pleasure (i.e., change in facial expression or body posture) when a parent initiates a sound-gesture routine.

- By 7 months, the infant anticipates the game when the adult produces the verbal component alone (independent of any gesture).

- The 8- to 9-month-old baby initiates as well as participates in the game (e.g., crawls behind the door and peeks his head out while smiling).

For slightly older babies, the clinician can utilize the "Picture-Book-Reading Routine" (Ninio & Bruner, 1978) with the baby seated next to or on the adult's lap. Select an enjoyable picture book and follow this sequence:

A: Say "Look" (attentional vocative) and point to picture

C: Touches or looks at the picture (response)

A: Say "What are these?" (query)

C: Vocalizes, smiles, or names the picture (response)

A: Say "Yes, that is a _____" or "No, that's not a _____, it's a _____" (feedback)

Vocalizations. The first year of life is characterized, in part, by rapid physical growth and neuromuscular maturation. As a result, the infant gains increasing control over the speech mechanism and exhibits significant expansion in the quality and variety of vocalizations. Infant vocalizations proceed through a series of predictable developmental stages as outlined in Table 4-2.

Expansion of an infant's vocal repertoire can be promoted by increasing the frequency, variety, or quality of the vocalizations produced by the infant. The clinician can stimulate vocalization by talking to the infant, singing, humming, cuddling, tickling, or playing sound-gesture games such as peekaboo. Clinicians may also imitate the infant's vocalization in a playful manner to initiate a repetitive imitative exchange. Action-identification tags are playful sounds that infants enjoy listening to and may attempt to reproduce, such as the motor sound ("vroom"), cow sound ("moo"), telephone ("dingaling"), dog barking ("ruff ruff"), or car horn ("beep beep").

Communicative Intentions. The meaning that a speaker wishes a message to convey is known as a **communicative intention**. At about 9 months of age, infants discover intentional communication and begin to express their communicative intentions through gesture and vocalization (see Table 4-3).

TABLE 4-2
Stages of Vocal Development in Infancy

Age	Behavior	Description
0–2 months	Reflexive	Undifferentiated crying and vegetative sounds (e.g., coughing, burping, sighing)
2–4 months	Cooing	Vocal signs of pleasure, primarily vowel and vowel-like sounds
4–6 months	Laughter	Sustained combination of cooing and crying features to produce audible "ha ha ha"
	Vocal play	Exploration of mouth with tongue, producing sounds such as squeals, growls, lip smacking, raspberries, and clicks
	Early babbling	Self-initiated sound play; combines stop consonants with vowels to produce isolated CV or VC syllables (e.g., /ba/ or /ɔk/)
6–8 months	Reduplicative babbling	Series of CV or VC syllables each identical to the other and frequently initiated with a /ə/ (e.g., /ədadada/)
8–10 months	Nonreduplicative babbling	Consonants and vowels may differ from one syllable to the next within a single string (e.g., /bawada/)
10–12 months	Jargon	Conversational intonation contours are imposed on longer strings of sound combinations; real words may be interspersed
	Protowords	Invented sound sequences that are used consistently to refer to a specific item or event (e.g., /na/ used to mean "Give [object] to me")

Sources: Adapted from Oller (1980) and Stark (1980).

Requests and statements are among the earliest communicative intentions to emerge. Requests represent the infant's intentional use of a listener as an agent or tool in achieving some end (e.g., a desired object). Statements are the infant's attempts to direct an adult's attention to some event or object in the environment. As children begin to acquire an initial vocabulary, they express communicative intentions through single-word utterances (see Table 4-4). Evidence suggests that the *rate* of preverbal communication in young children with developmental delays is a strong predictor of later vocabulary usage (Calandrella & Wilcox, 2000).

Intervention in the area of communicative intentions may be aimed at (1) increasing the number of different types of intentions a child can understand or express and/or (2) increasing the variety of forms (e.g., vocalization, gesture, word) understood or used to express a given intention. To elicit specific communicative intentions, the clinician should provide facilitating environments in which the intentions are obligatory or at least highly likely to occur (Spekman & Roth, 1984). Following are examples of facilitating environments for selected intentions:

Requests for action:	Introduce toys that cannot be operated without assistance from the clinician, such as a windup toy.
	Place highly desirable toys where child cannot gain access to them without assistance from the clinician.
	Present incomplete or broken materials such as puzzles with missing pieces or paints without brushes.

TABLE 4-3
Preverbal Communicative Intentions

Intention	Descriptive Example
1. Attention-seeking	
a. To self	Child tugs on mother's jeans to secure attention.
b. To events, objects, or other people	Child points to airplane to draw mother's attention to it.
2. Requesting	
a. Objects	Child points to toy animal that he wants.
b. Action	Child hands book to adult to have story read.
c. Information	Child points to usual location of cookie jar (which is not there) and simultaneously secures eye contact with mother to determine its whereabouts.
3. Greetings	Child waves "hi" or "bye."
4. Transferring	Child gives mother the toy that he was playing with.
5. Protesting/rejecting	Child cries when mother takes away toy. Child pushes away a dish of oatmeal.
6. Responding/acknowledging	Child responds appropriately to simple directions. Child smiles when parent initiates a favorite game.
7. Informing	Child points to wheel on his toy truck to show mother that it is broken.

Sources: Categories are derived, in part, from Bates, Camaioni, & Volterra (1975); Coggins & Carpenter (1981); Dore (1974); Escalona (1973); Greenfield & Smith (1976); Halliday (1975); and Wetherby, Cain, Yonclas, & Walker (1988).

TABLE 4-4
Communicative Intentions Expressed at the Single-Word Level

Intention	Definition
1. Naming	Common and proper nouns that label people, objects, events, and locations.
2. Commenting	Words that describe physical attributes of objects, events, and people, including size, shape, and location; observable movements and actions of objects and people; and words that refer to attributes that are not immediately observable such as possession and usual location. These words are not contingent on prior utterances.
3. Requesting object a. Present b. Absent	Words that solicit an object that is present in the environment. Words that solicit an absent object.
4. Requesting action	Words that solicit that an action be initiated or continued.
5. Requesting information	Words that solicit information about an object, action, person, or location. Rising intonation is also included.
6. Responding	Words that directly complement preceding utterances.
7. Protesting/rejecting	Words that express objection to ongoing or impending action/event.
8. Attention-seeking	Words that solicit attention to the child or to aspects of the environment.
9. Greetings	Words that express salutations and other conventionalized rituals.

Sources: Adapted from Dale (1900), Dore (1974), and Halliday (1975).

Requests for information:	Introduce novel or enticing toys for which the child is likely to request a label or information regarding its function, operation, or construction such as a transformer, spinning top, or a talking book.
Attention-seeking:	Pretend not to hear the child so that he or she must use the clinician's name, raise vocal pitch or intensity, or move closer to the clinician.

Nonsymbolic Play and Symbolic Play. Children learn through play and often practice their new acquisitions in play. Infants gain experience in both receptive and expressive language functioning by participating in play sequences. In addition, play is the most important context for the development of social communication skills and the natural context for early language learning (Johnson, Christie & Yawkey, 1987; Norris & Hoffman, 1990; Rivkin, 1986; Rogers & Sawyers, 1988). Some types of play do not require the use of symbolic agents and include activities such as running, filling and emptying receptacles, and water play. In symbolic forms of play, the child substitutes objects/events for other objects/events. Examples include pretending to talk on the telephone or using a stick as a sword. (See Appendix 4-B for stages of play development.)

Following are some suggested themes and activities for facilitating play, arranged developmentally:

- Exploring common objects such as blocks, rattles, spoons, pots, and pans through banging, mouthing, manipulating, and visual inspection

- Using toys appropriately such as Busy Box or See 'N Say

- Pretending to act out familiar single actions such as eating, sleeping, drinking

- Manipulating doll to perform familiar activities such as kissing, dancing, waving bye-bye

- Pretending to act out sequences of familiar actions such as pouring liquid into a cup, taking a sip, and then spilling the liquid onto the floor

- Using dough or clay to create "pretend" food such as hot dogs, pancakes

- Using miniature people, cars, dishes to act out daily routines such as taking a bath, going to the store, or having a birthday party

Initial Vocabulary. Infants begin to understand a few familiar words between 6 and 8 months of age. Production of first true words occurs around their first birthday. Early vocabulary development can be stimulated at the receptive and/or expressive level (McKeown & Curtis, 1987; Nagy & Herman, 1987; Whitehurst, Fischel, Valdez-Menchaca, Arnold, & Smith, 1991). Intervention aimed at the facilitation of a child's **receptive** vocabulary generally consists of repeated presentation of a target word as well as the use of exaggerated vocal intonation patterns to highlight salient aspects of an object or event. The following section presents two activities that can be used to stimulate comprehension of early vocabulary for a 12- to 24-month-old child with a language impairment.

- Engage the child in play with a large, lightweight ball. Demonstrate and say the following to the child:

    "Can you *throw* the ball to me? Put two hands over your head and *throw* it to me. That's right, let go and *throw* it over here. Great, you did it.

    "Now can you *drop* the ball? I'll *drop* it first and then you *drop* it again. Let me see you *drop* the ball. Good job.

    "Let me see you *kick* the ball. *Kick* the ball with your foot. *Kick* the ball as hard as you can. Good for you, you *kicked* the ball."

- Engage the child in play using a surprise box such as Disney Poppin' Pals. Say to the child:

    "Can you find Mickey's *ball*? Guess what? I see a *ball* right here. Oh look, there's another *ball* under Goofy. Do you see Dumbo's *ball*? That's not Dumbo, that's Donald. Donald has a really big *ball*. Touch Donald's *ball*."

The early **expressive** vocabularies of young children are not arbitrary. Initial lexicons are highly selective because children communicate about the social and physical events that are within their conceptual grasp and immediate

TABLE 4-5
Grammatical Classification of the First 50 Words Produced

Grammatical Function	Percentage of Vocabulary	Examples
Nominals	50	milk, dog, car
Action words	11–14	give, do, up, bye-bye
Modifiers	14–19	mine, no dirty
Personal/social	10	no, please
Functional	4	this, for

Sources: Based on Benedict (1979) and Nelson (1973).

environment. A grammatical classification of a typical initial lexicon is presented in Table 4-5. Expressive vocabulary growth is charted in Table 4-6.

Researchers also agree that children's early vocabularies express a basic set of semantic functions or intentions (Bloom, 1973; Brown, 1968; Nelson, 1973). Strategies for facilitating the acquisition of early lexical items are frequently based on semantic function rather than grammatical classification. Three main considerations in the selection of target vocabulary are (1) words that can be used in many different contexts during the child's daily activities; (2) words that are important to the child such as names of significant others or types of favorite foods or toys; and (3) words that represent dynamic rather than static states, especially referents that can be acted on or manipulated directly by the child such as ball or spoon versus tree or wall. Following are suggested contexts/activities that can be used to stimulate different types of semantic intentions at the single-word level.

Existence/naming: Introduce a container filled with interesting objects and reveal them to the child one at a time.

Nonexistence: Expose an attractive object to the child and then hide it from view.

Recurrence: Initiate a desirable activity and then stop.

TABLE 4-6
Expressive Vocabulary Growth

Age	Number of Words
15 months	4–6
18 months	20–50
24 months	200–300
3 years	900–1,000
4 years	1,500–1,600
5 years	2,100–2,200

Action:	Engage the child in an activity such as making pudding that will elicit a number of different actions (e.g., open, pour, stir, mix).
Possession:	Place a combination of the child's and clinician's belongings in a box, pull them out one at a time, and sort into separate piles.
Locative:	Engage the child in play with trucks or cars using props such as a Fisher-Price Garage that encourage changes in location.
Rejection:	Offer objects or activities that are known to be unappealing to the child.
Denial:	In a playful manner, intentionally misname objects or body parts that the child already knows.

Helpful Hints

1. Clinicians may want to incorporate some of the main characteristics of "motherese" in their speech to young children. These include exaggerated intonation, short utterance length, simple vocabulary and syntactic structures, frequent repetition of utterances, and talking about topics in the "here and now."

2. Clinician (CL) responses to child (CH) utterances should be framed in a way that encourages the exchange to continue and keeps the child in the interaction (sometimes referred to as **turnabouts**). For example:

   CH: dat?
   CL: Kitty cat. What does it say?
   vs.
   CH: dat?
   CL: It's a kitty.

3. Clinicians can maximize the effectiveness of intervention activities by selecting toys and materials that are developmentally appropriate for a particular child. (See Appendix 4-C for a developmental toy list.)

4. Clinicians need to be aware that many infants with communication impairments may exhibit concomitant impairments in other areas. Intervention programs must accommodate the infant's overall developmental profile. For example, tactile stimulation often elicits abnormal primitive reflexes in children with cerebral palsy and can significantly interfere with therapeutic programming.

5. Encourage parents to read books to their children. Ideal books for infants include things to touch, language that repeats over and over again, and colorful pictures of objects and words to match.

6. Clinicians should be prepared to address skepticism of other professionals and parents regarding the merits of language intervention with infants and very young children.

Intervention with Children (2 to 5 Years)

During this developmental period, children acquire the major portion of the linguistic system. This period is characterized by rapid growth in vocabulary. After the age of 18 months, children add approximately 9–10 new words to their lexicons each day or 3,000 words per year (Graves, 1986). Average utterance length continues to increase, and the acquisition of syntax has its onset as children begin to impose word order on their two-word combinations. Morphological forms emerge and become solidified, although complete mastery is not attained until the early elementary school years. This developmental period also is marked by children's ability to understand and produce a variety of simple and complex sentence forms. In addition, children in this age range demonstrate substantial development in the area of emergent literacy through exposure and interaction with print. See Tables 4-7 through 4-15 for a review of mean length of utterance (MLU) stages, two-word semantic intentions, acquisition of grammatical morphemes, auxiliary verb development, negation development, question development, sentence-type comprehension progression, hallmarks of literacy development, and developmental stages of early writing.

TABLE 4 7
Stages of MLU Development

Stage	MLU (morphemes)	Approximate Age
I	1.75–2.0	18–24 months
II	2.0–2.5	2–2½ years
III	2.5–3.0	2½–3 years
IV	3.0–3.5	3–3½ years
V	3.5–4.0	3½–4 years

Source: Brown (1973).

TABLE 4-8
Two-Word Semantic Relations

Relation	Examples
Agent + action	Daddy eat, mommy drive
Action + object	Eat cookie, throw ball
Agent + object	Daddy shoe, grandma hat
Attribute + entity	Big doggie, pretty lady
Possessor + possession	Daddy car, baby bottle
Recurrence	More juice, more cookie
Nonexistence	No bed, allgone milk
Demonstrative + entity	This cup, that doggie
Entity + location	Daddy chair, toy floor
Action + location	Go home, sit horsie

Sources: Bloom (1973), Brown (1973), and Schlesinger (1971).

TABLE 4-9
Brown's 14 Grammatical Morphemes: Order of Acquisition

Morpheme	Example	Stage
Present progressive -ing (no auxiliary verb)	Daddy sleeping	I–II
In/on	Doggie on table	II
Regular plural -s	Me have two shoes	I–III
Irregular past	Drank, came, fell, broke, ate	I–IV
Possessive 's	Daddy's chair	I–IV
Uncontractible copula (used as main verb)	This is hot.	II–IV
Articles (a/the)	Open the door.	II–V
Regular past -ed	Mommy walked the dog.	I–Post V
Regular third person -s	Mommy works.	I–V
Irregular third person	Does, has	II–Post V
Uncontractible auxiliary	The doggie is running.	II–Post V
Contractible copula	He is tall.	II–Post V
Contractible auxiliary	Daddy is coming home.	II–Post V

Source: Adapted from Brown (1973)

TABLE 4-10
Auxiliary Verb Development

Category	Form/Examples	Stage
Contracted form of "is"	's	Early II
Forms of "to be"	is, am, are, was	Late II
Early infinitives (catenatives)	hafta, gonna, wanna	Late II
Early modals	can, do, may, will	Stage III →
Subjunctive modals	could, would, should, might	Stage III →
Mood of obligation modals	should, must, have to	Stage IV →
Perfective	have . . . en	Stage V or later
Double expansion of auxiliary	has been, might have	Stage V or later

TABLE 4-11
Development of Negation

MLU Stage	Form	Example
I	Negative + utterance Utterance + negative	No drink; not hungry Mommy no; doggie not
II–III	Subject + negative + main verb Unanalyzed "don't/can't" (not true auxiliary forms)	Me no drink; he not sit Don't hit; You can't go
III–IV	Subject + auxiliary + negative + main verb	He is not running; Mommy cannot go

TABLE 4-12
Development of Question Forms*

MLU Stage	Form	Example
I		
Yes/no	Rising intonation	Me go?; See hole?
Wh	What NP** doing?	What daddy doing?
	Where NP going?	Where mommy going?
	Wh-word + NP	What that?
II–III		
Yes/no	Rising intonation in longer utterances	You see red ball?
Wh	Wh-word + sentence	Who you draw in book?
III–IV		
Yes/no	NP and auxiliary verb	Can I go?; Do you see me?
	Inversion of subject	
Wh	Wh-word + subject NP + auxiliary + main verb	Why he can ride?
IV–V		
Yes/no	Remains the same in longer utterances	Should I throw it over there?
Wh	Wh-word + auxiliary verb + subject NP + main verb	Why can he ride?

*Note: Wh-words emerge in the following sequence: (a) what, where; (b) who; (c) when, how, and why, in variable order.
**NP – Noun phrase.

Emergent Literacy Intervention (Birth through Preschool Years)

The overall goal of emergent literacy intervention is to promote those oral and print-awareness skills that are associated with the ability to successfully learn reading and writing skills. This goal addresses the positive relationship between early intervention and academic achievement. Speech-language pathologists may play a variety of direct and indirect roles in this area of intervention. SLPs would likely work directly on providing emergent literacy intervention to children with identified communication disorders. Indirect roles would encompass collaborative consultation with others, professional staff development, parent/community education, and curricular policy recommendations regarding the critical nature of emergent literacy skill acquisition for all children.

In addition to oral language, there are several other components of emergent literacy, each of which can be used as an avenue to increase a child's awareness of print. Below are five main areas accompanied by instructional guidelines (Roth & Baden, 2001):

- *Shared book-reading and sense of story*

    Expose child to quality literature that is developmentally appropriate with respect to complexity and content

    Select predictably patterned stories with repetitive themes and well-developed plot structure

TABLE 4-13
Developmental Sequence of Sentence Comprehension

Syntactic Structure	Example	Age of Comprehension between 75% and 90%
Simple imperative	Stop!	4-6 to 6-0
Negative imperative	Don't touch the stove!	5-6 to 7-0
Active declarative		
Regular noun and present progressive	The girl is walking.	3-0
Irregular noun and present progressive	The deer are running.	6-6 to 7-0
Past tense	The dog chased the cat.	5-6 to 7-0+
Past participle	The lady has spoken.	6-0 to 7-0+
Future tense	She will play the piano.	7-0 to 7-0+
Reversible	The man kisses the lady.	6-6 to 7-0+
Perfective	Daddy has been working.	7-0+
Interrogative		
Who	Who is on the bed?	3-0
What	What do we wear?	3-6 to 5-0
When	When do you sleep?	3-6 to 5-6
Negation	The man isn't swimming.	5-6 to 7-0+
Reversible passive	The dog is chased by the cat.	5-6 to 6-0
Conjunction		
If	If you're a teacher, point to the dog.	7-0+
Then	Look at the third animal, then point to the dog.	7-0+
Neither/nor	Show me the one that is neither the ball nor the dog.	7-0+

Source: Adapted from Carrow (1973); Scarborough (1989).

Direct the child's attention to the printed words rather than focusing solely on the pictures

Engage in dialogic reading; ask questions throughout the reading activity about what has been read and what might happen next

- *Alphabetic letter knowledge*

 Program instruction hierarchically in the following order: letters in which the sound represents the beginning of the letter name (e.g., b, p); letters in which the sound represents the end of the letter name (e.g., f, l); and finally, letters in which the sound is not related to the letter name (e.g., w, y)

 Call attention to the way letters are formed by the mouth (e.g., lip rounding for /w/ or tongue tip elevation for /t/)

TABLE 4-14
Hallmarks of Literacy Development

Stage	Description
Early Emergent	Awareness of some print conventions (e.g., front versus back of books; left-right directionality of writing; words versus pictures)
	Shows sustained interest during book reading
	Recognizes familiar environmental print (e.g., logo for McDonald's)
	Engages in random drawing and scribbling
Later Emergent	Pretends to read and write
	Demonstrates a sense of "story" (i.e., beginning/middle/ending)
	Recognizes and produces predictable language patterns of familiar stories
	Attempts to write letters using scribbles and wavy lines
Early Beginning Reader	Attempts to read words by matching each letter to its corresponding sound (early decoding)
	Begins to develop a sight-word vocabulary which consists of highly familiar words
	Attempts to write words using primarily beginning and ending letters
Later Beginning Reader	Decodes familiar print easily; may struggle with new material
	Demonstrates large sight-word vocabulary
	Engages in self-correction during reading and writing
	Spells most familiar words accurately
	Shows awareness of writing conventions such as punctuation
Independent Reader	Reads fluently and focuses on understanding the meaning of text
	Uses text-based strategies such as predicting, summarizing, re-reading, and paraphrasing
	Demonstrates consistent use of spelling rules and writing conventions such as punctuation, paragraphing, and topic versus supporting sentences

Source: Adapted from Salinger (2001).

- *Adult modeling of literacy activities*

    Provide frequent opportunities for the child to observe adults engaged in reading and writing in natural contexts (e.g., preparing grocery list, following written instructions to assemble a toy)

    Engage child as a "helper" in everyday activities (e.g., hunting for items in a catalog or following a simple recipe to prepare a favorite food)

TABLE 4-15
Developmental Stages of Early Spelling

Stage	Description/Example
Drawing	Child scribbles using wavy and circular lines
Pre-phonemic	Random combination of pictures, squiggles, letters, and numbers with no connection between letters and sounds (e.g., Az4Esu7)
Semi-phonemic	Writes 1–3 letters to stand for a word (e.g., P = piano, PTE = pretty)
Phonetic/letter name	Spells words the way they sound (e.g., LETL = little, EGL = eagle)
Transitional	Within-word patterns include vowels in each syllable (e.g., EGUL = eagle)
Conventional	Basic rules of spelling are mastered (e.g., EAGLE = eagle)

Source: Adapted from Bear & Templeton, 1998; Gentry, 2000.

- *Experience with writing materials*

    Provide materials that permit children to write by themselves (e.g., pens, pencils, markers, crayons, rudimentary keyboarding)

    Facilitate all forms of writing (e.g., drawing, scribbling, basic letter formation) (See Table 4-15 for stages of writing development)

    Encourage child to dictate a "story" given visual stimuli (e.g., word-list picture books, cartoon frames)

Example Profiles

Following are two typical profiles of preschool children with language disorders. These examples have been designed to illustrate the selection of intervention targets, as well as specific therapy activities and materials. Most of the chosen activities are easily implemented in either individual or group therapy settings.

PROFILE 1

Austin is a 3-year, 1-month-old male child who presents with moderate delays in receptive and expressive language skills. Birth and developmental history are unremarkable, and hearing acuity is within normal limits. The results of a recent speech-language evaluation indicate that Austin's language comprehension abilities approximate the 24-month level, while expressive language skills fall at the 18- to 20-month level. Numerous articulation errors also were noted. Family members and the preschool teacher report that Austin is a socially interactive child who understands simple directions and communicates mainly through single words and occasional gestures.

Selection of therapy targets. The areas to be targeted are the comprehension of two-step commands, production of action + object utterances, and comprehension of early developing wh-questions. These targets were selected for two primary reasons: (1) these behaviors represent the next logical steps in the normal developmental sequence, and (2) they are highly relevant to the majority of Austin's daily activities. In addition, shared book-reading was selected as an instructional focus to enhance the development of emergent literacy.

Sample Activities

1. Gather 20 common objects with which the child is familiar. Develop a list of 10 two-step commands, each containing four linguistic elements in V + O constructions (e.g., *"Give me* the *car* and *push* the *spoon"*). Place three objects at a time on the table in front of the child. Verbally present the corresponding two-step command and encourage the child to perform each part as it is spoken. If the child is successful, repeat the same stimulus but instruct the child to refrain from responding until the entire two-stage command has been presented. Following are sample commands:

   Pick up the *cup* and *give me* the *shoe.*

   Throw the *spoon* and *wave bye-bye* to the *doggie.*

   Give me the *cup* and *push* the *car.*

   Drop the *spoon* and *point* to the *ball.*

   Give me the *brush* and *pick up* the *shoe.*

   Push the *doggie* and *throw* the *ball.*

   Open the *book* and *drop* the *cup.*

   Close the *box* and *give me* the *car.*

   Hug the *doggie* and *bang* the *spoon.*

   Pick up the *block* and *close* the *book.*

2. Develop a list of 20 two-word action + object utterances containing vocabulary words that are already part of the child's spontaneous expressive repertoire. Try to develop sets of two or three utterances that are topically related to one another to provide a meaningful context. Examples include the following:

open juice	throw ball
pour juice	kick ball
drink juice	roll ball
open book	wash baby
read book	brush hair
close book	kiss baby

   Gather toy replicas of each of the objects and any other toy props that may be required to perform the action sequences (e.g., for the utterance, "pour juice," a juice container and a cup will be needed). Place the objects in a large bag or pillowcase. Shake the bag to solicit the child's attention. Instruct the child to close or cover his eyes and to pull one of the objects from the bag. Depending on the child's abilities, either label the object or ask the child to name it. Then ask the child to perform one of the actions on the object (e.g., "Open the juice") and say, "What are you doing?" or "What's happening?" Following the child's correct production of the target utterance "open juice," reinforce the response with a comment such as "I like the way you opened the juice so carefully" or an expansion such as "You opened the juice." Then ask the child to perform another action with the same object (e.g., "Pour the juice"). Repeat the same training sequence with the other action + object combinations. If the child does not produce a verbal response or responds with a single-word utterance (e.g., "open"), model the target two-word utterance and repeat the item. After two unsuccessful attempts with a given utterance, model the target response and proceed to the next item.

3. Obtain a theme toy such as a farm, house, car wash, airport, or hospital and four toy people that can serve as a "mommy," "daddy," "sister/brother," or "baby," based on the composition of the child's family. Place the theme toy (e.g., house) on the floor in front of the child and put the "family" in front of the house. To ensure understanding of the lexical items, ask the child to point to each of the locations in and around the house and the family members when named. Examples of locations include the following:

kitchen	patio
bedroom	stairs
bathroom	laundry room
den/family room	backyard
basement	dining room

Instruct the child to place one of the people in a location about the house (e.g., "Put mommy in the living room") and say, "*Who* is in the living room?" Following the child's correct response, query the child: "*Where* is mommy?" Reinforce a correct response with a comment, expansion, or other scaffolding utterance. If the child responds incorrectly to either or both of the wh-questions, provide a prompt such as "Who? Mommy. That's *who* is in the living room. Mommy." Then ask: "*Who* is in the living room?"

4. Select a simple story from children's literature (e.g., The Three Bears) to read to the child. Throughout the reading of the book, engage the child in the PEER picture book reading routine (Burns, Griffin, & Snow, 1999):

P = *P*arent/adult initiates exchange about the book (e.g., "What are the three bears doing?")

E = Parent/adult *e*valuates child's response (e.g., "Yes, Poppa Bear is tasting the porridge.")

E = Parent/adult *e*xpands child's response (e.g., "And what is Momma Bear doing?")

R = Parent/adult *r*epeats initial question to check child's comprehension (e.g., "What are the three bears doing? Do you remember?")

PROFILE 2

Keisha is a 5-year, 7-month-old female child who demonstrates a mild receptive language delay and a moderate expressive impairment. Birth and medical history are unremarkable except for chronic middle ear infections during the first two years of life. At present, Keisha exhibits normal hearing acuity bilaterally. Her current communicative status is characterized by a six- to nine-month delay in most areas of language comprehension. Her language production abilities are more impaired, approximating the 3- to 3½-year level and consisting primarily of three-word utterances that tend to be telegraphic in nature (e.g., It my book; Daddy sleeping bed). Keisha's pragmatic use of language is essentially age appropriate and her speech intelligibility is judged to be good.

According to her kindergarten teacher, Keisha seems to understand most classroom activities but experiences a great deal of difficulty with reading readiness skills such as sound-letter correspondence.

Selection of therapy targets. The areas to be targeted are the auxiliary verb "is," regular plural "-s," and rhyme recognition. This auxiliary form was chosen for two reasons: (1) the progressive "ing" form is already occasionally observed in Keisha's spontaneous speech, and (2) the productive use of this auxiliary form would significantly decrease the telegraphic quality of her utterances. The plural marker "-s" was selected because Keisha grasps the concept of plurality but lacks the means for coding this information linguistically. Finally, rhyme recognition was targeted because it is a basic phonological awareness skill that contributes to early reading success.

Sample Activities

1. Collect 20 pictures or drawings of single agents performing various actions and attach each picture to an index card or other durable surface. Appropriate actions may include the following:

eating	kissing
drinking	reading
sleeping	hugging
laughing	painting
crying	washing
kicking	driving
throwing	swimming

   Cut basic shapes of laundry items (e.g., shirts, pants, socks) out of construction paper and mark an X on several of them. Loosely attach one picture card to the back of each laundry item cutout. String a clothesline between two chairs and hang the cutouts on the line with clothespins. Explain that the laundry items will be removed from the line one at a time. As the child removes an item from the line, the clinician models an appropriate sentence incorporating the "is _____ing" construction (e.g., "The boy is swimming"; "He is sleeping") and instructs the child to imitate it. Following a correct response, the child can remove the picture card from the cutout to look for an X on the back of the laundry item. If an X is found, the child receives a sticker or other reinforcer. Repeat this sequence for all 20 action pictures.

2. Gather materials including paper, marker, small paint bottle with sponge top (i.e., bingo marker), pictures or drawings of 10 single and 10 multiple objects, index cards, and a Colorforms kit. Using the marker, make a 20-square bingo board template (four rows of five squares each) on a large piece of paper. Laminate the pictures to the index cards and stack them randomly in a deck. Instruct the child to select the top card from the deck and name it three times. Remind the child that plural "s" must be added to the end of a word whenever more than one object is pictured (e.g., shoes). If all three productions are correct, the child uses the bingo marker to place a dot in one of the squares on the bingo board. Each time a row of five dots is completed, the child is given a Colorform piece. After the final row is completed, the child is allowed to create a picture using all the accumulated Colorform pieces.

3. Write the numbers 1 to 10 on 3-by-5-inch index cards. Construct a list of 20 word rhyme pairs, two of which rhyme with each number (adapted from B. Baden, personal communication, March 1994). Examples of rhyme pair stimuli are as follows:

1 = sun-done ton-won	6 = kicks-fix mix-sticks
2 = clue-blue shoe-moo	7 = heaven-leaven Evan-Kevin
3 = see-knee tree-free	8 = date-gate wait-mate
4 = store-pour sore-wore	9 = dine-line fine-mine
5 = dive-hive chive-drive	10 = men-pen then-den

Review the concept of rhyming with the child by explaining that rhymes are words that end in the same way. Give some examples of words that do and do not rhyme (e.g., hat-bat, shoe-blue, map-cap, cat-cow, top-tall), explaining why each does or does not rhyme. Place the number cards in a row on the table or floor in front of the child. Ask the child to name each of the numbers aloud. Explain that the clinician will say words that rhyme with or sound like the numbers on the cards. Instruct the child to listen carefully as the clinician says each rhyme pair and to hold up or point to the corresponding rhyming number. For example, the clinician says "store-pour" and the child holds up the number 4. Following a correct response, say, "That's right, store-pour-four all rhyme with each other." Instruct the child to repeat the verbal sequence.

Note: A variation of this activity is to substitute color words for number words with children who have reliable color word vocabularies.

Helpful Hints

1. It may be useful to teach the agent + action and action + object semantic relations sequentially because it generally provides an easy transition into three-word utterances (i.e., agent-action-object constructions).

2. Clinicians can encourage families to engage children in activities to promote emergent literacy. These may include the following:

   - Reading aloud to a child who is in a comfortable position. Ideal books for children at this age range include objects to identify, language that repeats and has rhyme, and activities that are highly familiar to the child.

   - Adult reads a story and has child draw a picture to go with it.

   - Have child plan a party for four to six people. Look in the food section of the newspaper for ideas of what to serve.

   - Adult and child look through newspaper and clip out articles about events in different parts of the world and attach each article to its location on a map or globe.

3. It may be more effective to repeat or expand a child's utterance than to directly correct the child's form.

4. Parents of children with severe language impairments often overestimate their child's level of ability, particularly in the area of language comprehension. Effective counseling may require that the clinician carefully guide parents to a more realistic perception of their child's true language skills.

CONCLUSION

This chapter has presented basic information, protocols, and procedures for intervention for early childhood language disorders at an **introductory** level This information is intended only as a starting point in the reader's clinical education and training. For more in-depth coverage of this area, the following readings are recommended:

Nelson, N. W. (1998). *Childhood language disorders in context: Infancy through adolescence.* Boston: Allyn & Bacon.

Owens, R. E. (2004). *Language disorders: A functional approach to assessment and intervention.* Needham Heights, MA: Allyn & Bacon.

Paul, R. (2001). *Language disorders from infancy to adolescence: Assessment and intervention.* Boston: C. V. Mosby.

ADDITIONAL RESOURCES

The Psychological Corporation
19500 Bulverde
San Antonio, TX 78259
Phone: 800-872-1726
Fax: 800-232-1223
Web site: www.psychcorp.com—go to Speech and Language section

Pictures, Please: Picture Gallery Articulation, Language, and Adult Language
More than 1,000 black-and-white illustrations on CDs, for clients from 3 years through adult. Drawings of common objects, actions, and situations covering

24 consonants and 19 vowels/diphthongs. Search by vocabulary level, word length, and various clinical features and select whether you want the picture, the word, or both to appear.

Pro-Ed

8700 Shoal Creek Boulevard
Austin, TX 78757-6897
Phone: 800-897-3202
Fax: 800-FXPROED
Web site: www.proedinc.com

Books Are for Talking Too!
A compendium of suggested books for preschool through twelfth grade. For each book, the following information is provided: 1) synopsis of the book, 2) the target area for therapy, 3) suggested strategies for teaching targets, and 4) suggested grades and interest level.

Classroom Listening and Speaking: Early Childhood
Reinforce target vocabulary by engaging children in active learning. Eight thematic units including kitchen, vegetables, numbers, colors, shapes, bedtime, farm animals, and water. Each thematic unit includes planning pages, reproducibles, language activities, annotated list of children's books with coordinated activities, and suggestions for field trips.

LinguiSystems

3100 4th Avenue
East Moline, IL 61244-9700
Phone: 800-776-4332
Fax: 800-577-4555
Web site: www.linguisystems.com

Maxwell's Manor: A Social Language Game
This game teaches students the social skills needed to get along with others, be more accepted by their peers, and be successful in the classroom. A dog named Maxwell leads the way as students practice positive social language skills. Six card decks offer practice in nonverbal communication, conversational skills, being a friend, practicing self-control, being polite, and following the rules.

Just for Me! Series: Concepts
Teaches basic concepts in four areas: spatial, attributes, quantity, and temporal. The activities include coloring, cutting, and creating an example of each concept.

Great Wave Software

5353 Scotts Valley Drive
Scotts Valley, CA 95066
Phone: 408-438-1990
Fax: 408-438-7171

Daisy Quest and Daisy Castle
Computer program for children 4 to 7 years old. Daisy Quest focuses mainly on the phonological awareness skill of rhyming while Daisy Castle targets sound blending and sound counting. It is a learning adventure where a wizard guides children through a medieval fantasy castle and on a quest.

Speech Bin
1965 Twenty-Fifth Avenue
Vero Beach, FL 32960
Phone: 800-4-SPEECH
Fax: 888-FAX 2 BIN
Web site: www.speechbin.com

Practicing Individual Concepts of Language (PICL)
Board game that reinforces skills in language content and use. Two to six players learn target structures in 30 categories including vocabulary, qualitative concepts, pronouns, plurals, and verb tenses.

Silly Sentences
Card games to learn: subject + verb agreement, S + V + O sentences, humor and absurdities, speech sound articulation, questioning and answering, and present progressive verbs. Includes three color-coded decks of 40 cards each.

Creatures and Critters: Barrier Games for Referential Communication
Language barrier games using dinosaurs and other "critters" to teach children how to take turns, listen for details, follow and give directions, and understand listeners' needs. Five decks of full-color cards, manual and data sheets included.

Speech and Language Handouts
Two-sided fact sheets to answer parents' questions about speech/language development at specific ages and regarding topics along several speech/language parameters such as developing pragmatic skills, fostering listening skills, increasing vocabulary, keeping a healthy voice, reading to your child, etc.

Super Duper Publications
P.O. Box 24997
Greenville, SC 29616-2497
Phone: 800-277-8737
Fax: 800-978-7379
Web site: www.superduperinc.com

Webber Classifying Cards
Large, colorful card pack in carrying tote with seven decks including animals, food, around the home, occupations, clothing, transportation, colors, shapes, and numbers.

Look Who's Listening
Ages 3 and up. Ten auditory games in one. Includes auditory skill card decks to target auditory discrimination, auditory memory, and auditory integration.

Students take turns listening carefully, following card directions, rolling the die, and placing tokens on game board.

Language Development Lessons for Early Childhood
Lessons in a reproducible book including three basic techniques for increasing oral responses from children in grades K–3: yes/no answers, choosing between two answers, and sentence completion. Each lesson has a student worksheet with three pages of lesson plans.

Paul H. Brookes Publishing Company
P.O. Box 10624
Baltimore, MD 21285-0624
Phone: 800-638-3775
Fax: 410-337-8539
Web site: www.brookespublishing.com

Road to the Code
Developmentally sequenced 11-week program designed to give kindergarten and first-grade students repeated opportunities to practice and enhance beginning reading and spelling abilities. Contains 44 lessons, each featuring three activities.

Miscellaneous

Burns, M. S., Griffin, P., & Snow, C. E. (1999). *Starting out right: A guide to promoting children's reading success.* Washington, DC: National Academy Press.

Clinician- and parent-friendly guide to the development of reading and spelling skills in young children. Includes specific activities to promote emergent and early literacy from infancy through mid-elementary school.

Griffith, L., & Olsen, M. A. (1992). Phonemic awareness helps beginning readers break the code. *The Reading Teacher, 45,* 516–523.

This article contains a list of books that involve sound play for young children.

Ratner, N. B., Parker, B., & Gardner, P. (1993). Joint book reading as a language scaffolding activity for communicatively impaired children. *Seminars in Speech and Language, 14,* 294–313.

At the end of this article, there is a lengthy appendix that contains the names of books that can be used to facilitate development in different areas of language. The books are listed according to the language structure that can be targeted (e.g., present progressive, past tense, copula, and so on). The selection of books is geared toward preschool children.

Torgesen, J. K., & Bryant, B. R. (1994). *Phonological awareness training for reading.* Austin, TX: Pro-Ed.

Focuses on training in four areas: sound blending, sound segmenting, reading, and spelling. Skills are taught in a sequential manner through a variety of games. It includes a detailed description (script) for each activity as well as precise instructions for implementation.

Yopp, H. K. (1992). Developing phonemic awareness in young children. *The Reading Teacher, 45,* 696–703.

This article focuses on the use of songs and melodies for training phonological awareness and provides specific suggestions.

Yopp, H. K., & Yopp, R. H. (2000). Supporting phonemic awareness in the classroom. *The Reading Teacher, 54,* 130–143.

This article provides sample phonological awareness activities appropriate for preschool, kindergarten, and first-grade classrooms within a developmental hierarchy of difficulty.

DEVELOPMENTAL LANGUAGE MILESTONES: BIRTH TO 5 YEARS

Age	Milestones
Receptive	
1 month	Startle response to loud or sudden sound Sound arrests activity; human voice usually has quieting effect Generally looks at speaker
2 months	Alert to surroundings Direct regard of speaker's face Visually and auditorily recognizes mother Beginning response to human voice Anticipates bottle
3 months	Localization: turns head when hears a voice; may not be in direction of sound Frightened by angry voices Excited when favorite toy is presented (increased kicking, arm waving) Resists adult who playfully tries to remove toy from grasp Aware of strange people and situations
4 months	Cessation of crying upon hearing human voice Reciprocal gaze (4–8 months) Responds to name by turning head (4–6 months)
5 months	Localization: horizontal plane to right or left depending on sound source Responds to "no" when said with inflection Distinguishes meaning of warning, anger, and/or friendly voices (changes in facial expression and/or body gestures) Responds to gesture stimulus with a gesture response (e.g., come up) Recognizes familiar environmental sounds (e.g., doorbell, running bath water) Reciprocal gaze (4–8 months) Responds to name by turning head (4–6 months)
6 months	Localization: two-step behavior, horizontal scan then vertical scan (6+ months) Begins to understand a few familiar words such as "mommy," "daddy," "bye-bye," and phrases such as "Daddy's coming," "Do you want the bottle?" (change in behavior) Responds to name by turning head (4–6 months) Reciprocal gaze (4–8 months)
8 months	Responds to "no" said without inflection Ceases activity when name is called Recognizes names of a few common objects Responds to scary faces; "stranger anxiety" Pats image in mirror Reciprocal gaze (4–8 months)

(continues)

Appendix 4-A (continued)

Age	Milestones
9 months	Gives toy in hand on request Follows simple verbal directions when accompanied by a gesture (e.g., Get ball, Open door) Uses gesture in response to a verbal "bye-bye" stimulus
11 months	Responds to music with body movements Says "bye-bye" on request
12 months	Responds to simple commands without an accompanying gesture (e.g., Get ball, Come here) Identifies one body part Selects object in a two-way object discrimination task Understands up to 10 words
14 months	Responds to verbal direction "Give me + object" without an accompanying gesture cue
15 months	Pats pictures in a book Points to common objects when named
16 months	Identifies object in a four-way object discrimination task
18 months	Completes one-stage commands containing two linguistic elements in a four-way object discrimination task (e.g., *Throw* the *car*) Responds to some question forms: What-doing?; Where-object? (18–24 months) Points to three body parts Attends to pictures and identifies one or more Understands up to 50 words
21–22 months	Understands some personal pronouns
24 months	Follows one-stage commands containing three linguistic elements in four-way object discrimination task (*Give me* the *car* and the *spoon*) Responds to some question forms: What-doing?; Where-object? (18–24 months) Points to at least four body parts Points to five or more pictures Understands prepositions "in" and "on"
3 years	Follows two-stage commands containing four linguistic elements in a four- to five-way object discrimination task (e.g., *Give me* the *spoon* and *push* the *car*) Understands some simple wh-questions Recognizes basic colors Understands concepts of same and different Categorizes items into basic groups (e.g., toys)
4 years	Understands 5,600 words Responds correctly to most questions about daily activities Uses word-order strategy to understand message Understands most wh-questions Understands concept of rhyming and alliteration

(continues)

Appendix 4-A (continued)

Age	Milestones
5 years	Understands 9,600 words
	Understands temporal concepts (e.g., before/after; yesterday/tomorrow)
	Follows three-stage commands with six linguistic elements in a four- to five-way object discrimination task (e.g., *Throw* the *shoe*, *give me* the *baby*, and *kiss* the *cup*) (4–5 years)
	Recognizes some alphabet letters
	Understands short paragraph-length material
5½ years	Understands 13,500 words
	Understands subordinating conjunctions "if," "because," "when," in most contexts
	Understands most simple and some complex sentence constructions; understands reversible passive sentences (e.g., The dog is chased by the cat).

Expressive

Age	Milestones
1 month	Produces undifferentiated crying and vegetative sounds (e.g., cough, sneeze, burp) (0–1½ months)
	Produces differentiated cry (e.g., pain, anger, hunger) (1½–2 months)
	Cries if adult removes pacifier
2 months	Gurgles and coos when played with
	Produces two or more syllables
	Produces vowels with consonant-like sounds (gu, nu) that are one second in duration
	Cries if adult removes toy
	Does not cry if adult removes pacifier
	Social smile (2–4 months)
3 months	Vocalizes in response to speech
	Produces pleasure sound (e.g., nasal "mmm")
	Coos without external stimulus
	Social smile (2–4 months)
4–5 months	Produces early babbling sounds; frequently heard consonants: p, b, d, h, w
	Produces some intonation during sound making
	Produces vocal play when playing with toys (e.g., squeals, growls, raspberries, trills: sounds produced in front of mouth)
	Produces approximately four different sounds
	Produces a displeasure sound
	Social smile (2–4 months)
	Takes turns with sounds
6 months	Produces reduplicative babbling
	Responds to name 50% of the time by vocalizing
7 months	Vocalizes upon seeing bottle
	Produces more consonant sounds such as t, n, d

(continues)

Appendix 4-A (continued)

Age	Milestones
8 months	Vocalizes to threaten, persuade Produces five or more consonants Shakes head for "no"
9 months	Produces "uh oh" exclamation
10 months	Produces nonreduplicative babbling Tries to imitate sounds
11 months	Produces three or more words or protowords Produces and imitates sounds and correct number of syllables
12 months	Produces five or more words (12–14 months) Produces true words during sound play Uses voice and gesture to get objects (12–14 months) Uses jargon; mixes words with jargon Most words are one and two syllables (12–18 months) Speech is 25% intelligible to the unfamiliar listener (12–18 months) Imitates animal noises (12–15 months)
14–16 months	Produces four to seven words Communicates using gesture + words/vocalizations Uses jargon and words in conversation Most words are one and two syllables (12–18 months) Speech is 25% intelligible to the unfamiliar listener
16–18 months	Produces 6 to 12 words Uses words to express wants and to communicate Imitates most words Uses jargon Most words are one and two syllables (12–18 months) Speech is 25% intelligible to the unfamiliar listener
18–24 months	Produces 10 to 20 words Begins to combine words into two-word utterances Uses jargon Names one picture in a book Imitates two- and three-word sentences Names some body parts Enjoys humming and singing
20–22 months	Produces 20 to 30 words Uses question intonation (e.g., Me go?)
22–24 months	Produces most vowels and the consonants: m, b, p, k, g, w, h, n, t, d Uses 50 to 200 words by 24 months 65% of speech is intelligible Uses two- and three-word combinations to express a variety of semantic relationships Names at least three of these objects: car, chair, box, key, fork Says "no" Uses some pronouns but not necessarily correctly

(continues)

Appendix 4-A (continued)

Age	Milestones
3 years	Produces 900 to 1,200 words Produces multiword utterances Routinely uses subject-verb-object forms Asks what, where, and who questions Overregularizes past tense (e.g., goed) Begins to use complex sentences
4 years	Produces 1,500 to 1,600 words Names primary colors; counts to five Uses complex sentence constructions more frequently Uses personal pronouns more accurately Uses negative and question forms correctly Uses conjunctions (e.g., and, but) correctly Uses relative pronouns (e.g., who)
5 years	Produces 2,100 to 2,200 words Has mastery of most syntactic rules and can converse easily Formulates short, well-structured stories Uses past and future verb tenses correctly
5½ years	Produces 2,300 words Continues to master irregular morphological and syntactic forms

APPENDIX 4-B

STAGES OF PLAY DEVELOPMENT

Age Range	Description and Examples
6–8 months	Nonmeaningful manipulation of objects (e.g., mouthing, banging, dropping).
8–12 months	Purposeful exploration of objects. Child shows knowledge of the appropriate use of objects (e.g., bangs toy drum; winds up jack-in-the-box).
12–18 months	Self-related symbolic play. Play behavior mimics daily activities involving only the child and uses only real objects (e.g., child picks up an empty cup and pretends to drink).
18–24 months	Other-related play. Child's symbolic play behaviors begin to involve other recipients of actions, but still uses only real objects (e.g., child uses his spoon to feed a doll). At the end of this period, the child begins to combine action sequences by (1) performing a single action on a variety of different recipients (e.g., feeding a doll, then feeding mommy, and finally feeding self) and (2) performing a series of actions on a single recipient (e.g., feeding a doll, putting it to bed, and kissing the doll goodnight).
24–30 months	Planned symbolic play. Play behaviors are characterized by (1) child uses one object to represent another (e.g., a stick for a spoon); (2) evidence of planning prior to engaging in the play sequence (e.g., child verbalizes or searches for props before initiating play schema); and (3) use of a doll or other object as the agent of the play action (e.g., the doll feeds the baby).
3–5 years	Socio-dramatic play. Pretend play sequences involve at least two or more children who (1) select a theme (e.g., going to the doctor); (2) assign roles (e.g., nurse, patient, doctor); and (3) use language appropriate to the different roles. (At this point, language begins to become an integral part of symbolic play).

Source: Adapted from Nicholich (1977) and Katz (2001).

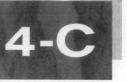

APPENDIX 4-C

DEVELOPMENTAL TOY LIST

Birth to 3 Months
rattles
stuffed animals
textured materials (i.e., smooth, scratchy, fuzzy, and soft objects) for rubbing on hands, arms, or feet
mobiles
plate designs (pictures or drawings on paper plates)

3 to 6 Months
rattles
stuffed animals
textured objects that the baby can hold onto
mobiles
mirrors
play gym
dolls
book of faces

6 to 9 Months
blocks
rings on a cone
stacking cubes
vinyl books

9 to 12 Months
ball
containers (to put objects in and out of)
small switches, dials, and slides
busy box
bath toys

12 to 15 Months
pull and push toys
ball
book
floating water toy
playdough
large boxes

15 to 18 Months
toy garage set
zoo set
telephone
bubbles

tape recorder and tapes
Styrofoam boats

18 to 24 Months
books
containers that open and close
puzzles
indoor slides
farm set
mini sandbox
pretend painter's set
push and pull toys
water toys

24 to 36 Months
tricycle/Big Wheels
interlocking block systems
puzzles
Legos
toy house
tea set
kitchen set
cars, trucks, road signs
windup plane

36 to 48 Months
tricycle
wagon
board games (Candy Land, Hi-Ho Cherry-O)
shape sorter
wooden beads for stringing
medical kit
swings, slides
sandbox
concentration picture matching game

48 to 60 Months
ball
magnetic letters
dominoes
alphabet game
musical instruments (drum, tambourine, castanets, bells)
playing cards
art materials

Source: Schwartz & Miller (1996).

CHAPTER 5

Intervention for Language in School-Age Children through Adolescence

Several advancements in oral language occur during this period. Children's vocabularies increase in size and in depth of word knowledge (e.g., shades of meaning: red versus crimson; steal versus embezzle). Utterance length increases by an average of one word per year until about nine years of age, when the length of oral language utterances begins to taper off. Syntactic growth is marked by the increased use of low-frequency structures (e.g., passive sentences) and an increased use of complex sentences (e.g., relative clause constructions). Another important advance in oral language development during this period occurs in the area of *metalinguistic awareness*. Metalinguistic awareness involves explicit knowledge and the ability to manipulate the structural aspects of language independently from the meaning conveyed by the message. Many language activities require this ability to focus on language as an entity unto itself, including the phonological awareness tasks of segmenting and blending speech sounds or syllables (metaphonology); provision of formal definitions; appreciation of humor, metaphors, idioms and other figurative language forms (metasemantics); and the ability to make grammatical judgments (metasyntax). Of particular significance is the refinement of children's phonological awareness knowledge to the level of phonemic awareness (i.e., ability to segment and blend *individual* speech sounds in words). It has been determined that phonemic awareness, and specifically the ability to segment words into phonemes, is the strongest predictor of early reading and writing skills (Torgesen, Wagner, & Rashotte, 1994; Wagner & Torgesen, 1987; Wagner, Torgesen, & Rashotte, 1994). Thus, there is a developmental relationship between oral language skills and literacy, and further, this relationship is reciprocal. That is, phonemic awareness skills promote early reading ability, and early reading skill furthers the development of phonemic awareness (see Chapter 4 for additional information regarding phonological awareness and its development).

In addition to progress in oral language, children acquire basic literacy skills during the elementary school years as they begin to receive formal instruction in reading and writing. In reading, they first learn to *decode* printed words (and nonwords) by making sound-letter correspondences (i.e., use the alphabetic principle). As children gain word recognition accuracy, their reading *fluency* improves and they begin to read connected text with greater ease and automaticity. By middle elementary school, the focus of reading and reading instruction shifts to *reading comprehension*, or reading for meaning. Thus, third to fourth grade represents a critical transition because "learning to read" becomes "reading to learn." See Table 5-1 for definitions and stages of reading development.

Third to fourth grade is also the point at which children's writing development progresses in both *spelling* and written *composition* (writing at the text level). By mid- to late elementary school, children reach the stage of conventional spelling and can correctly spell a large number of words automatically (see Chapter 4 for the developmental stages of spelling) and can spell with enough fluency to compose sentence-length text. Thus, they display advances in both the *processes* and *products* of writing. Writing processes include planning (prewriting), drafting, revising, and editing written text (Hayes & Flowers, 1987), in addition to forming letters and combining letters into words. Writing products are the output of writing processes, and occur at the word level (e.g., word selection, spelling), sentence level (e.g., grammatical complexity), and text level (e.g., cohesion, discourse type). Writing conventions such as punctuation and capitalization are also aspects of writing products.

TABLE 5-1
Definitions of Reading Processes and Stages of Reading Development

Terms	Definition/Description
Decoding	Word recognition processes that convert print into words
Comprehension	Processes by which printed language is understood and interpreted
Stages of Development	
Word-Level Reading	
Logographic/ Pre-alphabetic	Association of spoken words with environmental print without knowledge of letter-sound correspondences (alphabetic principle); e.g., logos, brand names, street signs
Transitional	Partial knowledge of sound-letter correspondences; e.g., use of initial or final letter to guess the word; sight-word vocabulary for highly familiar words
Alphabetic	Full knowledge of alphabetic principle; i.e., ability to decode both familiar and unfamiliar words
Orthographic	Use of spelling patterns to recognize and pronounce commonly recurring letter patterns as units (e.g., root words, prefixes, suffixes, syllables); builds large reading vocabulary
Automatic word recognition	Proficient and fluent reading of most words by sight
Text-Level Reading	
Phase 1, 4th–6th grade	Can read familiar content (i.e., narratives); consolidates reading fluency and speed; not reading to gain new information so can concentrate on the print
Phase 2, 7th–8th grade	Reads text to learn new information (reading becomes a source of ideas); reads materials that contain one point of view to obtain facts, concepts, how to do things, rather than for nuance; begins to bring prior knowledge/ experience to written text; growing importance of vocabulary/word meanings
Phase 3, 9th–12th grade	Can read multiple points of view, more than one set of facts, and can acquire new concepts and viewpoints from text (textbooks, reference works, mature fiction, newpapers, magazines)
Phase 4, 12th+ grade	Mature reading stage; reads for greater detail and completeness; reading becomes more qualitative, as reader constructs own knowledge using analysis, synthesis, and evaluation of information from different sources; reads at different levels to obtain desired level of detail, such as skimming versus studying text

The development of written text structures proceeds from the narrative form to various types of expository writing. Narrative discourse involves story or story-like forms in which the events occur in a chronological order. Expository texts present nonchronologically sequenced events and generally convey information that is novel to the reader. Examples of different types of expository text structures are description, comparison/contrast, and persuasion/ argumentation. See Table 5-2 for the differences between narrative and expository texts.

TABLE 5-2
Narrative and Expository Text Differences

Narrative	Expository
Purpose to entertain	Purpose to inform
Familiar schema content	Unfamiliar schema content
Consistent text structure	Variable text structures
Focus on character motivations, intentions, goals	Focus on factual information and abstract ideas
Often requires multiple perspective taking—understanding the points of view of different characters	Expected to take the perspective of the writer of the text
Can use pragmatic inferences, i.e., inference from similar experiences	Must use logical-deductive inferences
Connective words not critical—primarily *and, then, so*	Connective words critical—wide variety of connectives, e.g., *because, before, after, if-then, therefore*
Each text can stand alone	Expected to integrate information across texts
Can use top-down processing	Relies on bottom-up processing

Adapted from Westby, C. (1999). Assessing and facilitating text comprehension problems. In H. W. Catts & A. G. Kamhi (Eds.), *Language and reading disabilities* (pp. 154–219). Boston: Allyn & Bacon.

TREATMENT FOR SCHOOL-AGE CHILDREN

Intervention for school-age students revolves, in large part, around the relationship between oral language and literacy. Language therapy goals are programmed to address the demands and expectations of the educational curriculum. Therefore, service delivery is often accomplished through a variety of models including classroom consultation and collaboration, in addition to more traditional individual therapy sessions. Approaches to goal selection still may include a developmental focus, especially for younger school-age clients. However, strategies designed to facilitate functional performance are used increasingly with preteens and adolescents. Many approaches to language therapy have been designed for the wide variety of communication deficits exhibited by this population. Regardless of theoretical orientation, all intervention goals should be guided by well-designed studies that demonstrate their instructional effectiveness. See Stone, Silliman, Ehren, & Apel (2004) for a compendium of research-based practices in language instruction/intervention. Clinicians should remain sensitive to the cultural and linguistic background of each client throughout all stages of the intervention process.

Example Profiles

PROFILE 1

Willy is an 8-year, 3-month-old male child with normal nonverbal intelligence who demonstrates a moderate broad-based language impairment. His receptive language is notable for a reduced vocabulary, difficulty understanding complex sentence constructions, and difficulty monitoring the adequacy of a speaker's message. Willy's expressive output is characterized by use of simple sentences; omission of grammatical markers; overuse of nonspecific referents; and difficulty relating information in a logical, sequential order. Willy's teacher reports that he continues to experience significant problems with simple grade-level reading materials and word problems used in mathematical instruction (i.e., addition and subtraction).

Selection of therapy targets. Due to the broad-based nature of Willy's language impairment, multiple components of the linguistic system will be targeted for treatment. In the area of semantics, categorization skills will be taught to strengthen Willy's vocabulary and concept knowledge. Coordinating conjunctions will be targeted to facilitate his use of syntactically more complex utterances. Present, past, and future verb tense markers will be included in the therapy program because Willy consistently omits these morphological forms in his spontaneous speech (although he evidences understanding of these time concepts). In the area of pragmatics, therapy will focus on increasing Willy's ability to recognize inadequate messages from other speakers and implement appropriate repair strategies. Instruction also will be provided in the metalinguistic area of phonemic awareness (i.e., sound blending) to facilitate the acquisition of early reading skills (i.e., decoding). Finally, specific vocabulary will be taught to address Willy's curriculum goals in mathematics.

Sample Activities

1. Collect 15 picture cards depicting items in each of two semantic categories (e.g., clothes and birds) and 10 unrelated picture cards to serve as foils (e.g., book, car, horse). Provide the child with a simple definition of both target concepts. For example: A bird is an animal that has feathers, two legs, and two wings; clothes are things that you wear to cover your body, arms, and legs. Shuffle the cards and place them in a deck on the table. Instruct the child to sort the cards into two piles according to category (e.g., "Find all the birds"). As each card is sorted by the child, the clinician explains why the card belongs in either the birds or clothes category (e.g., "It's a bird because it has wings"). For unrelated foils, the clinician explains why the item should be excluded from the two primary categories (e.g., "It doesn't have feathers, and you can't wear it").

   Note: Categorization activity can be made conceptually more sophisticated by modifying the task according to the following progression:

   a. Sort objects by function (e.g., things we eat, things we use as furniture, things we play with, things we use in a hospital).

b. Sort objects according to semantic relationships (e.g., What goes together? bat and ball, milk and cookies, hammer and nail).

c. Sort objects by dimensions or attributes such as size, shape, color, or texture (e.g., find all the ones that are big versus little, round versus square).

d. Sort objects within a single category according to whether they are central or peripheral instances of the concept (e.g., robin versus emu, shirt versus ascot, respectively).

2. Develop a list of 20 sentences, each of which contains the coordinating conjunction "and," "or," or "but." Print each sentence on a long strip of paper (approximately 2 inches by 11 inches) with the conjunction word represented by a blank line. Write each of the three conjunction words on small triangular pieces of paper. Following are example sentences:

The waitress said, "You can order salad, rice, _____ a potato with your meal."

Ed likes basketball, _____ he likes baseball more.

Which one do you want: soda, hot chocolate, _____ lemonade?

For breakfast, you can have an omelette _____ scrambled eggs.

John _____ Billy went to the movies together.

For lunch, Dion had a hamburger _____ french fries.

Mary had to decide whether to go to New York by train _____ plane.

The dentist drills _____ fills cavities in teeth.

Rita wants to go to the movies _____ she has no money.

Bill wants to be a lifeguard _____ he cannot swim that well.

We ate all the donuts _____ one.

Place sentence strips facedown in a pile in the center of the table. Position the conjunction triangles in a row in front of the child. Define the conjunctions by explaining when each is used:

"And" is used to connect things together.

"Or" is used to indicate a choice of one thing over others.

"But" is used to mean "except," "with the exception of," or "on the other hand."

Instruct the child to turn over one sentence strip. The clinician reads the sentence aloud and instructs the child to choose the triangle that best finishes the sentence and place it on the blank line. The clinician then reads the completed sentence aloud and instructs the child to imitate the model.

Task difficulty can be increased by eliminating the conjunction triangles, thereby changing the multiple-choice format to a spontaneous generation task.

3. Print 25 third-person singular active sentences on separate index cards. Develop three cue cards for present progressive, past, and future verb tenses in the following manner:

Yesterday	Right Now	Tomorrow
-ed	is _____ ing	will

Place the cue cards in a row on the table approximately three inches apart in the order as illustrated. Place the deck of sentence cards on the table. Instruct the child to read each of the cue words aloud or to repeat each word following the clinician's model. Review the three verb tense forms with the child. Explain as follows:

a. When something has already occurred and is no longer happening, we attach "-ed" to the end of the action word. For example, you would say "Yesterday, the boy order*ed* the pizza."

b. When something is happening right now, we say "is" before the action word and attach "-ing" to the end of the action word. For example, you would say "The boy *is* order*ing* the pizza."

c. When something has not yet happened but will happen in the future, we say the word "will" before the action word. For example, you would say "Tomorrow, the boy *will* order the pizza."

Instruct the child to select the top card from the sentence deck and to inflect the sentence correctly as the clinician points to each of the cue cards. Example sentences include the following:

The girl talks on the phone.

Jose plays his guitar.

Sam walks to school.

The dog chases the cat.

Daddy paints the house.

The teacher points to the chalkboard.

Jamie washes her hair.

Maria wishes for a puppy.

Joey kicks the football.

Mom picks apples from the trees.

Lee cheers for his team.

Monique laughs at the funny clown.

Tim practices his spelling words.

Grandma cooks dinner for the family.

The dog barks at the mailman.

As the child begins to master the past and future tense markers, the cue cards can be modified to include other lexical items that denote these concepts (e.g., last week, when I grow, next summer, two days ago).

4. Prepare a list of 20 directions for completing a variety of simple tasks and gather the necessary props. Some directions should contain ambiguous, incomplete, unintelligible, or absurd information, while others are clearly worded. Examples may include the following:

Direction	*Context*
Give me the red block.	There are no red blocks on the table.

Direction	*Context*
Give me the pencil with the eraser.	All three pencils on the table have erasers.
Give me the #$%$#% un(intelligible).	There are three different objects on the table.
Place the pencil next to the book.	There is a book and a pencil on the table.
Put the money in the brown wallet.	There are three wallets on the table, none of which are brown.
Give me the ingredients for making pizza: dough, sauce, cheese, picture frame.	All these objects are on the table.
Cut a big hole in the white piece of paper.	There are red and white pieces of paper on the table, along with scissors and tape.
Give me three (mumble rest of message).	There are three paper clips, six pencils, and five pennies on the table.

Explain that the child will be asked to carry out directions using props and that some of the messages will be inadequate and require more information. This activity focuses on two strategies for obtaining this additional information: (a) asking for repetition of the direction (e.g., "Huh?" or "What did you say?") and (b) requesting clarification of the message (e.g., "Which book?" or "What color?"). Instruct the child to listen to the clinician's messages and think carefully about what is being said. After each direction is presented, instruct the child to identify whether the message was "OK" or inadequate. If the direction is identified as unclear, instruct the child to request a repair using one of the two target strategies. The clinician then revises the original message according to the type of repair requested and the child performs the task. If the child does not recognize the need for repair, prompt with one or more of the following: "Is that clear?"; "Did I say that right?"; or "Do you get it?"

5. Print a list of 25 monosyllabic words with initial continuant sounds on index cards and segment each word into phonemes (see following examples). Draw a game board of a bridge that consists of 20 blank spaces and draw a pot of gold at the end of the bridge. Place a small wrapped "prize" on the pot of gold. Shuffle the cards and place them facedown in a pile in the center of the board. Obtain a game piece that can be moved from space to space on the board and place it at the footpath to the bridge. Explain to the child that, in this game, there is a troll who lives under the bridge and who talks in a very funny way; he says all his words one sound at a time (Lundberg, Olofsson, & Wall, 1980). Tell the child that he has to figure out the words and say them to move his game piece to the end of the bridge and find the hidden prize. Instruct the child to pick up the top card and give it to the clinician. The clinician plays the role of the troll and produces the segmented word, phoneme

by phoneme. (Always produce the actual sound rather than the alphabet letter name.) The child blends the sounds together and "guesses" the troll's message. Following a correct guess, the clinician repeats both the segmented word and the "whole" word. The child is then permitted to move the game piece one space on the board. Following are some sample words:

f—or—k

s—u—n

z—oo—m

v—o—te

m—a—p

s—ou—p

v—e—s—t

n—o—se

f—u—ll

m—a—tch

Note: There are several issues regarding difficulty level that require consideration in programming for phonological awareness skills. Three are presented as follows, each organized in a progression from least to most difficult.

a. *Phonological awareness skills* (Adams, Foorman, Lundberg, & Beeler, 1998; Blachman, Ball, Black, & Tangel, 2000; Swank & Catts, 1994; Troia, Roth, & Graham, 1998; van Kleeck & Schuele, 1987)
   1) Rhyming/alliteration
   2) Blending
   3) Segmenting
      a) Categorization (e.g., Which one begins with a different sound: "feet" "five" "soup" "fat"?)
      b) Deletion (e.g., Say "trip" without the /t/)
      c) Substitution (e.g., Replace the /m/ in "man" with /f/)
      d) Manipulation (e.g., Say the word "stop." Now move the /s/ to the end of the word and say it again).

b. *Task mode*
   1) Matching (e.g., Show me the one that rhymes with "hat")
   2) Elimination (e.g., Show me the one that doesn't rhyme with the other two words)
   3) Judgment (e.g., Do "hat" and "bat" rhyme?)
   4) Production (e.g., Tell me a word that rhymes with "hat")

c. *Stimuli level for segmenting/blending*
   1) Sentences into words
   2) Words into syllables (compound words such as "blackboard" are easier than noncompound words because each syllable is a common word)
   3) Syllables into phonemes (polysyllabic words and/or consonant clusters increase task difficulty)

d. *Phoneme class for segmenting/blending*
1) Continuant sounds such as fricatives and nasals are easier than non-continuant sounds such as stops (continuants are longer in duration and acoustically more discrete; they can be produced in isolation and emphasized by overarticulation)

6. Make two lists of the following words/phrases on separate poster boards and attach to wall:

Addition Words	Subtraction Words
in all	how many more
more	how many are left
altogether	difference
sum	less
total	fewer

Write 10 to 20 simple word problems, half of which require addition and half subtraction, on 3-by-5 inch index cards. Obtain two containers into which the cards can be sorted. Label one container with a large (+) sign; label the other container with a large (−) sign. Provide a highlighter and game board. Explain to the child that the words on the two wall charts are clues for solving math word problems. Review each clue word on the addition chart and remind the child that these are "adding" words; then review each clue word on the subtraction chart and remind the child that these are "take away" words. Shuffle the index cards and place them facedown in a pile on the table. Explain that the top card should be turned over and read aloud. Instruct the child to highlight any clue words that are recognized from the wall charts and state whether the problem requires addition or subtraction. Then have the child place the index card in the correct container. Repeat this procedure for all cards in the deck.

Example Addition Problems

a. Juan has 3 jelly beans and Eddie gives him 3 more. How many does Juan have altogether?
b. Ilana has 5 pencils on the desk and Eli put 4 more on the desk. What's the total number of pencils on the desk?
c. There were 7 birds sitting on a fence. Five more birds joined them. How many birds are there in all?
d. Mary put 6 blue beads on a string. Kayla put 5 red beads on the string. What is the total number of beads on the string?
e. Ali drove 8 blocks to Steve's house and then both boys drove 9 blocks to the store. Find the sum of the blocks they drove.

Example Subtraction Problems

a. Kate has 10 stickers and Shawna takes 4. How many are left?
b. John has 5 green crayons and Daron has 9 yellow crayons. How many more yellow crayons are there?
c. Marsha put 12 cards in a pile and Kim put 7 in another pile. What's the difference between the two piles?

d. Kathy has 9 books and Stacy has 6 fewer books. How many books does Stacy have?

e. Jean drank 14 cups of water. Nan drank 8 cups of water. How much less water did Nan drink?

Note: This activity can be extended to computation using a game board with spaces color coded for plus and minus. The child rolls the dice and moves a game piece the appropriate number of spaces. If the piece lands on an "addition" space, instruct the child to remove a card from the (+) container and solve the problem. Follow this same procedure for subtraction.

PROFILE 2

Vivian is a 9-year, 1-month-old female child with normal nonverbal intelligence who has been diagnosed with a learning disability. She demonstrates a significant reading deficit characterized by the inability to decode written words. Weaknesses in the area of receptive language include comprehension of connected oral text such as stories. Expressively, Vivian experiences notable difficulty with assignments that require formulating definitions for vocabulary known to be within her receptive repertoire. According to the classroom teacher, these difficulties are exacerbated by Vivian's inability to sustain focused attention. As a consequence, her academic performance across the entire fourth-grade curriculum is adversely affected.

Selection of therapy targets. Vivian's profile of oral language and literacy deficits warrants intervention in a variety of areas necessary to effectively learn from teacher discourse and textbook information. In the area of semantics, the structure and elements of formal definitions will be targeted to strengthen Vivian's network of higher-order semantic knowledge. The framework of narrative structure will be taught to promote recall, comprehension, and production of oral and written text-level material often incorporated into fourth-grade curricula. Finally, intervention will target the phonemic awareness skill of sound segmentation in conjunction with letter-sound correspondence training (alphabetic principle) to improve Vivian's reading decoding ability.

Sample Activities

1. Create a "Jeopardy" game, including stimulus cards, a buzzer, and play money. Use curriculum materials (e.g., textbooks, homework assignments) to develop a list of 10 to 15 familiar vocabulary words in three or four different semantic categories (see following sample list with definitions).

Science

a. microscope: A *microscope* is an *instrument* that makes *small objects look bigger.*

b. solar system: A *solar system* is a *group of planets* that *revolve around a sun.*

c. volcano: A *volcano* is a *mountain* that *explodes with lava and ash.*

Math

a. number: A *number* is a *symbol* that *shows how many.*

b. fraction: A *fraction* is a *number* that *compares small pieces or parts to the whole.*

c. calculator: A *calculator* is a *machine* that *does arithmetic.*

English/Language Arts

a. paragraph: A *paragraph* is *two or more sentences* about *a single idea.*

b. topic sentence: A *topic sentence* is a *statement* that *gives the main idea of a paragraph.*

c. comma: A *comma* is a *mark* that *shows a small break between parts of a sentence.*

Miscellaneous

a. bicycle: A *bicycle* is a *vehicle* that has *two wheels.*

b. dog: A *dog* is an *animal* that *barks.*

c. house: A *house* is a *building* that *people live in.*

For each category, print the words on the face of index cards and write increasing dollar values on the back (e.g., $100, $200, $300). Attach the cards to a wall in category columns with the dollar amounts facing out. Construct a wall chart that shows the three key elements of a formal definition, i.e., the word, the superordinate category name, and a relevant function/attribute of the referent, in a style that the child can understand.

Explain to the child that this activity is a Jeopardy game, in which the child will select a category and dollar level. The clinician will read the vocabulary item and the child must sound the buzzer and respond using the formal definition structure. Correct responses receive the play money in the amount listed on the back of the card; incorrect responses result in the subtraction of specified dollar amounts from the total.

Teach the child that a definition explains the meaning of a word by (a) stating the word, (b) identifying the larger category it belongs to, and (c) describing how it looks or what it does. Encourage the child to use the wall chart as a visual cue to remember all three components. For example:

Child: I'll take "living things" for $200, please.

Clinician: Spider.

Child: A *spider* is a *bug* that has *eight legs.*

Clinician: Great definition. You win $200. What category do you want next?

Note: The activity works particularly well in a small group setting.

2. Write or identify a short story that contains at least one episode. The story should clearly illustrate the following components:

Setting: Information regarding characters and physical, social, and/or temporal environment

Problem: Occurrence that influences the character(s) to act; precipitating event

Actions: The character's overt attempt to solve the problem

Resolution: The character's success or failure in solving the problem and resultant thoughts or feelings

See the following sample story:

The Cookie Jar Incident

Once there was a stubborn young lady named Leigh-Anne who lived in New York City. Late one afternoon, she was really hungry and wanted a chocolate chip cookie. She knew that she wasn't allowed to eat sweets before dinner, but that didn't stop Leigh-Anne. She sneaked into the kitchen, stood on her tiptoes, and reached for the cookie jar. As she grabbed it, the jar fell on the floor and broke into a thousand pieces. As she heard her mother's footsteps, Leigh-Anne felt guilty about doing something she wasn't supposed to do.

Setting
Character: Leigh-Anne
Environment: New York City
              late afternoon

Problem
hungry
no cookies before dinner

Actions
sneaked
stood
reached
grabbed

Resolution
jar broke
felt guilty

Obtain a large poster board and small self-stick notes. Draw a story map like the one in Figure 5-1. Explain that this map will help the child identify the main parts of a story. Using the definitions provided previously, teach the child each of the four story parts and where they belong on the map. Instruct the child to listen as the clinician reads the story aloud. Upon completion, ask the child to identify the components of each story part on the map, beginning with the setting and ending with the resolution. The clinician writes each of the child's responses on a self-stick note and has the child place it on the map in the correct box. Then jointly retell the story using the map as a visual guide.

Note: The difficulty level of this activity can be adjusted in a variety of ways. To branch down to an easier level, the response mode can be a multiple-choice format, in which the child's task is to select the appropriate piece of

FIGURE 5-1
Story Map

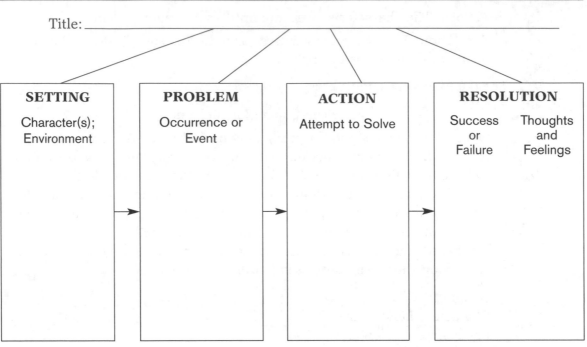

Title: _____

SETTING	PROBLEM	ACTION	RESOLUTION
Character(s); Environment	Occurrence or Event	Attempt to Solve	Success or Failure Thoughts and Feelings

Source: Adapted from Thomas (1971).

story information from an array of completed self-stick notes. To branch upward, the clinician can increase the number of episodes in a given story.

3. Make a list of 30 two- and three-phoneme words that are picturable and within the child's expressive vocabulary repertoire. To incorporate exposure to the alphabetic principle, choose words with CV, VC, or CVC patterns. Avoid words that involve digraphs (e.g., h*ea*t; s*oa*p; th*ie*f) and silent vowels (e.g., gat*e*; bon*e*; sam*e*). Following is an illustrative word list:

top	cab	up
cup	bus	in
sad	sit	hi
mat	tag	go
jam	red	on
van	mop	no
fog	nut	ma
dad	nap	me
dot	pot	us
bag	pig	he

Attach the picture for each word to a "playing card." Gather six small blocks and individual alphabet letters (can be written, plastic, or cut from foam).

Tell the child that this game involves breaking words down into smaller parts. Explain that the point of the game is to figure out which words have more sounds. The cards are dealt into two equal decks. The clinician and child simultaneously turn over the top card from each deck (clinician = Deck 1; child = Deck 2). The clinician verbally segments the word from Deck 1 and lines up one block for each sound. Instruct the child to do the same for the card from Deck 2. Tell the child to identify which of the two words has more sounds. The clinician then adds the appropriate alphabet letters on top of the blocks and sounds out that word again. If the child correctly chose the word with the most sounds, the child wins both cards and sets them aside. If the choice was incorrect, the clinician wins both cards. Repeat this sequence until all cards from both decks have been played. (If the two words have the same number of sounds, each player wins one card). The player with the most cards at the end of the game is the winner.

Note: The difficulty level of the activity can be increased or decreased according to the phonological awareness hierarchy on page 175.

Helpful Hints

1. Whenever possible, conduct phonological awareness activities in a group setting to encourage interaction and avoid a sense of drill/rote memorization. In addition, a group setting is beneficial because it encourages interaction and participation.

2. Visualization is an effective strategy for some children to enhance semantic categories. For example, a child might be instructed as follows: "Close your eyes and imagine that you are in (*a particular location*) (e.g., classroom, supermarket). Look all around and tell me all the things you see."

3. A referential communication task is a good instructional mechanism for facilitating the development of a variety of pragmatic skills. It involves a speaker who is responsible for describing something (e.g., objects, shapes) so that a listener can identify the correct object or replicate the pattern. This task can be manipulated in numerous ways to focus on communicative intentions, perspective taking, and conversational discourse abilities. (See Spekman & Roth, 1984, for specific intervention suggestions.)

4. Another aspect of metalinguistic skills that can be trained is humor. The appreciation of humor requires the ability to detect ambiguity. There is a developmental progression that the clinician can keep in mind when programming targets in this area.

Nonverbal (up to 6 years): Recognition of the absurdity or incongruity in a situation

> *Example:* A cartoon picture of a rabbit dressed in a velvet smoking jacket, holding a pipe

Phonological (6 to 9 years): A sound sequence can be interpreted in more than one way

> *Example:* Why was the doctor upset? He was out of patience (patients).

Lexical (9 to 12 years): A word has more than one meaning

> *Example:* Why didn't the skeleton cross the road? It didn't have the guts.

Syntactic (13+ years): Words in a sentence can be grouped differently

Example: What is the difference between a running dog and a running man? The man wears trousers and the dog pants.

Metalinguistic: Develops throughout the age range depending on the complexity of the "meta" twist

Example: Where does Thursday come before Wednesday? In the dictionary.

5. Whenever appropriate, supplement an activity with the provision of written word or sound cues as an indirect means of facilitating word recognition skills in children who are beginning readers.

6. The information-giving aspect of counseling may involve educating parents about the purpose and procedures of the IEP process so that they can effectively participate in decision making for appropriate educational placements and services.

7. An important aspect of counseling with this age group often is apprising the family of the potential impact of oral language disorders on the acquisition of early reading and writing skills.

8. Story frames can facilitate a child's generation of a well-formed story. See the following example:

Once upon a time _____

Suddenly _____

Luckily _____

In the end _____

INTERVENTION WITH ADOLESCENTS (10 TO 18 YEARS)

Adolescence is the developmental period during which youngsters (1) develop a stable identity, (2) acquire independence from family, (3) develop career plans, and (4) develop moral and ethical values consistent with those of society (Erikson, 1968). There are three main stages of adolescence, and the intervention goals for each stage differ slightly. In early adolescence (10 to 14), the primary focus is on developing communication skills for academic and personal-social purposes. The goals for midadolescence (14 to 16) involve facilitation of communication skills for academic, personal-social, and vocational aims. By late adolescence (16 to 20), language intervention is concentrated on developing communication skills for personal-social and career purposes.

In the adolescent period, communication skills are refined and higher-order language abilities undergo significant development as the child's linguistic system reaches the adult form. Significant growth occurs in the metalinguistic area of nonliteral or figurative uses of language, including idioms, metaphors, proverbs, and humor. These are considered higher-order language forms because they require the ability to go beyond the conventional meaning of language for correct interpretation or use. Figurative language forms increasingly appear in both oral and written language materials beginning in middle and upper elementary school years. In fact by eighth grade, at least 20% of teacher talk and written text consist of nonliteral uses of language (Nippold, 1991).

During adolescence, continued development also occurs in conversational maturity, utterance length, comprehension/production of complex sentences and linguistic cohesion devices, and low-frequency syntactic structures (language forms that occur in literate texts, spoken and written, with greater frequency than in oral conversational speech such as expanded noun phrases and expanded verb phrases). Semantic knowledge also undergoes further growth both with respect to vocabulary size and depth of word knowledge. Word knowledge reflects an increased understanding of multiple meaning words (e.g., block, cold) and the literate lexicon (words that commonly occur in scholarly contexts such as textbooks, lectures, and seminars).

In addition to oral language, students demonstrate advances in the written language domain as they become mature readers and skilled writers/authors by the end of this developmental period. In both reading and writing, there is a shift in focus from content facts (simple propositions conveyed by a text, such as information about a character in a story or facts about mammals) to content schema (macrostructures that represent the organization of a text structure, such as a story, compare/contrast essay). Children are reading longer and more complicated texts (see Table 5-1, page 169 for stages of reading development) and can increasingly concentrate on obtaining/synthesizing new information from a variety of print materials (i.e., textbooks, essays, poems, reference sources). Their written expression shows steady gains in the use of planning and organizational strategies, ability to reflect on and revise/edit initial drafts for grammar, punctuation, and word choice, and the ability to meet the organizational and structural demands of different discourse genres. See Table 5-3 for different types of text structure and their characteristics.

A final area of importance during this developmental period is *metacognitive/ executive functioning*. Metacognitive abilities involve an awareness of one's own problem-solving abilities and include self-regulation behaviors that are used to guide, monitor, and direct the success of one's performance (Barkley, 1996; Borkowski & Burke, 1996). They include planning, attending selectively to certain aspects of a situation, shifting attention as necessary, inhibition of behavioral impulses, setting goals, and organizing one's behavior and work. Children show marked advances in metacognitive functioning beginning at about fourth grade, and as a result, they gradually become more strategic learners. Metacognition is considered a higher-order ability area because these "meta" strategies must be invoked from the outset of a task and require task analysis and a great deal of planning. Knowledge of metacognitive development and deficits is necessary for SLPs because these skills and strategies are largely mediated through language. Students engage in "self-talk" throughout the school day about the nature of a task/assignment, how and why they are doing it, the effectiveness of their strategies, and ways to change their behaviors and strategies, etc.

At least two potential problems may be encountered when working with adolescents: (1) resistance to dependent relationships with adults because they

TABLE 5-3
Expository Text Types and Characteristics

Text Type	Function	Key Words
Descriptive	Does the text tell me what something is?	No key words
Sequence/procedural	Does the text tell me how to do or make something?	first . . . next . . . then; second . . . third . . . following this step; finally
Cause/effect	Does the text give reasons for why something is/happens?	because, since, then, therefore, for this reason, results, effects, consequently, so, in order, thus, then
Problem/solution	Does the text state a problem and offer solutions to the problem?	a problem is; a solution is
Comparison/contrast	Is the text showing how two things are the same or different?	different, same, alike, similar, although, however, on the other hand, but, yet, still, rather than

Adapted from Westby, C. (1999). Assessing and facilitating text comprehension problems. In H. W. Catts & A. G. Kamhi (Eds.), *Language and reading disabilities* (pp. 154–219). Boston: Allyn and Bacon.

are striving to achieve and demonstrate their own independence and (2) rejection of the idea of being flawed or different in any way from their peer group. For intervention to be successful with the adolescent, the teen has to be a fully cooperative partner in the therapy program. The teen should be consulted regarding the selection of specific therapy objectives, and the clinician must clearly explain the rationale for each target behavior. This allows the student to take ownership of the problem, take primary responsibility for achieving the goals, and recognize that it is the student who will lose out if follow-through does not occur.

Example Profiles

PROFILE 1

Pedro is a 12-year, 6-month-old male who presents with a moderate language learning disability. He demonstrates particular difficulty with higher-order language skills. Specifically, Pedro performs poorly on confrontational naming tasks as well as tasks that require the comprehension of figurative language forms. His oral and written narratives omit essential story information and lack a logical sequence. According to direct observation and teacher report, Pedro exhibits difficulty initiating and maintaining conversational exchanges, as evidenced by his tendency to talk about inappropriate topics and interrupt ongoing conversations. Although some minor grammatical errors were observed during timed tasks, comprehension and production of syntax and morphology were noted to be relative strengths.

Selection of therapy targets. Based on Pedro's overall profile, the areas to be targeted involve semantics as well as narrative and conversational discourse. With respect to semantics, idioms were selected because they are among the earliest developing forms of figurative language. In addition, word finding was chosen to accommodate the increasing demand at the middle school level for accurate retrieval of specific vocabulary words in different academic subject areas. Narrative discourse was targeted to improve Pedro's knowledge of the organization of extended text because text is the primary vehicle for transmitting academic knowledge. The area of conversational initiation was selected to address the negative effects/perceptions that Pedro's verbal interaction style has on peers and adults in his environment.

Sample Activities

1. Select five idioms and write three different short story contexts for each. For each story, include three written alternative response choices (see following examples). Duplicate these materials for the client. Define an idiom for the child by explaining that idioms are expressions in which a new meaning is given to a group of words that already has a meaning. For example, the expression "over the hill" can be interpreted literally *or* as an idiom meaning that someone is old. Explain that the clinician will be reading stories containing idioms and that the client will be asked to select the most appropriate meaning from three choices. Recite the first short story aloud as the client reads along silently. Depending on the client's skill level, instruct him or her to listen to or read the choices and select the response that best fits the context of the story. After the three stories for a particular idiom have been successfully completed, ask the client to brainstorm at least one personal experience to which the specific idiom could have been applied. Examples include the following:

   Kick up our heels:

   John made the football team. He was so happy and excited. He wanted to kick up his heels.

   Does this mean? He wanted to celebrate.
                   He kicked his feet in the air.
                   He was upset.

   Hannah sat in her classroom and waited for the announcement. The principal finally came on the public-address system and said: "Students, the winner of the school spelling contest is Hannah Smith. Congratulations!" Hannah felt like kicking up her heels.

   Does this mean? She took off her shoe.
                   She was thrilled.
                   She was very disappointed.

   Larry wanted to get an A in math. He was a good math student but always got Bs. The final exam was last week and he studied harder than ever.

When the mail came, Larry ran to see his report card. He opened it up, saw an A next to math, and felt like kicking up his heels.

Does this mean? He did not do well in math.
He lifted his legs in the air.
He wanted to cheer.

Shake a leg:

Sue forgot to set her alarm for the swim meet. Her mom woke her up and said, "We have only 10 minutes to get to the pool, so shake a leg."

Does this mean? Sue has to hurry.
Sue's leg is hurting.
Sue's mom shook her leg.

Bobby wanted to win the bicycle race. He had trained hard for it all summer. But now he was in fourth place with just one mile to go. He told himself that he'd better shake a leg if he wanted to win.

Does this mean? Bobby has to slow down.
Bobby has to ride faster.
Bobby does not want to win.

Mom and Dad are going out to dinner for their anniversary. It's time to go, but Dad is still shaving. Mom says, "Honey, shake a leg; our reservations are in 20 minutes."

Does this mean? They will probably be early.
Dad should move his leg while shaving.
Dad should hurry up.

A fish out of water:

Mariah was very excited about the school dance. She wanted to look really cool. She decided to wear her new faded blue jeans and her favorite flannel shirt. When she walked into the gym, all of the girls were wearing party dresses. Mariah felt like a fish out of water.

Does this mean? Mariah doesn't like to swim.
Mariah was not wet.
Mariah felt different from everyone else.

Joan was going to sleep-away camp for the first time. She kissed her parents good-bye after checking in. When she walked into her cabin, all the other girls seemed to know each other. They laughed and talked like old friends. Joan felt like a fish out of water.

Does this mean? Joan felt like she didn't fit in the group.
Joan wanted to go swimming.
Joan likes to go fishing at the lake.

Jason just moved to the city and was starting his senior year in high school. Jason rode his bike on the first day of school. As he entered the parking lot, he noticed that all the seniors were driving cars. Jason felt like a fish out of water.

Does this mean? He felt like he couldn't breathe.

He felt like he didn't belong.

He felt very happy.

All thumbs:

Jack was helping his dad build a birdhouse in the maple tree. Jack hammered the nail into the wood but kept missing it. His dad said, "Son, you're all thumbs today."

Does this mean? Jack was clumsy.

All of Jack's fingers look like thumbs.

Jack put his thumb on the nail.

Kate and Nika decided to bake some chocolate chip cookies. Nika took the eggs out of the refrigerator and dropped one on the floor. Then she spilled the flour all over the table and knocked over the milk. She said to Kate, "I guess I'm all thumbs."

Does this mean? Nika was finished with the cookies.

Nika was klutzy.

Nika's thumbs were all sticky.

The period bell rang and David raced to his locker to get his English book before the next class. He held his books in one hand and turned the combination, but the lock wouldn't open. He tried again and dropped all his books onto the floor. He said to himself, "I'm all thumbs."

Does this mean? David wished that all his fingers were thumbs.

David's locker opened easily.

David was clumsy.

2. Develop a list of 20 names of objects or people. Write a synonym, category name, or other semantic cue for each word on an index card. In addition, write the initial sound (not letter) of each word on another set of index cards. Examples include the following:

Word	*Semantic Cue*	*Phonological Cue*
cook	chef	/k/
gloves	mittens	/g/
jacket	coat	/dʒ/
comb	brush	/k/
tissues	Kleenex	/t/
van	vehicle	/v/
pencil	writing utensil	/p/
shoe	sneakers	/ʃ/
lamp	light	/l/
soda	Coke	/s/
hat	cap	/h/
pocketbook	purse	/p/
painting	picture	/p/
carpet	rug	/k/
car	automobile	/k/

Word	*Semantic Cue*	*Phonological Cue*
notebook	binder	/n/
jeans	clothing	/dʒ/
backpack	knapsack	/b/
sailboat	kind of boat	/s/
dollar	money	/d/

Explain that the client will be asked to guess a specific word based on two clues provided by the clinician. Further explain that the two clues represent different strategies that the client can use when trying to retrieve specific vocabulary words. Instruct the client to use the first clue to create a visual image of the object and the second clue to identify what the mystery word sounds like. For example, the clinician says, "I'm thinking of a word. It's like a 'chef' and starts with /k/." Encourage the child to refrain from responding quickly, but rather to pause reflectively and think about the cues. After each item, instruct the client to produce the target word in a sentence that describes its function.

3. Write the main elements of a story on separate index cards along with short definitions of each part (Stein & Glenn, 1979). For example:

Setting: The main characters in the story (who the story is about) and where the story takes place

Problem: The main event or problem that the main character faces

Response: The way that the main character feels about the problem

Attempt: What the main character actually does to try to solve the problem or achieve the goal

Outcome: What happens at the end of the story; whether or not the character achieves the goal

Reaction: How the main character feels about the outcome (success or failure at attaining the goal)

In addition, write one or more question cues for each of the main story parts on separate index cards. For example:

Setting: Who is the story about?
Where does the story take place?

Problem: What happened to the main character?
What caused the main character to act?

Response: How does the main character feel about the problem?

Attempt: What does the main character do to solve the problem?

Outcome: What happens at the end of the story?
Does the main character achieve the goal?

Reaction: How does the main character feel at the end of the story?

First, review the story part definition cards with the client. Then explain that the clinician will tell a short story aloud as the client follows the written text.

EXAMPLE STORY

Once upon a time, there was a 12-year-old boy named Jacob who lived in a town called Wallston. He lived about one mile from school and rode his bike there every day. Last week for his birthday, his parents gave him a new bike, the one he'd been asking for since June. On Wednesday morning, Jacob grabbed his backpack and headed for school. As he approached the front gate, he immediately noticed that his new bike was gone. Jacob thought to himself, "Oh no! I forgot to chain the bike last night. Somebody probably stole it. Mom will ground me for a month. I promised to take care of it." Jacob thought all day about what to do. After school, he went to the police station and spoke to one of the officers. The policeman suggested that Jacob put up signs in lots of places such as the police station, the post office, and in store windows. The signs should include Jacob's name, telephone number, and a description of the bike. So Jacob made the signs, put them up all over town, and walked home to wait by the telephone. At about 5:30 P.M., it rang and Jacob jumped up to answer it.

A woman named Mrs. Ramirez said, "I just saw a bike at the grocery story that matches the description on the signs." Jacob thanked the lady and ran to the market as fast as he could. Sure enough, it *was* his bike. His initials were on the bottom of the seat just as he had scratched them on. Jacob was so happy and relieved. As he rode home, he promised himself that he would never leave his bike unlocked again.

After the story is completed, instruct the client to answer the cue card questions either verbally or in writing. Review and discuss each answer with the client to ensure a correct response.

Then instruct the client to use the cuing questions to construct a story of his or her own. During the initial stages of therapy, the clinician may want to provide the client with a set of choices for each part of the story to facilitate story construction. For example, the clinician might say: "Your story needs a setting. Do you want it to be about a boy named Joe or a teacher named Mr. Petry?"

Task difficulty can be increased by requiring the client to generate a spontaneous story and use the question cues as a self-monitoring strategy to check the quality of the finished product. The task also can be made more sophisticated by decreasing the number and specificity of question cues. A final set of questions might include the following:

Are all of the story parts included?

Does my story have a beginning, middle, and end?

Are the story parts in the correct order?

Note: This activity can be adapted to facilitate the client's production of written narratives. Mnemonic devices are effective tools for helping clients remember and sequence ideas in a logical manner (e.g., SPACE: *S*etting, *Pro*blem, *A*ction, *C*onsequent *E*vent) (Harris & Graham, 1996). Other acronyms can be used to revise and/or proofread written text (e.g., COPS: *C*apitalization, *O*verall appearance, *P*unctuation, *S*pelling) (Schumaker et al., 1982).

4. Tell the client that today's session will focus on how to start a conversation. Explain that there are four sequential steps in initiating a conversation: (a) choosing the setting, (b) selecting the topic, (c) getting the listener's attention, and (d) introducing the topic. Design at least six scenarios for each of the four steps, most of which are conversationally inappropriate. Explain that the clinician will read the scenarios for each step aloud. Instruct the client to show a thumbs-up or thumbs-down gesture to identify the appropriateness of each event. Example scenarios include the following:

Choosing the Setting

Your friend is on the telephone. (thumbs down)

Your friend is sitting next to you on the bus. (thumbs up)

Two classmates are sitting in the corner and whispering to each other. (thumbs down)

You are watching a movie in a theater. (thumbs down)

A new classmate is sitting by himself in the cafeteria. (thumbs up)

You are in science class during a lecture. (thumbs down)

Selecting the Topic

Do you have any brothers or sisters? (thumbs up)

Why is your hair so short? (thumbs down)

What kind of music do you like? (thumbs up)

I heard that your parents are getting a divorce. (thumbs down)

Does your father make lots of money? (thumbs down)

You're not invited to my party. (thumbs down)

Getting the Listener's Attention

Saying: "Hey, how's it going?" to the church pastor. (thumbs down)

Saying: "Good morning, Mr. Web" to the school principal. (thumbs up)

Saying: "Know what?" to a group of teachers in the lounge. (thumbs down)

Saying: "Come here" to an upper classman. (thumbs down)

Saying: "Excuse me" to an adult who is reading a book. (thumbs up)

Saying: "Here I am" to a group of classmates talking in the cafeteria. (thumbs down)

Introducing the Topic

Starting a conversation with: "Did you see where he went?" (thumbs down)

Starting a conversation with: "I wanted to talk to you about, you know, the assignment we . . . Remember what Ms. Jones said yesterday . . . You know what I'm talking about?" (thumbs down)

Starting a conversation with: "Everyone says that you didn't make the school play." (thumbs down)

Starting a conversation with: "I lost my doohickey, the thing I need to do the math homework problems." (thumbs down)

Starting a conversation with: "Can I talk to you about the party on Saturday night?" (thumbs up)

Starting a conversation with: "Wanna shoot hoops at recess with me?" (thumbs up)

PROFILE 2

Paul is a 17-year-old high school junior with a long-standing history of language deficits and persistent academic difficulties in the absence of overall intellectual impairment. He presents as an outgoing and friendly individual who demonstrates basic conversational competence in the areas of semantics, syntax, and morphology. Significant deficits are noted in his knowledge of higher-level abstract language forms, especially multiple meaning words, metaphoric uses of language, and inferential comprehension. Recent test results indicate that Paul is reading and writing at approximately the eighth-grade level. According to classroom observation and teacher report, Paul is "disorganized" and demonstrates ineffective study habits and test-taking strategies, poor time management, and poor follow-through on class assignments. These traits are indicative of limited metacognitive functioning (i.e., the awareness of one's own problem-solving strengths and weaknesses, how to apply them, and when to use them effectively). Recently, Paul met with his guidance counselor to discuss his academic status and explore his options following graduation. He expressed a clear preference for career training over college education.

Selection of therapy targets. The areas to be targeted are semantics, metalinguistics, metacognition, social communication skills, and academic language skills and strategies. With respect to semantics, inferencing was chosen as a means of improving Paul's ability to derive intended meaning from oral and written material. In the area of metalinguistics, metaphors were selected because this figurative language form occurs frequently in the academic environment. Metacognitive training will focus on goal setting, self-monitoring, self-evaluation, goal outcome, and reflection. Both Paul's age and current academic status indicate he would benefit from therapy activities that focus on social-communication skills in a vocational setting. Finally, the intervention program will target language-mediated study skills to provide Paul with the requisite tools for improving his academic performance.

Sample Activities

1. A metaphor is a nonliteral use of language in which one element (**topic**) is compared to another element (**vehicle**) on the basis of one or more common features (**ground**). Develop a list of metaphors and write each on an index

card. Each should contain an explicitly stated topic, vehicle, and ground. Each card also should contain two alternative meanings for each metaphor. Following are examples, with the correct choice indicated by an asterisk (Nippold, Leonard, & Kail, 1984).

The sun was a basketball sitting in the sky.

This means that the sun:

a. was orange and round.*

b. was very hot.

The giraffe was a flagpole living at the zoo.

This means the giraffe:

a. was tall.*

b. was on top of the flagpole.

The skater was a top spinning on the ice.

This means the skater:

a. was twirling very fast.*

b. had a top next to her on the ice.

David's nose was a grapefruit sitting on his face.

This means that David's nose:

a. was big.*

b. was bleeding.

The girl's smile was a ray of sunshine on a cloudy day.

This means that the girl's smile:

a. was bright.*

b. was big.

The man was a pumpkin walking down the street.

This means that the man:

a. was fat.*

b. was orange.

Matt's arms were broom handles hanging at his sides.

This means that Matt's arms:

a. were long and skinny.*

b. were hairy.

John's teeth were kernels of corn growing in his mouth.

This means that John's teeth:

a. were yellow.*

b. were chipped.

The soldiers were cornrows going down the road.

This means that the soldiers:

a. were straight lines.*

b. were tall.

The runner was a jet plane flying in the sky.

This means that the runner:

a. was fast.*

b. was getting on an airplane.

Explain that a metaphor is a comparison between two things that are alike in some way. For example, in "The girl's hair is spaghetti," the two things that are being compared are "hair" and "spaghetti." Both are thin and long. So this metaphor means that the girl's hair is thin and long. Explain that the client will read each metaphor aloud and, along with the clinician, identify the two things that are being compared. The client will then be presented with two choices and asked to pick the "best" meaning.

Note: Similes are easier to understand than metaphors because they have the syntactic markers "like" or "as" to signal the comparison. These markers can be used as a transition to metaphors (e.g., "The sun was [like] a basketball sitting in the sky").

2. Gather two 5-by-7-inch index cards in each of five colors for a total of 10 cards. Write goals and target behaviors from the following list on one card of each color. Follow color coding and write corresponding self-questions on the remaining cards.

Goals and Target Behaviors	*Self-Questions*
a. **Goal-Setting/Planning**	
Think before acting/speaking.	What do you want to do? What message do you want to send? How do you want this to come out?
b. **Self-Monitoring**	
Think about how the task is coming along. Are you devoting enough time/effort/attention?	How does your work look? Are there any problems? Do you need new or different strategies? How is your progress?
c. **Self-Evaluation**	
Rate the overall quality of the finished product and effectiveness of your performance.	Did you solve the problem(s)? Were the strategies useful? Was your work correct? Was it efficient?
d. **Goal Outcome**	
Evaluate the result of your work.	Did you achieve the goal? Was the goal realistic? Should it have been modified in some way?
e. **Reflection**	
Think about what the experience taught you.	Would you do things differently next time? What did you learn about your ability to solve problems?

Explain that this activity is designed to help the client approach problems or tasks in a systematic, organized manner. Jointly review the client's current course requirements and select a relevant assignment. For example, a civics class assignment might be a group project to develop a campaign to change some aspect of school board policy or local government ordinance. This client's group chose to petition the county council to install a stop sign at a busy intersection. As a group member, the client's responsibility is to write a persuasive letter to the appropriate government officials.

Introduce and discuss each of the goals and target behaviors in the order in which they were listed previously. Provide several examples for each component. Then have the client generate additional examples. Once the client demonstrates reliable recall of the five goals and target behaviors, begin the task by implementing the first goal (planning). Introduce the self-questions as instructional cues to facilitate achievement of the target behavior. When goal-setting is finalized, proceed to each subsequent component in the hierarchy using the self-questions to support the client's performance at each phase.

Note: The ultimate aim of this metacognitive training procedure is for the client to internalize the self-questions and use them as strategies for problem-solving across tasks.

3. Teach social communication skills in the context of vocational settings by using the training sequence of explanation, demonstration, and role playing. As each activity is mastered in the therapy session, the clinician can ask school personnel to participate in simulated work environments to provide the client with practice and promote generalization of the newly learned skills. For example, the school librarian, principal, or cafeteria staff could play the role of "employers" or "potential employers" to provide the student with opportunities to practice the skill in quasi-work environments (i.e., library, office, restaurant). "Debriefing" sessions can be held on a regular basis to review performance and improve the student's self-monitoring skills. Following are suggested tasks/contexts:

Telephoning to request a job interview

Undergoing a job interview

Accepting a suggestion from an employer

Accepting criticism from an employer

Providing constructive criticism to a coworker

Explaining a problem to a supervisor

Complimenting a coworker

Accepting a compliment from a coworker

4. Develop 20 situations that have clear logical inferences and write each on the top portion of an index card. Explain that an inference is a conclusion reached by using information that you know to be true to make a "good guess" about what is also likely to be true. For example, Mr. Jones made several jokes in class today, so I **inferred** that he was in a good mood. Instruct the client

to read each situation and write one logical inference. After each response, discuss with the client the reason that it was a correct/incorrect inference. Examples include the following:

> The principal usually makes the announcements, but today the vice principal gave them.
>
> Tyler blushed when he saw Emily.
>
> Tony picked up his baseball bat and walked out to the plate.
>
> Joe hammered the nail and yelled "Ouch!"
>
> Ken walked into his apartment and his CD player and TV set were gone.
>
> Chad walked by his best friend Steve without saying "Hello."
>
> Hank rented a tuxedo for Saturday night.
>
> Ashley is making a salad for dinner. Her eyes are stinging and tears are rolling down her cheeks.
>
> Noah made sure to put on gloves and a hat.
>
> Wanda put the book down after reading only half of it.
>
> The boss walks by and gives you a pat on the back.
>
> Alex looked at the clock and ran out of the room.
>
> The sand burned Madison's feet.
>
> Danny took one bite of the apple and threw it away.
>
> Mrs. Jensen frowned as she handed Tim his math exam.
>
> Jack smiled as he left his basketball game.
>
> Allison took the cookies out of the oven and threw them in the trash.
>
> Sam walked into the backyard to get some tomatoes and peas.
>
> Mia could hear the waves from her bedroom window.
>
> Fred searched for a quarter and called a tow truck driver.

5. The development of language-mediated study skills is particularly critical for successful academic performance at the junior high and high school levels. A compendium of important skill areas is included in Table 5-4 on page 197. Training can be accomplished most effectively by using the students' actual classroom materials (e.g., lecture notes, textbook readings, homework assignments, and term projects). One effective school-based service delivery model for study skill training is the provision of a course that meets regularly and is taken for academic credit.

Helpful Hints

1. With adolescents, it is important to use written materials that are relevant and chronologically age appropriate (e.g., magazines on topics of interest, newspaper advertisements). Also engage the teen in relevant writing tasks such as making shopping lists, copying recipes, writing letters of inquiry about housing.

2. When using role playing as a technique for fostering the development of social skills, it may be useful to portray examples of both appropriate and inappropriate behaviors to highlight the differences between more and less socially acceptable behavior.

3. To facilitate peer relationships through small group settings, it may be helpful to include a normally achieving peer who can model appropriate skills. This strategy may also buffer the effects of low acceptance and rejection that may occur in larger peer groups.

4. Inferencing can be trained in the context of paragraph-length material using a multiple choice response format. For example:

> Hal was watching a movie on TV. It was about a man who was crossing a desert. Hal could almost feel the hot sun. Soon, Hal ran to get something he wanted very much. What do you think it was?

   a. Something to ride on
   b. Something to drink
   c. Something to play with

5. To reinforce meaning and foster generalization over time, it is preferable to use several different contexts for the same figurative language form rather than introducing several different expressions.

6. Introduce new figurative language forms in matching and multiple choice tasks because they are easier than explanation tasks.

7. Certain types of idioms, metaphors, and so on are easier to understand than others because their meaning is more transparent or closer to the literal meaning. For example, the idiom "keep a straight face" is more explicit than "come apart at the seams." The following examples are from Schweigert (1986), pp. 33–45.

Examples of Transparent Idioms	Examples of Opaque Idioms
on the other hand	asleep at the switch
pain in the neck	finger in the pie
hit the road	fine kettle of fish
burned out	big frog in a small pond
on the tip of his tongue	upset the applecart
coast is clear	iron in the fire
over his head	shout from the housetops
hit the sack	build a fire under
have a ball	paddle his own canoe
big head	clip his wings
up the creek without a paddle	know which side his bread is buttered on

8. Begin with predictive metaphors because they are easier to understand than proportional metaphors. Predictive metaphors are based on similarity and contain only one topic and vehicle. Proportional metaphors contain two top-

ics and two vehicles and express an analogical relationship with usually one topic left unstated (e.g., The bird's nest was a piggy bank that had no coins). The analogy is: *nest* is to *piggy bank* as **eggs** are to *coins* (leaving the topic eggs to be inferred).

9. Dictionaries of English figurative language forms are commercially available. Two examples are: (a) R. L. Chapman, (Ed.). (1998). *Dictionary of American slang.* New York: Harper Collins; and (b) D. M. Gulland & D. G. Hindes-Howell (2001). *Dictionary of English idioms.* New York: Penguin.

10. Adolescent clients may demonstrate significant behavioral problems that are, in fact, related to their language impairment. Clinicians may need to provide counseling to help students function more effectively in classroom as well as clinical settings.

11. Instruction that addresses linguistic cohesion devices can significantly improve a student's comprehension and production of oral and written text. See Appendix 5-A for examples of the most common types of cohesion.

TABLE 5-4
Language-Mediated Study Skills for Older Children and Adolescents

STUDY SKILLS

1. *Time Organization*
   Budgeting time for completion
   Establishing daily homework and study schedules
   Breaking assignments into smaller units
   Planning for deadlines
   Organizing notebook

2. *Text Analysis*
   Table of contents
   Glossary
   Legends, maps, diagrams, tables

3. *Note-Taking*
   Importance of taking notes
   Different methods: mapping, outlining, abbreviating, summarizing, webbing

4. *Study Strategies*
   Active thinking method
   Scanning versus skimming versus reading
   Memory strategies: mnemonic devices, chunking, peg words, acronyms, brainstorming, visualizing

5. *Test-Taking Strategies*
   Preparation: establish study schedule; inquire as to type of questions that will be on test
   Review terms often used on tests: for example, prove, review, summarize, compare, contrast, criticize
   Strategies for different types of tests: fill-ins, multiple choice, matching, true/false, essay

6. *Reference Skills*
   Library and media center skills: alphabetical order, catalogue skills, cross-referencing
   Review different types of reference sources: dictionary, encyclopedia, atlas, thesaurus, internet

(continues)

Table 5-4 Language-Mediated Study Skills for Older Children and Adolescents (continued)

CRITICAL THINKING

1. *General Thinking Behaviors*
   Observing and describing
   Developing concepts
   Hypothesizing
   Generalizing
   Predicting outcomes
   Explaining an event
   Offering alternatives
   Inferencing

2. *Problem-Solving*
   Teach steps in decision making: define problem, break into small parts, develop options, choose
   option, predict outcome, critique decision made

3. *Higher-Thinking Skills*
   Teach inductive and deductive reasoning
   Teach solving analogies

LISTENING/READING

1. *Prelistening/Reading*
   Strategies for "getting ready" to listen, for example, review material beforehand

2. *Listening/Reading*
   Teach recognition of organizational cues and phrases, for example, in the beginning, the first point,
   the key point, three main areas are, in summary
   Reading: teach identification of topic sentence, supporting sentences, details

3. *Evaluative Listening*
   Teach distinction between fact and opinion, for example, propaganda, commercials, prejudice,
   absurdities

ORAL AND WRITTEN EXPRESSION

1. *Organization*
   Ways in which to ask questions
   Strategies for organizing paragraphs
   Teach forms of expository writing, for example, description, explanation, compare/contrast

2. *Craftsmanship*
   Sentence and paragraph construction, for example, S-V agreement, tense agreement, topic versus
   supporting sentences, coherence
   Editing
   Proofreading: spelling, peer proofing

Source: F. Roth and E. Fye, personal communication, July 1991.

CONCLUSION

This chapter has presented basic information, protocols, and procedures for intervention for childhood language disorders at an **introductory** level. This information is intended only as a starting point in the reader's clinical education and training. For more in-depth coverage of this area, the following readings are recommended:

Nelson, N. W. (1998). *Childhood language disorders in context: Infancy through adolescence.* Boston: Allyn & Bacon.

Owens, R. E. (2004). *Language disorders: A functional approach to assessment and intervention.* Needham Heights, MA: Allyn & Bacon.

Paul, R. (2001). *Language disorders from infancy to adolescence: Assessment and interventions.* Boston: C. V. Mosby.

ADDITIONAL RESOURCES

Miscellaneous

Burns, M. S., Griffin, P., & Snow, C. E. (1999). *Starting out right: A guide to promoting children's reading success.* Washington, DC: National Academy Press.

> Clinician and parent-friendly guide to the development of reading and spelling skills in young children. Includes specific activities to promote emergent and early literacy from infancy through mid-elementary school.

Glazer, S. (1990). *Creating readers and writers.* Newark, DE. International Reading Association.

> This book contains a section that describes the types of books that are appropriate for children in four different age ranges between infancy and 12 years of age.

Torgesen, J. K., & Bryant, B. R. (1994). *Phonological awareness training for reading.* Austin, TX: Pro-Ed.

> Focuses on training in four areas: sound blending, sound segmenting, reading, and spelling. Skills are taught in a sequential manner through a variety of games. It includes a detailed description (script) of each activity as well as precise instructions for implementation.

Yopp, H. K., & Yopp, R. H. (2000). Supporting phonemic awareness in the classroom. *The Reading Teacher, 54*, 130–143.

> This article provides sample phonological awareness activities appropriate for preschool, kindergarten, and first-grade classrooms within a developmental hierarchy of difficulty.

APPENDIX 5-A

TYPES OF COHESION

> Cohesion: Linguistic devices for connecting sentences to one another so that text is coherent and "hangs together" (Halliday & Hasan, 1975)

Ellipsis: Redundant words are eliminated from the utterance.

Examples: The *roses* were red. There were twelve.
Have you been swimming? Yes.

Conjunction: Connective words link two independent clauses.

Examples: She was never happy here. *So* she's leaving.
Harry left *because* the party was over.
Sally ran downstairs, *but* she missed the bus.

Lexical: General nouns or repetitions link two sentences.

Examples: Joe stayed awake three nights in a row. The *man* is crazy.
There was a caterpillar in the forest. The *caterpillar* was green.

Reference: Pronouns, demonstratives, the definite article, and comparative terms are used to refer back to a referent.

Examples: John went to the store. *He* bought a sweater.
I went to New York City. Guess what I did *there*?
My grandfather had a clock. *The* clock had chimes.
Two birds sat in a tree. *Another* came along.

CHAPTER 6

Intervention for Adult Aphasia, the Dysarthrias, and Apraxia of Speech
(with Introduction to Dysphagia)

This chapter will cover three major types of adult neurological communication disorders: (1) aphasia, (2) the dysarthrias, and (3) apraxia of speech. Aphasia is a language-based disorder, while apraxia and dysarthria are considered motor speech impairments. These deficits may occur alone or coexist in the same individual. There is a lack of consensus concerning many issues related to each of these disorders, including basic terminology. To minimize confusion, the technical vocabulary used in this chapter was selected for its common usage and clarity. Traumatic brain injury, dementia, right hemisphere dysfunction, and dysphagia are beyond the scope of this chapter. Selected references are provided at the end of this chapter for readers interested in these topics.

APHASIA

Aphasia is a language disorder due to brain damage that results in impairment in the comprehension and/or formulation of language and can affect both the spoken and written modalities. The major cause of aphasia is cerebrovascular accident (CVA) or stroke. Other etiologies include tumors; head trauma; and certain disease processes, such as encephalitis. Aphasia is associated with damage to the dominant hemisphere for language in the brain, which is the left hemisphere in most individuals. It frequently is accompanied by motor and sensory deficits. As the left hemisphere controls the contralateral (or opposite) side of the body, these motor and sensory impairments are most often right-sided in individuals with aphasia. A common motor impairment is **hemiplegia** or **hemiparesis**, which refers to paralysis or weakness on one side of the body, respectively. **Hemianopsia** is a visual field deficit in which an individual cannot see to the right or left of midline in one or both eyes. (Other pertinent medical terms are located in a glossary in Appendix 6-A).

Classification of Aphasia Syndromes

Historically, there has been an enormous amount of effort devoted to the classification of aphasic types and syndromes. This work has resulted in the development of several different approaches to classification, including site of lesion taxonomies (e.g., Goodglass, Kaplan, & Barresi, 2000; Kertesz, 1979); linguistic structure paradigms (Jakobson, 1964); and modality-oriented systems that address behavioral symptoms of language impairment (e.g., Schuell, Jenkins, & Jimenez-Pabon, 1964). A detailed discussion of the similarities and differences among the various aphasia taxonomies is beyond the scope of this chapter. (The reader is referred to Johns [1985] for comprehensive reviews of classification issues and approaches.) From a treatment-oriented perspective, we find it clinically useful to adopt the Boston group's (Goodglass, Kaplan, & Barresi, 2000) approach to classification, which includes two main categories of aphasia: **nonfluent** and **fluent**. This classification system is based on quality of output and involves both oral and written modalities. Within each category, the degree of severity may range from mild to profound.

The profile of nonfluent aphasias is one of poor output with relatively spared comprehension. It generally is characterized by reduced vocabulary; agrammatism; and impairments of articulation, rate, and prosody (rhythm, stress, and into-nation) resulting in labored and effortful production.

Fluent aphasias consist of impairment in language comprehension with maintenance of normal melodic speech contour. The main characteristics are word-retrieval difficulties, paraphasias (phonemic and semantic), neologisms, perseveration, and the maintenance of normal melodic speech contour.

Definitions of key terms related to language deficits in aphasia are presented in Table 6-1. The major categories of fluent and nonfluent aphasia can be further divided into selected subtypes as shown in Table 6-2.

Treatment Efficacy/Evidence-Based Practice

As part of the natural recovery process, the brain regains some of its speech, language, and motor functions. The greatest amount of this **spontaneous recovery** occurs during the first two months after injury. However, changes may be seen

---

TABLE 6-1
Terminology Related to Language Deficits in Aphasia

Term	Definition
Agrammatism	Syntactic deficit characterized by omission of function words and grammatical inflections. Semantic aspects of language remain intact. Speech output consists primarily of content words. Example: When asked to describe a picture of a picnic with someone sleeping in a hammock, the client responds, "Food . . . man bed . . . he sleep."
Word-retrieval problems	Difficulty accessing a word from one's mental vocabulary. Severe naming difficulty is termed **anomia**. Example: When asked to name a picture of a hammock, the client responds, "It's to sleep in . . . under trees . . . you know, with a rope."
Paraphasia	Errors in speech output characterized by the production of unintended sounds, syllables, or words. The two main types are (1) phonemic and (2) semantic. **Phonemic paraphasias** (also known as literal paraphasias) consist of extraneous or transposed sounds and syllables and substitution of one correctly articulated phoneme for another. Example: When asked to name a picture of a hammock, the client may respond with one of the following: "hammerock," "hackamm," "pammock," respectively.
Semantic	Involve the unintended substitution of one word for another, usually within the same semantic category (also known as paraphasias). Example: When asked to name a picture of a hammock, the client responds, "It's a bed."
Neologism	Invented words that have no true meaning but that adhere to the phonological rules of a given language. This error tends to occur primarily with nouns and verbs rather than function words. Example: When asked to name a picture of a hammock, the client responds, "That's a blick."
Perseveration	Inappropriate continuation of a response after the presentation of a new stimulus. Example: After successfully naming a picture of a hammock, the client continues to respond "hammock" when shown the next three pictures of a chair, key, and glove.

TABLE 6-2
Classification of Aphasia Syndromes

Syndrome Type	Characteristics
Nonfluent Aphasias	
Broca's	Agrammatism; effortful articulation of phrase-length utterances; impaired prosody and intonation; concomitant apraxia of speech; good comprehension; lesion in the posterior inferior frontal lobe, as well as central and inferior parietal regions
Transcortical motor	Little to no initiation of spontaneous speech; output similar to Broca's but excellent imitation (even of long utterances); relatively intact comprehension; lesion in the medial-frontal cortex, involving the supplementary motor area
Global	Severe deficits in all areas of language comprehension and production; output may be limited to stereotypic utterances; lesion encompasses both pre- and postrolandic speech zones
Fluent Aphasias	
Wernicke's	Fluent but often meaningless speech (jargon); good articulation, intonation, and prosody; impaired comprehension; lesion in the posterior portion of the first temporal gyrus of the left hemisphere
Conduction	Relatively fluent speech; frequent phonemic paraphasias; marked difficulty with imitation; good language comprehension; lesion in the arcuate fasciculus, deep supramarginal gyrus, or superior temporal gyrus
Anomic	Significant word-finding difficulties in the presence of otherwise fluent and grammatical speech; good comprehension; lesion in the angular gyrus region

Source: Adapted from Hegde (1995).

in some individuals even after six months or longer. Following the period of spontaneous recovery, individuals will continue to demonstrate some degree of chronic impairment. Several factors influence the degree of spontaneous recovery and ultimate prognosis. These include the size, location, and etiology of the lesion; type and severity of the initial aphasia (particularly verbal comprehension); age at onset; and overall health of the client (Kertesz, 1979; Kertesz & McCabe, 1977). In general, lesions located in the temporo-parietal region are associated with a poorer prognosis. Studies also indicate that hemorrhagic strokes have a more remarkable recovery pattern than those due to blockage of cerebral blood flow (i.e., embolism or thrombosis). As a rule, prognosis is more favorable for younger clients and for those without additional medical problems. During spontaneous recovery, the initial aphasia syndrome may evolve into a different (usually milder) classification type.

Historically, there is controversy over the efficacy of aphasia therapy. Some studies have suggested that any objective improvement seen in a client's status is attributable to the brain's spontaneous recovery rather than a result of treatment effects (e.g., Sarno, Silverman, & Sands, 1970). Others contend that aphasia treatment results in measurable gains in communicative functioning through both traditional and group treatment models (e.g., Elman & Bernstein-Ellis, 1999; Wertz et al., 1981). In part, this controversy is a result of methodological problems associated with obtaining matched subject samples and the ethical dilemma of withholding treatment from individuals assigned to control group conditions.

To confound the issue further, disagreement also exists regarding the optimal time to initiate therapy. The main source of contention is whether to initiate therapy immediately or wait until the spontaneous recovery process has run its course. The available data do not adequately solve the problem of separating spontaneous recovery changes from treatment effects. Several studies have reported that delaying initiation of treatment had no significant negative impact on client progress (Sarno et al., 1970; Sarno & Levita, 1971; Wertz et al., 1986). However, most clinicians advocate early intervention based on the premise that treatment may serve to accelerate the natural process of spontaneous recovery.

In 1996, Holland, Fromm, De Ruyter, and Stein published a comprehensive summary of available data on treatment efficacy for aphasia. They reviewed large and small group studies, single-subject studies, and program evaluation data from several rehabilitation sites throughout the country. Their overall conclusion was that aphasia therapy is efficacious in that treated clients make significantly more improvement than untreated clients. The analysis also resulted in several additional conclusions:

- Most of the large group studies indicated that treatment benefits are greatest for individuals with a single, left-hemisphere stroke.

- Small group and single-subject studies suggested that treatment is effective for clients with chronic aphasia well beyond the period of spontaneous recovery.

- Client improvement is greatest when therapy is provided on a frequent basis over a period of at least five to six months.

- Program evaluation data from inpatient rehabilitation settings suggested that the greatest amount of functional improvement occurs in receptive language skills, followed by speech production and expressive language skills.

- The literature is unclear regarding the extent to which severity of aphasia, type of aphasia, or client age influence treatment outcome.

- Further research is needed to determine which treatment techniques are most efficacious for specific types of aphasic impairment.

More recently, Robey (1998) conducted a meta-analysis of 55 multiple-subject studies to examine clinical outcomes in the treatment of aphasia. His findings, which confirm and extend those of earlier studies, include the following:

- In all stages of recovery, clients who receive treatment demonstrate outcomes superior to untreated individuals. This is particularly true when treatment is initiated during the acute phase of recovery.

- Clients who receive two or more hours per week of intervention during the acute and post-acute stages exhibit greater gains than those receiving services on a less intense schedule.

- Even individuals with severe aphasia benefit substantially from intervention provided by speech-language pathologists.
- Outcome information is still needed regarding the effects of different intervention approaches on different types of aphasia.

Treatment for Aphasia

The overall goal of aphasia therapy is to improve a client's communication skills to the highest degree possible within the constraints of the neurological damage. The majority of individuals with aphasia will experience at least some residual language deficits throughout their lifetime. For this reason, clinicians must decide when to shift the focus of treatment from a "cure" to "care" orientation. The goal of treatment changes from recovery of premorbid language skills to establishing compensatory/maintenance strategies for functional language skills. To devise an appropriate and effective intervention program, the clinician must have thorough knowledge of prognostic variables as well as familiarity with the most predictable patterns of recovery that are associated with the different aphasia subtypes. For example, one common recovery pattern is for a global aphasia to evolve into a chronic Broca's aphasia. There are few well-designed studies that evaluate aphasia therapy in terms of optimal frequency, duration, or the relative value of different methods. This is especially true in the area of fluent aphasia. Therefore, speech-language pathologists (SLPs) should design intervention programs in accordance with individual clients' presenting clinical profiles as well as premorbid status factors such as intellectual level, education, and reading ability. In addition, cultural and linguistic differences should be considered across instructional and interpersonal aspects of therapy. Very few individuals with aphasia are completely unable to comprehend auditory information, and conversely, few have perfectly preserved auditory comprehension skills. The goal of the SLP is to recognize both spared areas of function in clients with severe aphasia and subtle areas of weakness in clients with mild aphasia.

There are four main theoretical orientations to aphasia treatment:

1. **Stimulation-facilitation:** This approach is based on the assumption that an individual's ability to access his own linguistic knowledge has been disrupted and that these language processing pathways can be strengthened through direct stimulation (Schuell, Jenkins, & Jimenez-Pabon, 1964). The main emphasis of this approach is the use of intensive and repeated sensory stimulation, particularly through the auditory channel, to reorganize the client's language system.

2. **Deblocking:** This approach is also based on the premise that linguistic pathways have been disrupted. However, rather than attempting to directly stimulate damaged channels, this treatment paradigm focuses on language systems that remain intact. These are used to trigger improved function in the impaired modalities (Luria, 1970). This approach may involve intrasystemic reorganization of language function, that is, within a single modality (e.g., use of singing to facilitate verbal output) or intersystemic reorganization using one modality to stimulate another (e.g., use of signs or gestures to improve verbal expression).

3. **Operant conditioning:** The main assumption of this approach is that brain injury has resulted in a loss of linguistic knowledge rather than a disruption of access to that knowledge. This treatment strategy focuses on relearning lost language skills through the use of reinforcement contingencies. (See Chapter 1 for detailed discussion of operant conditioning.) The procedures associated with an operant approach are similar to those used in stimulation-facilitation. However, in operant programming, the clinician uses systematic reinforcement to directly shape language behaviors rather than relying on intensive repetition to facilitate disrupted pathways (LaPointe, 1985).

4. **Functional/compensatory:** This approach also is based on the premise that language function has been lost in the individuals with aphasia. However, the focus of therapy is on establishing functional communication. The procedures are designed to encourage use of whatever modalities are available to the individual to convey messages to listeners (Byng, Pound, & Parr, 2000; Davis & Wilcox, 1981; Simmons-Mackie, 2000, 2001). These may include speaking, gesturing, signing, writing, facial expressions, drawing, and so on. The selection of functional therapy goals can be guided by the communicative behaviors identified in the Functional Assessment of Communication Skills (FACS) developed by the American Speech-Language-Hearing Association (Frattali, Thompson, Holland, Wohl, & Ferketic, 1995). This framework specifies 43 communicative behaviors that are grouped according to four domains: (a) social communication; (b) basic needs; (c) reading, writing, and number concepts; and (d) daily planning. Therapy goals also can be selected based on the functional end points of aphasia treatment suggested by Holland (1995), which are outlined in Table 6-3.

In summary, stimulation-facilitation, deblocking, and operant conditioning are traditional approaches to treatment in that they focus on structural language forms (i.e., semantics and syntax). Functional communication therapy is a more recent development that emphasizes the exchange of communicative messages rather than the form of those messages. The unit of analysis in this treatment paradigm is always the dyad (speaker + listener) rather than the client as an individual. Typical goal areas in functional communication therapy include turn taking, topic initiation, and communicative intent.

Guidelines for Programming and Implementing Therapy. Therapy may focus on improving a client's abilities in listening, speaking, reading, and writing. For the first three therapy approaches outlined previously, intervention is programmed according to hierarchies of difficulty (refer to Chapter 1 for detailed information on basic therapy programming). The hierarchies are based on neurolinguistic research that has explored how adults with and without aphasia comprehend and produce language (e.g., Berndt, Mitchum, & Wayland, 1997; Goodglass & Wingfield, 1998; Hillis, 2001; Mitchum & Berndt, 2001). Following is a sample hierarchy for the selection and sequencing of therapy targets in the area of verbal expression. This general therapeutic progression also can be applied to each of the other language modalities.

TABLE 6-3
Functional Long-Term Goals for Aphasia Therapy

1. Communicate to obtain assistance in emergency situations.
   Example: Call 911.

2. Express feelings.
   Example: Make attitudes and emotions known.

3. Convey basic needs.
   Example: Communicate hunger, thirst, fatigue.

4. Follow simple directions.
   Example: Set alarm clock.

5. Engage in social relationships or situations.
   Example: Enjoy social interactions to the degree commensurate with pre-aphasia status.

6. Declare autonomy and independence through action, thought, or opinion.
   Example: Indicate disagreement or difference of opinion.

7. Resume activities that were pleasurable prior to onset of aphasia.
   Example: Enjoy hobbies or grandchildren.

8. Take on some routine responsibility.
   Example: Put out trash, water plants.

9. Keep up with news events.
   Example: Read headlines, watch TV news.

10. Function as an individual independent of the aphasic impairment for at least brief time periods.
    Example: Attend a concert or sports event.

Source: Adapted from Holland (1995).

1. Intervention may begin at the nonverbal level by establishing pointing responses.
2. Single-word tasks can then be introduced in the form of responsive or confrontation naming. In responsive naming, a clinician provides a verbal descriptive phrase to elicit a target label (e.g., The object that we use to sweep the floor is called a _____). A confrontation naming task is more difficult because it requires the client to name a visual stimulus (e.g., picture or object) without any contextual support.
3. Phrase-length responses can then be targeted through sentence completion activities that require the client to fill in a word or phrase that accurately completes a sentence stem.
4. Finally, sentence-level formulation may be required in which a client might be asked to describe pictures or the function of objects or respond to direct questions posed by the clinician.

This hierarchy of difficulty focuses on utterance length as the critical factor. However, aphasia therapy entails much more than simply increasing the length of a target response. Several factors can be manipulated while maintaining the same response length. For example, a clinician may decrease the amount of support provided in the form of modeling, cues, and prompts to encourage a client to become a more independent communicator. In addition, therapy can be designed to elicit responses at more sophisticated levels of linguistic complexity (e.g., maintaining a phrase-length response while moving from literal language forms to figurative forms such as idioms, metaphors, and humor). At the single-word level, more complex language forms such as antonyms and synonyms can be elicited through the use of word association tasks. Further, the latency between clinician stimulus and client response also can be manipulated. Once the accuracy of a target behavior has been established, task difficulty can be boosted by increasing the speed of the expected response without altering either the length or linguistic complexity of the utterance. In contrast, preliminary data from single-subject research on individuals with agrammatic aphasia suggest that generalization of sentence production is facilitated when the direction of therapy progresses from more complex to less complex syntactic structures (Thompson, Shapiro, Kiran, & Sobecks, 2003).

Another important component of intervention programming for aphasia is the use of **group therapy** as well as individual sessions. An ideal model allows a client to learn new communication behaviors in individual sessions and provides group settings for opportunities to practice and expand these skills in an interactional situation. Group settings also provide a milieu in which clients can socialize and identify with peers who have problems similar to their own. In addition to therapy groups, intervention for aphasia often includes group sessions for family training and counseling. Family members can facilitate the aphasic individual's everyday communication performance by learning and implementing the techniques used by the clinician in therapy sessions. Family counseling is an essential aspect of aphasia therapy. Families may require guidance about how to talk to the affected family member. Specific suggestions are provided in Appendix 6-B. Of all communication disorders, aphasia is the one that causes the most severe adjustment problems for families because of its sudden and abrupt onset. Virtually overnight, a family member experiences dramatic changes in health and personality as well as in the ability to communicate.

Finally, one common technique used with clients who present with word-retrieval deficits is **self-cuing**. These are strategies that can be used by a client to trigger the verbal production of a specific word and include the following:

1. Automatic sequences (e.g., days of the week)
2. Paired verbal associates (e.g., bread and _____ [*butter*])
3. Sentence completion (e.g., We use a broom to sweep the _____ [*floor*])
4. Idiomatic expressions (e.g., Look before you _____ [*leap*])
5. Alternative words (e.g., synonyms and antonyms)
6. Rhyming words (e.g., sounds like *fall*)
7. Phonemic cues (e.g., initial sound/syllable of target word)
8. Writing the initial letter, syllable, or entire word
9. Subordinate category cues (e.g., Pizza and hot dogs are types of _____ [*food*])
10. Air tracing (i.e., writing a word in the air with one's finger)
11. Gesture or pantomime cues (e.g., pretending to drink from a cup)
12. Object or action attributes (e.g., present two or more pictures and ask questions such as "Which one is sharp?" and "Which one is slow?")

Specific Intervention Procedures. Numerous procedures have been used in the rehabilitation of individuals with aphasia. This section briefly describes six of the most common programs identified in the clinical research literature.

Stimulation-Facilitation. (Schuell, Jenkins, & Jimenez-Pabon, 1964). Stimulation-facilitation is not a specific procedure but rather a general approach to aphasia treatment that incorporates the basic principles of competent intervention (Duffy & Coelho, 2001). Specific characteristics of this approach, as advocated by Schuell, are as follows: (1) the focus of therapy is intensive auditory stimulation to elicit language; (2) a client's incorrect responses are met with increased stimulation rather than corrective feedback; (3) the highest possible number of responses should be elicited in each session; (4) target behaviors are elicited through continual repetition of the clinician's stimulus rather than via direct instruction; and (5) therapy tasks are focused mainly on the semantic and syntactic components of the linguistic system.

Melodic Intonation Therapy. (Albert, Sparks, & Helm, 1973). Melodic Intonation Therapy (MIT) is a deblocking technique that utilizes "intoning" to facilitate verbal expression in clients who demonstrate severely restricted verbal output and relatively good speech comprehension. This approach uses variations in pitch, tempo/rhythm, and stress to recruit participation of the right hemisphere to improve verbal production in clients with damage to the language-dominant left hemisphere. The MIT program consists of a 15-step hierarchy (Helm-Estabrooks & Albert, 2004; Helm-Estabrooks & Holland, 1998; Sparks, 2001; Sparks & Holland, 1976), which is presented in a condensed form as follows:

- Client taps out rhythm while listening to clinician's hummed and intoned utterance.
- Client and clinician intone utterance in unison.
- Clinician fades out of unison production.
- Client independently imitates clinician's model of intoned utterance.
- Client's response is no longer intoned but produced in unison with exaggerated inflection and then gradually shaped to approximate more normal speech prosody.
- Clinician fades out of unison production.
- Client independently imitates clinician's model of spoken utterance.
- Client fades imitative response and spontaneously produces the spoken utterance in response to clinician questions.

MIT generally begins with utterances consisting of two- and three-syllable words and short, commonly used phrases. Longer and more complex utterances are gradually introduced at later stages in the program. There are specific scoring procedures for each step in the program. At all levels of stimulus difficulty, it is recommended that the utterance should be produced slowly and with continuous voicing.

The most suitable candidates for MIT are aphasic individuals who demonstrate the following characteristics:

1. Unilateral stroke in the left frontal lobe (Broca's area), often extending to the parietal region
2. Severely limited verbal output with poor speech articulation
3. Extremely poor speech imitation skills
4. Relatively spared comprehension of verbal input
5. Emotionally stable with good attention span

Amer-Ind. (Skelly, Schinsky, Smith, & Fust, 1974). Amer-Ind is a gestural system based on American Indian Hand Talk in which the gestures stand for basic concepts rather than words. Each signal can represent several different English words. Each gesture is very concrete and easily recognizable (i.e., highly transparent) (Campbell & Jackson, 1995). This system is telegraphic in nature in that there is no grammar; rather, the signals are sequenced in a logical order. Amer-Ind can be used as an alternative communication system or as a facilitator of other communication modalities (Coelho, 1990; Rao, 2001). When used as an intersystemic deblocking technique, this therapy approach consists of the following main steps:

- Extensive imitation is used to establish comprehension and production of very common and easily recognized (iconic) gestures such as head nods and shoulder shrugs.
- Imitation is gradually faded in favor of more spontaneous and communicatively meaningful use of the signs.
- Client is then taught a group of topic signs that can be used to provide the communication partner with a context for interpreting an upcoming message.
- Clinician begins to pair the signs with spoken words after client has mastered several signs.
- Client is required to produce the sign in unison with the clinician and is encouraged to pay close attention to the clinician's production of the spoken word.
- Client is asked to produce both the sign and the word in unison with the clinician.
- Clinician then fades out of unison production and provides a model of the sign + word combination for the client to imitate.
- The imitative nature of the client's response is gradually shaped to spontaneous production of the sign + word combination in response to clinician questions.

The ultimate aim of this program is for the client to meaningfully use sequences of sign + word combinations (see Rao, 2001, for a treatment hierarchy in which Amer-Ind is implemented as an *alternative* method of communication).

The most appropriate candidates for Amer-Ind are individuals with severely restricted verbal repertoires resulting from aphasia or apraxia. It also is most effective with clients whose gestural skills are better than their verbal skills.

Visual Action Therapy. (Helm-Estabrooks & Albert, 2004). Visual Action Therapy (VAT) is a functional/compensatory approach to aphasia intervention that enhances an individual's functional communication skills through the use of representational gestures rather than speech. This nonvocal strategy is designed for severely impaired or globally aphasic individuals and focuses on the production of messages at the single gesture level. VAT is a hierarchically structured three-level program that utilizes objects, realistic line drawings of the objects, and action pictures depicting a figure appropriately manipulating the objects. Ultimately, the client progresses from matching pictures and objects to the spontaneous use of symbolic hand/arm or mouth/face gestures to communicate simple messages. Currently, there are three VAT program variations: (1) **proximal limb** (focuses on gestures composed of gross movements of the shoulder, arms, and fingers, e.g., sawing); (2) **distal limb** (focuses on gestures composed of finer movements of the hand and fingers, e.g., turning a screwdriver); and (3) **bucco-facial** (focuses on gestures composed of movements of the mouth and face, e.g., whistling). All three VAT variations follow the same basic training sequence, summarized as follows:

Level I

- Client matches then points to objects and pictures in four different seven-way discrimination tasks.
- Client is taught to demonstrate appropriate use of each object through clinician modeling and shaping until spontaneous performance is achieved.
- Clinician points to a specific action picture and client is required to pick up the corresponding object from an array of seven and demonstrate its use.
- Client locates or points to a specific object from an array of seven in response to pantomime gestures produced by the clinician.
- Client is required to produce an appropriate pantomime gesture when shown each of the seven objects.
- Client is shown two randomly selected objects, which are then hidden; one object is then returned to view and the client is encouraged to self-initiate the correct gesture for the one that remains hidden.

Levels II and III

For both of these levels, the use of real objects is discontinued. In Level II, the training begins at the point in which pantomime gestures are introduced by the clinician and stimuli consist solely of the action pictures. Level III training begins at the same point in the hierarchy and utilizes only object pictures. The most appropriate candidates for VAT demonstrate the following characteristics:

Limb VAT	*Bucco-Facial VAT*
Unilateral damage to left hemisphere, especially primary language zones	Unilateral damage to left hemisphere, especially anterior language areas
Global aphasia; severe impairments in spoken and written language modalities; moderate to severe limb apraxia	Severely impaired verbal output with relatively intact verbal comprehension

Alert and cooperative with good   Alert and cooperative with good
attention span   attention span

Promoting Aphasics' Communicative Effectiveness (PACE). (Davis, 1993; Davis & Wilcox, 1981). Promoting Aphasics' Communicative Effectiveness is another example of a functional/compensatory approach to aphasia intervention. Therapy is conducted in the context of naturalistic conversation between the clinician and client. The goal is to improve a client's ability to convey intended messages using whatever means of communication available to the individual. In 1981, Davis and Wilcox identified four principles that underlie the implementation of PACE.

1. The clinician and client are to be egalitarian communication partners and take an equal number of turns as speaker and listener. The purpose is to create an interaction pattern that adheres to the turn-taking rules of everyday conversation. It also provides a built-in natural mechanism for the clinician to model a range of appropriate communication styles that the client can incorporate into subsequent messages.
2. The messages that are communicated must contain new information rather than information that is already known to both communication partners. This requirement encourages the speaker to reformulate or revise messages that initially meet with listener confusion.
3. Messages can be exchanged using any vocal or nonvocal modality or combinations of modalities.
4. The clinician provides feedback regarding the communicative effectiveness of messages conveyed by the client; errors in linguistic form of messages are not addressed.

Implementation of these four principles is accomplished through a picture description task in which the clinician and client take turns acting as the sender of a message. The designated sender chooses one picture from a facedown pile (being careful to keep it from the listener's view) and describes it using any available communication modalities. Unlike most intervention programming, PACE requires that the clinician be unaware of the specific stimulus items selected by the client from the pile. The aim of this task is for the speaker to successfully transmit the intended information to the listener.

PACE is a flexible treatment technique that has been used with individuals with various types and degrees of aphasia. These include both fluent aphasic adults (Pulvermuller & Roth, 1991) and nonfluent aphasic adults (Newhoff & Apel, 1990). According to Davis and Wilcox (1981), the pragmatic orientation of PACE makes it a suitable component of any aphasia treatment program regardless of the severity of linguistic impairment (Carlomagno, Losanno, Emanuelli, & Casadio, 1991).

Life Participation Approach to Aphasia (LPAA). (Elman & Bernstein-Ellis, 1999; Lyon, 1998; Simmons-Mackie, 2000, 2001). This approach broadens the functional/compensatory orientation to aphasia intervention. The overriding philosophy of LPAA is to maximize the client's re-engagement in life and base all therapeutic decision-making on the life concerns identified by clients and their families. Therapeutic goals are designed explicitly to help clients translate newly learned skills to everyday life experiences. The main emphases of this intervention model are that:

- All individuals with aphasia are entitled to receive services as needed at all stages of recovery.

- Both personal/intrinsic and environmental/extrinsic factors should be incorporated into therapeutic programming. These range on a continuum from obstructive to facilitative and should be identified on a case-by-case basis.

- Success is measured by documented changes in life areas defined as important by clients and their families.

In addition to these five specific intervention approaches, BASE-10 Programmed Stimulation (LaPointe, 1985) provides a general framework for data collection and record keeping within an operant conditioning paradigm of aphasia therapy. It involves the clear specification of therapy tasks, pretreatment baseline measures, and session-by-session recordings of client responses. BASE-10 Response Forms are used to document each of the following components of treatment:

- Tasks and their level of difficulty are determined by client performance on diagnostic/baseline measures and by degree of functionality and relevance to a client's daily life.

- Task criterion and response scoring can be binary in nature (e.g., correct versus incorrect) or multidimensional (e.g., an eight-point rating scale).

- Clinician then chooses 10 stimulus items that are likely to evoke the desired target behavior.

- Clinician employs key teaching strategies (see Chapter 1) to improve client performance on the selected 10 stimulus items.

- Reinforcement contingencies are systematically applied.

- A separate Response Form is used to chart progress on each task over 10 sessions.

The BASE-10 program provides a highly structured, systematic approach to stimulus selection and presentation. It also incorporates an ongoing visual record of daily progress. This allows the clinician to quickly identify any need for task modification and provides the client with concrete feedback regarding therapy performance. LaPointe (1985) suggests that programmed stimulation can be used with a wide range of philosophies and approaches to aphasia therapy.

In conclusion, although each of the six treatment procedures described represents a distinct approach to aphasia therapy, they are frequently used in combination with one another. When determining goals and criterion for therapy, consideration must be given to premorbid skills and level of functioning, including educational level, age of onset, intelligence, and so on. Finally, it is more important to identify individual strengths and weaknesses and to treat the presenting symptoms than to design treatment according to a diagnostic label.

Example Profiles

Below are three profiles representative of the communication problems exhibited by individuals with different types of aphasia (i.e., Wernicke's, Broca's, and global). These examples have been designed to illustrate the selection of intervention targets as well as specific therapy activities and materials. Most of the chosen activities can be implemented in either individual or group therapy settings.

PROFILE 1

Mr. Chang is a 39-year-old right-handed male who presented with a severe-profound fluent aphasia (Wernicke's) after sustaining a left parietal CVA nine months ago. His initial status was characterized by intelligible verbal output and frequent semantic and phonemic paraphasias. No evidence of dysarthria or apraxia of speech was observed. It was noted that the content of Mr. Chang's output was often unrelated to the topic at hand. He demonstrated severe word-retrieval difficulties and significant auditory comprehension deficits, including an inability to answer yes/no questions. Mr. Chang did not demonstrate the ability to point to objects, pictures, or body parts named, nor did he follow any single- or multiple-step commands. His automatic writing of the alphabet was incomplete, although Mr. Chang accurately wrote his name and the numbers 1 to 20. Reading comprehension was poor; he did demonstrate the ability to match written word stimuli to objects and pictures.

Mr. Chang received speech-language intervention services for several months poststroke. His current communication status is characterized by occasional semantic and phonemic paraphasias and moderate word-finding deficits. His auditory comprehension skills have improved; Mr. Chang correctly answers simple questions, identifies objects named by others, and inconsistently follows simple single-stage commands, such as, "Put the pencil next to the book." Writing is Mr. Chang's strongest communication modality as evidenced by his ability to write paragraph-length passages with minimal difficulty. Reading comprehension skills are also relatively strong in the areas of word recognition and sentence comprehension.

Mr. Chang's verbal description of the "cookie theft" picture from the *Boston Diagnostic Aphasia Examination* (Goodglass, Kaplan, & Barresi, 2000) is as follows:

> All right well there's a rolly dolly, whatever it is. And the dirl and be and the willy it fall and the fell and he fall down into the drom. And well the waver, water it's all out off for the end. And the mon, mother doing the dibs all the way and she's for the wauby be.

Selection of therapy targets. The areas to be targeted are word retrieval and auditory comprehension. These were selected for two main reasons. First, word retrieval and comprehension are Mr. Chang's most impaired language skills and continue to have the greatest negative impact on his ability to communicate effectively in everyday situations. Second, these areas have shown improvement with therapeutic intervention in the past, suggesting the potential for continued growth.

Sample Activities

1. Assemble a pile of 20 pictures of common objects and place them facedown on a table. Based on the PACE approach, explain that the clinician and client will take turns selecting pictures from the pile and describing them. Instruct the client to use any means of communication to convey the contents of each selected picture (e.g., verbal naming, verbal description of physical appearance of the object, pantomime the function of the object, draw the object, write the name of the object). Emphasize that the purpose of this activity is to successfully communicate the intended message rather than to retrieve a specific label. When a strategy is ineffective and results in listener confusion, encourage the client to reformulate the message using another communication mode. The clinician should use his or her turn as speaker to model various communication strategies. The client's communication effectiveness is measured by the clinician's ability to accurately identify the object pictured.

2. Identify a topic that is meaningful or of interest to the client (e.g., favorite hobby, job, family) and collect 25 identical pairs of picture cards that relate to this theme. Based on pretreatment baseline data, select two self-cuing strategies that will be taught to facilitate the client's retrieval of each verbal label (e.g., air tracing and sentence completion). Demonstrate each technique several times and ask the client to imitate these strategies. Shuffle the deck and deal seven cards to each player. Explain that the object of the activity is to make pairs for all the cards in a player's hand by asking the other player(s), "Do you have a _____?" Instruct the client to use one or both of the self-cuing strategies for every request. The clinician continues to model the tracing and sentence completion procedures during his or her turn.

3. Collect five common objects (e.g., pencil, book, cup, spoon, comb). With these objects in mind, develop a list of 20 single-stage commands that contain three linguistic units (e.g., "Put the *spoon* in the *cup*"; *Give me* the *book* and the *pencil*"). Place the objects on the table and explain that the client will be given short instructions involving the manipulation of the objects. Instruct the client to write down the first letter of each important word in the direction as a strategy to facilitate comprehension of the verbal command. If the client demonstrates significant difficulty, the clinician can implement the following modifications: (a) reduce speech rate during presentation of stimulus commands, (b) increase redundancy by stating each direction twice before the client responds, and (c) increase the acceptable latency period between the clinician's stimulus presentation and the initiation of the client's response. These strategies will provide the client with needed extra processing time and can be faded gradually as performance improves.

PROFILE 2

Mr. Sanders is a 63-year-old right-handed male who presented with a moderate-to-severe nonfluent aphasia (Broca's) after suffering a left frontal intercranial hemorrhage two months ago. Currently, Mr. Sanders's verbal output is characterized by one- and two-word utterances in which the subject noun phrase and verb phrase are often separated by distinctive pauses. His output consists mainly of content words with the frequent omission of grammatical markers. Significant word-retrieval difficulties are not noted. Ability to imitate verbal utterances is poor even at the single-word level. Mr. Sanders's output is pragmatically appropriate and reflects relatively intact comprehension of verbal material. He demonstrates the ability to identify many objects and pictures when named by the clinician and follows one- and two-step commands with minimal difficulty. Articulation is awkward and labored with phoneme distortion errors most prevalent. However, it was noted that Mr. Sanders consistently articulated his last name correctly. Minimal use of stress and intonation patterns results in a notable lack of speech melody. Writing skills are consistent with verbal output with regard to both vocabulary and syntax; reading comprehension skills are mildly impaired.

Mr. Sanders's verbal description of the "cookie theft" picture from the *Boston Diagnostic Aphasia Examination* (Goodglass, Kaplan, & Barresi, 2000) is as follows:

> uh . . . mother . . . uh . . . she talking to the . . . uh . . . the . . . uh . . . I don't know . . . two cup . . . cookie in jar . . . fall down . . . wash . . . and stool . . . uh . . . tipping . . . boy . . . uh . . . get hurt

Selection of therapy targets. The areas to be targeted are utterance length and syntactic complexity as well as speech prosody. Because the content and use components of Mr. Sanders's linguistic system are relatively intact, utterance length and complexity were chosen to improve the form component of his verbal repertoire. Speech prosody was targeted because it is an essential component of intelligibility. Improved function in this area will facilitate listeners' ability to predict the content of Mr. Sanders's messages despite his articulatory deficits.

Sample Activities

1. (For MIT Level II, Step 1). Arrange seating to ensure that the client can readily see the clinician's mouth. Select stimulus items for this level of MIT with the following considerations in mind: (a) the stimuli must be meaningful and useful to the individual client; (b) stimuli in this early stage of the program should include a heavy concentration of sounds that are easy to visualize (i.e., bilabials); (c) short simple phrases should be used (e.g., imperatives such as "Stand up," "Open the door"); and (d) an extensive list of high-probability items is necessary so that any given stimulus utterance is not presented too often. Following is a sample list of stimulus items for Mr. Sanders at this MIT level:

watch TV	salt and pepper
take a nap	good morning
bowl of soup	peach pie
make the bed	cup of coffee
read the paper	start the car

Graphically, plot the intonation patterns for each stimulus item before the session begins. (See the following example.)

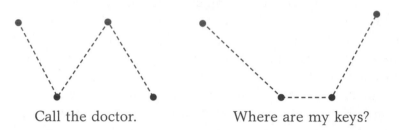

Call the doctor.   Where are my keys?

Set criteria for an acceptable response. The clinician takes the client's hand and hums the plotted intonation pattern for a stimulus while tapping the client's hand on the table once for each syllable. Next, the clinician intones (rather than hums) the same prosody pattern using words and continues to tap the client's hand once for each syllable. Avoid a staccato rhythm because continuous voicing facilitates verbal production. After a brief pause, repeat the intoned utterance with client hand tapping. Signal the client to join the clinician in unison repetition of the intoned phrase with assisted hand tapping. If the client's response is acceptable, carry this phrase to Step 2, in which the clinician fades the verbal model partway through the phrase so that the client must finish the utterance alone. The clinician continues to tap the rhythm with the client's hand. If the response is not adequate, pause for several seconds, choose the next item from the stimulus list and repeat the steps outlined previously. (For detailed information regarding the implementation of MIT, refer to Helm-Estabrooks & Albert, 2004; Sparks, 2001.)

2. Devise a list of 25 sentence pairs for a cloze task to train production of the regular plural form of nouns. Examples include the following:

> This is one book. These are two (*books*).
> He saw one cookie. He saw two (*cookies*).
> She washed a dish. She washed all the (*dishes*).
> I see the dog. I see lots of (*dogs*).
> The plant has one flower. This plant has many (*flowers*).

Gather two pictures that depict common objects for each sentence pair. One should contain a single exemplar of the object and the other multiple exemplars of the same object. Explain to the client that this activity focuses on the production of plural of nouns. Place the first pair of pictures on the table and demonstrate the activity by pointing to the singleton picture when saying the first sentence and pointing to the multiple picture while producing the second sentence with the correct plural noun form included. For the remaining sentence pairs, the clinician leaves the second sentence unfinished and instructs the client to complete the sentence fragment by supplying the plural noun form.

3. Create a conversational script like the following one according to the guidelines listed in Appendix 6-C.

   a. I can't watch the Orioles anymore.

b. This time they lost to Chicago.

c. And Chicago beat them by 10 runs.

d. They need to get a new coach.

Instruct the client to read the script aloud one sentence at a time. When the client encounters difficulties verbalizing the scripted information, suggest self-cuing strategies to facilitate production of the utterance. Examples include chunking utterances into shorter units, gesturing to convey meaning, and using techniques to trigger word retrieval. Next, videotape the client reading the script to a familiar listener who is unacquainted with its content. Coach the listener to concentrate on obtaining the gist of the message rather than focusing on specific words and details. The clinician, client, and familiar listener should evaluate the videotape according to the following parameters:

(1) How successful was the scripted interaction?

(2) What did the speaker/listener find most helpful?

(3) What did the speaker/listener find least helpful?

(4) What else could have been done by the client, listener, or clinician to facilitate the interaction?

Continue this cycle of coaching and evaluation with increasingly unfamiliar listeners.

4. Develop a list of 20 two-syllable word pairs that have dual intonation patterns. For these pairs, differential stress significantly affects meaning. Stress on the first syllable signals that the word functions as a noun, whereas stress on the second syllable indicates that the word is being used as a verb. Examples include the following:

present/pre**sent**	**con**tract/con**tract**
defect/de**fect**	**rec**ord/re**cord**
permit/per**mit**	**con**test/con**test**
convict/con**vict**	**ref**use/re**fuse**
produce/pro**duce**	**ob**ject/ob**ject**
rebel/re**bel**	**con**vert/con**vert**
contrast/con**trast**	**des**ert/de**sert**
discharge/dis**charge**	**proj**ect/pro**ject**
protest/pro**test**	**sub**ject/sub**ject**
survey/sur**vey**	**ad**dress/ad**dress**

Write each pair on a separate index card and underline or boldface the stressed syllable for each word. Develop a pair of questions or fill-in-the-blank statements for each word that are designed to elicit both noun and verb intonation patterns. For example, queries for the first pair might be: "What do you buy for somebody's birthday?" and "In honor of Frank Sinatra's great accomplishments, I now _____ him with this award." Instruct the client to choose one index card from the pile and practice both stress patterns in unison with the clinician. The clinician then presents the stimulus question/statement for the noun form and asks the client to look at the index card and spontaneously produce the target word with the appropriate stress pattern. Present the second question/statement to elicit the verb stress pattern indicated on the index card. Repeat this procedure for the remaining word pairs. Task difficulty can be increased by eliciting noun and verb forms in random order.

PROFILE 3

Mrs. Marshall is a 71-year-old right-handed female who presents with a global aphasia and a right hemiplegia and limb apraxia subsequent to a thrombosis of the middle cerebral artery resulting in extensive damage to the pre- and postrolandic areas six months ago. Her communicative status had not changed substantially since that time.

Currently, Mrs. Marshall demonstrates significant impairment in both language comprehension and language production in all modalities. She exhibits understanding of some simple yes/no questions, such as, "Is your name Polly?" and identifies body parts named by the clinician with approximately 50% accuracy. Mrs. Marshall does not appear to comprehend even simple one-step verbal commands. She relies heavily on nonverbal means to communicate, including facial expressions and head nods to indicate yes/no responses and a gross pointing gesture. Her speech output is limited to stereotypic utterances and neologisms that consist of both real and nonsense words. These are produced with differential stress and intonation and seem to express several communicative intentions. Reading comprehension is extremely poor even at the familiar single-word level. Writing skills are slightly better in that Mrs. Marshall can copy written words with occasional errors but does not exhibit the ability to generate legible written words spontaneously. Overall, she appears alert, attentive, and somewhat frustrated by her inability to communicate.

Mrs. Marshall's verbal description of the "cookie theft" picture from the *Boston Diagnostic Aphasia Examination* (Goodglass, Kaplan, & Barresi, 2000) is as follows:

> I can't. I don't think that . . . What is this? . . . I just don't have that. Oh yeah, right here. That's all.

Selection of therapy targets. Based on the severity of Mrs. Marshall's deficits, the areas to be targeted are auditory comprehension and functional communication skills. Auditory comprehension was chosen to establish a core receptive vocabulary that is meaningful within the context of her daily activities. Mrs. Marshall's verbal expression appears so limited that even after six months she does not represent a good candidate for intervention. Therefore, the compensatory approaches of PACE and Amer-Ind will be implemented to facilitate the effectiveness of her relatively stronger nonverbal communication skills. VAT was not considered an appropriate strategy for two reasons. First, the prescribed repertoire of gestural meanings was not deemed to be functional for Mrs. Marshall. Second, this approach requires the ability to perform a seven-way object and picture discrimination task as an initial level of training, which is clearly beyond her auditory comprehension abilities.

Sample Activities

1. Consult the client's family members and friends to identify vocabulary items that are most important to Mrs. Marshall. Items may include names of significant others, pets, favorite foods, terms for hobbies and other leisure interests (e.g., knitting, art, TV, and so on), frequently visited locations, and money terms. Select 20 of these items and gather large color pictures of each one (photographs are highly desirable). Complete the following three steps. Step 1: Place each picture card one at a time faceup on a table. Name each picture and then point to it to provide a model for the client. Step 2: Present each picture again, name it, and physically assist the client to point to the picture. Step 3: Place two pictures faceup on the table, name one, and signal the client to identify the target item by pointing. If the client experiences significant difficulty with the two-way discrimination task in Step 3, reduce the field to a single picture while still requiring a spontaneous pointing response.

2. Gather 25 colored photographs or easily recognizable pictures that depict activities or objects of daily living that are relevant for Mrs. Marshall. These may include brushing teeth, bathing, eating, sleeping, dressing, drinking, church, dentures, toilet, and doctor. Place the stack of pictures facedown on the table. Based on the PACE approach, select one picture from the pile and model several different strategies for communicating the contents of the picture to the client (e.g., verbal naming, description of activity/object characteristics, pantomime action or object function, drawing, rudimentary written cues). Repeat this modeling as necessary. Client and clinician take turns selecting pictures from the stack. The clinician should use his or her turn as speaker to emphasize that the purpose of this activity is to successfully communicate the intended meaning by whatever means possible rather than to elicit a particular lexical item. Encourage the client to reformulate a message using another communication strategy if the initial attempt is not successful. The client's ability to effectively convey messages is measured by the clinician's success in guessing the identity of the stimulus picture. It is important to recognize that the client's turn as listener requires an identification response. In the event that the client cannot provide a verbal label for the picture described by the clinician, an alternative response mode should be made available. This can be accomplished in the following manner: (a) provide a duplicate set of the 25 pictures; (b) display an array of three pictures, including the target and two foils; and (c) instruct the client to indicate the correct stimulus through pointing.

3. Identify three different communication situations that Mrs. Marshall encounters on a daily or weekly basis (e.g., neighbor visits, doctor appointments, and hairdressing appointments). From the concept illustration section in Skelly (1979), select five concrete and relevant Amer-Ind signals for each situation, such as the following:

Neighbor	*Doctor*	*Hairdresser*
hello/goodbye	pain	cut
sit	tired	okay
drink	medicine	comb
eat	nurse	thanks
walk	puzzled	money

(Mrs. Marshall's hemiplegia necessitates that the signals chosen can be executed with the left hand.)

Choose one scenario and gather objects and/or pictures that represent the signals to be trained. For the "neighbor" scenario, these might include a chair, a cup, a pretzel, a picture of people entering/leaving a room, and a picture of two women taking a walk. Demonstrate each signal with the corresponding object or picture several times. For example, the concept of "walk" is represented by the following signal: extend left arm in front of body with elbow at shoulder level; palm of hand is down and index/middle fingers are extended pointing down while the hand slowly advances to the right; the extended fingers alternate moving forward conveying the action of legs walking. Consult Skelly (1979) for explanations and visual illustrations of other Amer-Ind signals.

Place three of the referents on the table, model one of the signals, and encourage the client to identify the appropriate referent. Repeat this procedure until the client reliably recognizes the five target signals.

Place an object/picture on the table, model the corresponding gesture, and require the client to imitate it. If the client demonstrates difficulty with this task, provide physical assistance to shape the response. Once successful and unassisted imitation has been established for a given scenario, gradually fade the clinician's model and elicit more spontaneous and functional production of the signals through clinician questions or role playing.

Helpful Hints

1. Keep in mind that there is a basic hierarchy of difficulty with regard to picture difficulty. One can increase the complexity of a picture description task by progressing from object pictures to action pictures, to pictures denoting location, then to a series of pictures describing a logical sequence of events.

2. Remember that individuals with aphasia (particularly those of advanced age) often present with concomitant physical or emotional problems that may affect their ability to communicate. Poor performance on therapy tasks may not be attributable to the aphasia per se, but to any of several other factors, including hearing impairment, poor visual acuity or visual field deficits, medication imbalances or side effects, depression, and so on.

3. As a general rule, clients with auditory comprehension deficits benefit from substantial repetition and redundancy of verbal input.

4. Clinicians should consistently use a slower speech rate when interacting with clients with aphasia. Rate of speech may have a significant impact on these individuals' ability to process verbal information.

5. One unanimous comment from a survey of 50 recovered individuals with aphasia (Skelly, 1975) indicates that they understood much more of what was said in their presence and at a much earlier point in their recovery than the aphasia literature reports. Therefore, clinicians should ensure that their comments are respectful in both tone and content.

6. Individuals with global aphasia may benefit from the provision of a **communication book** that contains pictures of familiar objects, people, and events from their daily environment.

7. In the early stages of intervention, clinicians may have to rely heavily on yes/no questions to provide clients with a mechanism for expressing strong feelings of frustration, anxiety, or confusion.

8. Computerized programs for aphasia intervention are increasingly available from many sources. Clinicians are encouraged to seek out software with demonstrated efficacy or outcome data.

CONCLUSION

This section has presented basic information, protocols, and procedures for aphasia intervention at an introductory level. This material is intended only as a starting point in the reader's clinical education and training. For more in-depth coverage of this area, the following readings are recommended:

Brookshire, R. H. (2002). *An introduction to neurogenic communication disorders.* St. Louis, MO: Mosby-Year Book.

Chapey, R. (2001). *Language intervention strategies in aphasia and related neurogenic communication disorders.* Baltimore: Lippincott Williams & Wilkins.

Elman, R. J. (1999). *Group treatment of neurogenic communication disorders: The expert clinician's approach.* Woburn, MA: Butterworth-Heinemann.

Helm-Estabrooks, N., & Holland, A. (1998). *Approaches to the treatment of aphasia.* San Diego, CA: Singular Publishing Group.

Johns, D. F. (1985). *Clinical management of neurogenic communicative disorders.* Boston: Little, Brown.

Marshall, R. C. (1998). *Introduction to group treatment for aphasia: Design and management.* San Diego, CA: Elsevier.

Tanner, D. C. (1999). *The family guide to surviving stroke and communication disorders.* Needham Heights, MA: Allyn & Bacon.

U.S. Department of Health and Human Services. (1995). *Recovering after a stroke.* Washington, DC: U.S. Goverment Printing Office.

TREATMENT FOR MOTOR SPEECH DISORDERS

The optimal goal of therapy for motor speech disorders is to improve intelligibility within the limits of a client's neurological impairment. Articulation and prosody interact to exert a powerful influence on speech intelligibility. For this reason, therapy designed to improve intelligibility focuses primarily on the modification of these two parameters. Intervention tasks in this paradigm are programmed to progress along a continuum of difficulty from simple automatic responses (e.g., counting from 1 to 10) to more volitional and complex behaviors (e.g., responding to a question such as "What did you do last evening?"). Each client's unique characteristics will determine the most appropriate starting point along this continuum. In general, it is recommended that treatment be initiated as soon as possible to discourage a client's tendency to develop undesirable compensatory speech behaviors (e.g., pharyngeal fricatives).

The concept of drill is fundamental to any therapy program that seeks to directly modify motor speech behaviors in any of the communication subsystems (respiration, resonance, phonation, articulation, prosody). Because speech is a complex motor skill, intense repetitive practice is more successful in changing this behavior than a therapy approach that relies on cognitive learning (e.g., explanation, modeling). Drill activities are most effective when a single presentation of a stimulus is followed by multiple productions of the target response by the client. Re-presenting the stimulus to elicit each production breaks the cycle of the motor learning chain (Darley, Aronson, & Brown, 1975).

In some cases, improved speech intelligibility may not be a realistic goal. Certain neurologic conditions such as Parkinson's disease and multiple sclerosis are progressive and require that the treatment be aimed at slowing down the gradual deterioration of a client's speech. Sometimes the dysarthria is so severe or the disease process is so rapidly degenerative that speech cannot be the primary mode of communication. With these clients, the main goal of therapy is to provide a functional alternative method of conveying messages. This may include use of gestures, communication boards, or speech synthesizers.

THE DYSARTHRIAS

The dysarthrias represent a group of related motor speech disorders characterized by impaired muscular control over the speech mechanism as a result of central or peripheral nervous system damage. Apraxia is a deficit in the planning and sequencing of movement; dysarthria represents impaired ability to execute motor movement. Clients with either of these disorders will demonstrate inaccurate and/or labored performance on tasks that require rapid, repetitive movement of the articulators such as diadochokinesis (see Appendix 6-D for normative diadochokinetic rates).

The lack of neurological control with dysarthria can affect the motor speech subsystems of respiration, phonation, resonance, articulation, and prosody. Unlike apraxia, the dysarthrias involve paralysis, weakness, decreased tone, or incoordination of the speech musculature. Muscles can be impaired with respect to range, direction, strength, endurance, speed, or timing. Dysarthria can be manifested as a paucity or excess of any of these parameters (e.g., reduced range of motion versus involuntary or uninhibited movement). Dysarthria is a consequence of damage to the cortex, cerebellum, brainstem, or peripheral nervous system. Of particular significance are the cranial nerves, which consist of 12 pairs of neuron bundles emerging from the brainstem. See Table 6-4 for a list of the cranial nerves and

TABLE 6-4
Cranial Nerves

Nerve		Function	Type
I	Olfactory	Smell, taste	Sensory
II	Optic	Vision	Sensory
III	Oculomotor	Eye, eyelid, and pupil movement	Motor
IV	Trochlear	Eye movement	Motor
V	Trigeminal	Jaw movement; sensation from jaw, face, and mouth	Mixed
VI	Abducens	Eye movement	Motor
VII	Facial	Facial movement; sensation from anterior tongue	Mixed
VIII	Acoustic (vestibulocochlear)	Balance; hearing	Sensory
IX	Glossopharyngeal	Pharyngeal and palatal movement; sensation from posterior tongue	Mixed
X	Vagus	Movement and sensation from larynx, pharynx, esophagus, and internal organs; branches into inferior and superior laryngeal nerves	Mixed
XI	Spinal accessory	Larynx, chest, shoulder, and neck movement	Motor
XII	Hypoglossal	Tongue movement	Motor

Sources: Adapted from Brookshire (2003) and Duffy (1995).

their function. The major causes of dysarthrias include stroke, brain tumors, head trauma, toxins, and neuromuscular diseases, many of which are degenerative (e.g., Parkinson's, multiple sclerosis, myasthenia gravis). The degree of impairment secondary to dysarthria can range in severity from quite mild to devastatingly profound.

Impairment of the articulators (lips, tongue, mandible, velum) has a greater negative impact on speech intelligibility than disruptions of the respiratory or laryngeal systems. In dysarthria, the primary contributors to reduced intelligibility are distorted or omitted consonants and vowels, prolonged phonemes, and erratic articulation performance (Rosenbek & LaPointe, 1985).

Classification of the Dysarthrias

The most frequently cited classification system for the dysarthrias is based on the Mayo Clinic research studies conducted by Darley, Aronson, and Brown (1969a, 1969b, 1975). This work has resulted in the identification of the following seven major types of dysarthria based on differential patterns of neurological impairment and associated speech characteristics: (1) flaccid, (2) spastic, (3) ataxic, (4) hypokinetic, (5) hyperkinetic, (6) mixed, and (7) unilateral upper motor neuron. Table 6-5 presents a comparative outline of the dysarthrias.

TABLE 6-5
Classification of the Dysarthrias

Type	Cause	Site of Lesion	Neuromuscular Status	Speech Characteristics
Flaccid	Bulbar palsy; myasthenia gravis	Lower motor neuron	Weakness; low muscle tone	Indistinct and labored articulation; hypernasality; breathy voice quality
Spastic	Pseudobulbar palsy	Upper motor neuron	Increased muscle tone; reduced range of motion, strength, and speed	Slow, imprecise articulation; hypernasality; strained, strangled, harsh voice quality; monotonous pitch and loudness; short phrasing
Ataxic	Cerebellar disorders	Cerebellum	Inaccurate range, timing, and direction; low muscle tone; reduced speed of movement	Excess and equal stress; irregular articulatory breakdown; slow, inaccurate articulation; rhythm disturbances; phoneme prolongations; some excess loudness
Hypokinetic	Parkinsonism	Extrapyramidal (substantia nigra)	Markedly reduced range and speed of movement; marked muscle rigidity; rest tremors	Monopitch and monoloudness; slow speaking rate with short rushes of speech; long, inappropriate pauses; articulation accuracy fluctuates greatly
Hyperkinetic				
Quick	Chorea; Tourette's syndrome; Huntington's chorea	Extrapyramidal	Rapid, jerky, uncontrolled tic movements	Imprecise articulation; variable rate and loudness; harsh voice; inappropriate pauses; abrupt grunts and barks
Slow	Athetosis; dystonia; dyskinesia	Extrapyramidal	Slow, twisting, writhing movements and postures; variable muscle tone	Irregular articulatory breakdown; monopitch and monoloudness; harsh voice quality
Tremor	Organic voice tremor; myoclonus	Extrapyramidal	Involuntary, rhythmic movements	Voice tremors with rhythmic phonation breaks; choked-strained voice quality
Mixed	Amyotrophic lateral sclerosis (ALS); multiple sclerosis (MS); Wilson's disease	Multiple motor systems	Muscular weakness; reduced range and speed of motion; some intention tremors	ALS: severely defective articulation; slow rate; noticeable hypernasality; harsh voice quality; marked prosodic disturbances. MS: harsh voice quality; inconsistent rate and articulatory precision. Wilson's disease: similar to hypokinetic dysarthria without sudden bursts of speech
Unilateral upper motor neuron	Stroke	Posterior frontal lobe	Lower facial weakness; hemiparesis	Imprecise consonants; irregular articulatory breakdown; harsh voice

Sources: Adapted from Wertz (1985), Rosenbek & LaPointe (1985), Dworkin (1991), and Freed (2000).

No spontaneous recovery is associated with certain dysarthria etiologies, such as amytrophic lateral sclerosis (ALS), Parkinson's disease, and Huntington's chorea. However, some neuromuscular diseases, such as multiple sclerosis, do exhibit periods of remission in which symptoms abate. Prognosis for individuals with dysarthria is affected by many of the same variables that are associated with aphasia and apraxia recovery. In addition, there are two dysarthria-specific factors that significantly influence prognosis: (1) if the underlying neuropathology of the dysarthria involves a degenerative disease process, the prognosis for significant improvement is poor; and (2) the existence of a severe co-occurring aphasia will interfere with a client's ability to benefit from dysarthria therapy.

Treatment Efficacy

Experimental and clinical evidence indicates that therapeutic intervention is generally effective for individuals with dysarthria. Yorkston's (1996) and Kent's (2000) summaries of group-treatment studies, single-subject studies, and case profiles offer the following conclusions regarding treatment efficacy with various types of dysarthria:

- Individuals with Parkinson's disease derive greater benefit from treatment that targets both respiratory and phonatory function than treatment that focuses on respiratory function alone.

- A variety of behavioral therapy approaches are effective for individuals with stroke or traumatic brain injury, including feedback of acoustic information, respiratory and speech rate control, and physiological strategies such as biofeedback and reaction times.

- Devices such as palatal lifts result in gains in muscle strength and speech intelligibility for individuals with stroke or traumatic brain injury.

- Further research is needed to determine which intervention approaches are best suited for various types of dysarthria. Treatment studies using randomized clinical trials are required to generate reliable and valid efficacy/outcome information.

- Advanced measurement techniques such as neuroimaging should be increasingly utilized in efficacy studies with larger patient populations.

Treatment for the Dysarthrias

The overall goal of dysarthria therapy is to improve intelligibility and, if possible, speech motor control. Ultimately, goal setting is influenced by the type and degree of dysarthric impairment. For severely impaired individuals, establishing functional communication through the use of augmentative or alternative systems may be the focus of intervention. In contrast, the aim of therapy for clients with mild dysarthrias is to reestablish speech patterns that closely approximate normal production.

Types of Treatment. As outlined in Table 6-5, there are several different types of dysarthria with distinctive speech symptoms. However, the basic issues and approaches to treatment are similar across the dysarthria classifications. In general, there are four basic approaches to dysarthria therapy:

1. **Behavior modification:** The traditional approach in which progressively more difficult activities and feedback are used to improve client performance on nonspeech and speech tasks. This may include use of verbal reinforcement, metronome pacing, biofeedback, delayed auditory feedback, and pacing boards. Biofeedback involves electronic monitoring devices that are used to help a client gain some voluntary control over previously unconscious body functions such as respiration, nasality, and extraneous oral movements. Delayed auditory feedback (DAF) is a system in which a client's words are returned to him or her through headphones after an imposed electronic delay of a few milliseconds. A pacing board (Helm, 1979) is a series of divided colored squares used to reduce speech rate by requiring a client to touch one square per syllable or word uttered.

2. **Prosthetic devices:** The use of an artificial device or appliance to replace the function of a missing or impaired part of the speech mechanism. The most common prosthesis used in the treatment of dysarthria is a palatal lift. This is a mechanical device that elevates the soft palate toward the posterior pharyngeal wall to decrease hypernasal resonance in clients with velopharyngeal incompetence.

3. **Medical and surgical procedures:** The use of drugs and/or surgical procedures to ameliorate deficiencies in the speech production system. Pharyngeal flap and phonosurgery are examples of surgical intervention approaches. Pharyngeal flap surgery joins soft tissue from the posterior pharyngeal wall to the soft palate to improve velopharyngeal closure during speech. This procedure is used primarily with hypernasal clients for whom behavioral therapy and prosthetic interventions have been unsuccessful. There are three types of phonosurgery associated with treatment for unilateral vocal fold paralysis or paresis. These include (a) Teflon® or Gelfoam® injection in which material is injected into the compromised fold to increase its bulk. The additional mass shortens the distance that the healthy fold must travel across midline to make contact with the paralyzed fold; (b) repositioning of the impaired fold toward midline through surgical insertion of a plastic implant; and (c) reinnervation of the thyroarytenoid muscle through implantation of a nerve-muscle pedicle taken from an intact omohyoid muscle. (See Tucker, 1993, for detailed discussion of phonosurgical procedures.)

    Recently, intervention for parkinsonian-like disorders has included neurosurgical techniques such as *pallidotomy* which involves surgical sectioning of the globus pallidus (a portion of the basal ganglia). This procedure is designed to reduce major movement abnormalities by releasing inhibition in the thalamic and brainstem centers. With respect to speech, this surgical procedure has shown some positive impact on the phonatory and articulatory characteristics of patients with hypokinetic dysarthria (Schulz, Greer, & Freedman, 2000; Schulz, Peterson, Sapienza, Greer, & Freedman, 1999).

4. **Augmentative/alternative devices:** The use of a nonvocal mode of communication to supplement or replace speech. These may include communication boards, alphabet boards, gestural systems, computers, and speech synthesizers.

Dysarthria is an impairment that may affect all motor speech subsystems. Treatment of dysarthria is generally based on the hierarchical organization of these subsystems: respiration, phonation, resonance, articulation, and prosody. Following is a brief discussion of basic treatment programming for each of the subsystems.

Respiratory Subsystem. The main respiratory problem of clients with dysarthria is inefficient use of the breath stream for speech, rather than a reduction of vital capacity (total volume of air in the lungs). (Note: The normal rate of respiration is 16 breaths per minute.) The goal of intervention for this subsystem is to establish consistent, controlled exhalation of air to support speech production. Following is one basic treatment progression for behavioral training:

1. Establish a stable base for respiratory function through muscle relaxation and adjustments of body posture. For example, (a) progressive relaxation techniques (see Table 7-1) can be used to decrease muscle stiffness; (b) a supine (lying faceup) position may facilitate loudness. (Note: Modifications of posture and seating should always be implemented in consultation with other health care professionals such as physical therapists, occupational therapists, or physicians).
2. Decrease shallow inhalation and improve control of sustained exhalation by manipulating inspiratory and expiratory cycles in nonspeech breathing. For example, (a) ask the client to take a deep breath and hold it as long as possible while the clinician applies light counterpressure on the abdominal wall; (b) provide visual feedback of client's exhalatory pressure and duration through the use of devices such as manometers or oscilloscopes.
3. Further improve exhalatory control by establishing adequate loudness and voice quality while producing speech of increasing length and duration (beginning with isolated phonemes and progressing gradually to longer segments). For example, (a) ask client to produce and sustain a single phoneme (e.g., /s/) for as long as possible, gradually progress to consonant series (e.g., /s-s-s-s-s/), and add vowels and other consonants (e.g., /sa/, /sap/); (b) practice sound sequences with varying patterns of loudness, stress, and intonation, progressing systematically to the level of conversation.

Phonatory Subsystem. Individuals with dysarthria exhibit a wide range of phonatory abnormalities, which vary according to dysarthria type and underlying neurological damage. These problems can be classified into three main patterns of vocal fold movement: hyperadduction, hypoadduction, and incoordination. Hyperadduction refers to excessive laryngeal tension and overly forceful closure of the vocal folds, which produces a harsh or strained-strangled voice quality. Hypoadduction involves reduced laryngeal muscle tension and inadequate closure of the vocal folds, resulting in a breathy, hoarse voice quality with decreased loudness and pitch control. Incoordination can be defined as inconsistent fluctuations of vocal fold vibration cycles and can result in aphonia (no voice), asynchronous onset of exhalation and phonation, and inappropriate pitch and loudness breaks. In general, hyperadduction and incoordination of vocal fold movement have less overall impact on speech intelligibility than hypoadduction and are usually not the primary intervention targets for this subsystem.

The aim of intervention for hypoadduction is to achieve efficient vocal fold closure during speech. This goal may be accomplished through phonosurgical procedures or behavioral training. A behavioral training approach can proceed according to the following sequence:

1. Increase control of glottal closure through sustained breath holding. For example, instruct the client to take a deep breath and hold it for as long as possible with a closed-mouth posture.
2. Improve voluntary control of vocal fold abduction-adduction through physical maneuvers that elicit glottal closure (e.g., lifting, pushing, and pulling). For example, (a) instruct the client to assume a seated position, exhale slowly, and at each clinician signal, pull up as hard as possible on the sides of the seat while deliberately attempting to stop the exhalation; (b) introduce phonation by asking the client to produce /a/ at a comfortable loudness level on exhalation and employ the glottal closure maneuver described previously on each clinician signal.
3. Refine the client's control of vocal fold valving through the use of a continuum of speech activities. For example, (a) ask the client to use a physical maneuver to induce reflexive glottal closure (e.g., pull up on the seat) and, on clinician instruction, release glottal closure and produce an isolated vowel with a hard phonatory attack; (b) repeat this procedure with speech stimuli of increasing length and duration (e.g., syllable, word, phrase, sentence, conversation).

Resonance Subsystem. The two main symptoms of dysarthric impairment in this subsystem are hypernasality and accompanying nasal air emission due to impairment of the velopharyngeal musculature. The overall goal of intervention for resonance problems is to decrease hypernasality through the use of procedures designed to improve a client's ability to generate intraoral air pressure. Behavioral, prosthetic, and surgical approaches can be used to accomplish this goal. A behavioral regimen is most effective with clients who demonstrate mild resonance problems. Following is a basic behavioral treatment sequence:

1. Improve awareness of the degree of nasal resonance through the use of biofeedback devices. For example, instruct the client to produce single sustained vowels alternating between greater and lesser degrees of jaw opening, while using an instrument that measures and visually displays the differential amounts of nasal resonance.
2. Improve ability to generate intraoral air pressure during production of CV syllables that contain initial plosives. For example, instruct the client to alternately produce pairs of CV syllables that differ in the nasality of the initial consonant (e.g., me/be; no/go; my/pie).

3. Further refine control of velopharyngeal function during connected speech using biofeedback information. For example, instruct the client to maintain the target range of resonance while producing speech of increasing length and complexity (i.e., isolated words, short phrases, sentences, conversational speech).

For clients with moderate to severe impairments that significantly impact on speech intelligibility, a prosthetic or surgical approach may be recommended. A palatal lift is considered a reasonable treatment alternative under the following conditions: relatively isolated paresis or paralysis of the velum, lack of excessive spasticity or increased reflex activity in the velopharyngeal area, and adequate dentition to anchor the appliance. Pharyngeal flap surgery is generally instituted when behavioral and/or palatal lift approaches have been unsuccessful and when an adequate degree of lateral pharyngeal wall movement is available (see Dworkin, 1991; Freed, 2000; and Yorkston, Beukelman, & Bell, 1988, for detailed discussions of these procedures). Prosthetic and surgical interventions usually do not result in the restoration of "normal" function. Improvements gained from a palatal lift or pharyngeal flap must be considered in relation to a client's comorbid impairments in other speech subsystems.

Articulatory Subsystem. The overriding aim of articulation therapy for clients with dysarthria is to achieve improved speech sound production within the constraints of the underlying neuromuscular impairment. Intervention for the dysarthrias is similar to traditional articulation therapy with respect to both programming and procedures. However, the neuromuscular involvement associated with dysarthria necessitates an additional emphasis on oral-motor training. The following strategies can be used to facilitate improved function in the articulation subsystem:

1. Oral motor exercises to normalize muscle tone and increase strength and mobility of articulatory musculature (e.g., lip retraction and pursing, tongue elevation and depression, jaw opening and closing)
2. Phonetic placement through explanation, modeling, and tactile stimulation of correct positioning of the articulators (see Appendix 3-A and Dworkin, 1991, for specific training activities)
3. Phonetic shaping that entails the use of intact articulatory movements associated with one phoneme (e.g., /t/) to shape a different phoneme (e.g., /n/)
4. Overarticulation of speech sounds through exaggeration of some characteristic feature of a specific phoneme (e.g., aspiration, stridency, voicing) or the exaggerated production of a particular consonant in medial or final word position (e.g., ho*t*el, ha*pp*en, so*ck*, mu*d*)
5. Negative practice through the use of minimal pair stimuli (e.g., mat/pat, mob/mop; cook/took)

The pattern of articulatory errors, and therefore the specific targets selected for treatment, will vary according to the type of dysarthria. One basic sequence that can be considered in the selection of articulation targets mirrors the order of phoneme acquisition with regard to place of articulation. Therapy may begin with vowels and progress from bilabials → labio-dentals → lingua-dentals → lingua-alveolars → lingua-velars and culminate with lingua-palatals.

The following task hierarchy can be used to train identified phoneme targets (e.g., /b/) (LaPointe & Katz, 2002):

Final position of VC syllables:	/ab/
Final position of CVC syllables:	/tab/
Medial position of VCV syllables:	/aba/
Initial position of CV syllables:	/ba/
Initial position of CVC syllables:	/bag/

Varying positions in multisyllablic words and short phrases

Varying positions in sentences and conversational speech

Some clients with dysarthria may experience extreme difficulty producing particular phonemes (e.g., those that require tongue tip elevation). In such cases, it may be necessary to begin articulation therapy at the isolated phoneme level and/or develop compensatory movements to produce adequate approximations of these speech sounds.

Prosody Subsystem. The speech of clients with dysarthria is often characterized by prosodic and suprasegmental disturbances. Common manifestations include monopitch, monoloudness, excess and equal stress on each word, inappropriate phrasing and intonation contour patterns, and a tendency to attempt maintenance of premorbid speech rate although it is no longer appropriate. (Note: The normal speaking rate for adults is 150 to 250 words per minute or 4.4 to 5.9 syllables per second [Goldman-Eisler, 1968]. See Table 6-6 for comparative data regarding normal speech rate). The ultimate aim of intervention with any symptom in this subsystem is to increase a client's overall speech intelligibility. Following are basic intervention strategies for prosody problems:

1. Improve stress and intonation patterns through contrastive drills. This technique employs identical pairs of stimuli that change in emphasis or meaning as a result of differences solely in stress or intonation. Compound words, sentences, or longer units of connected language can be used. For example, "black board" versus "**blackboard**"; "Bill likes **baseball**" versus "**Bill** likes baseball"; or "Bill likes baseball" versus "Bill likes baseball?".
2. Reduce monopitch and monoloudness through the use of negative practice drills. In this procedure, a client is required to intentionally produce a target behavior using a habitual error pattern, thus highlighting the contrast between the habitual error and the desired response. For example, instruct the client to alternate between habitual and target productions of word pairs with respect to pitch or loudness (e.g., movie versus MOVIE). Stimuli can be systematically programmed to include more complex units of language. Negative practice drills can be used to highlight any aspect of prosody.

TABLE 6-6
Normal Speaking Rates for Adults and Children

Task	Average Speaking Rate	Study
Adults		
Uninterrupted discourse	220–240 words per min (wpm)	Weiner (1984)
Conversational speech	270 wpm 4.4–5.9 syllables per sec (sps)	Calvert & Silverman (1983) Goldman-Eisler (1961)
Oral reading	160–180 wpm 150–190 wpm	Calvert & Silverman (1983) Darley & Spriestersbach (1978)
Responses to questions	115–165 wpm 150–250 wpm	Andrews & Ingham (1971) Goldman-Eisler (1968)
Children		
Responses to questions	3 years: 116–163 syllables per min (spm) 4 years: 117–183 spm 5 years: 109–183 spm	Pindzola, Jenkins, & Lokken (1989)
Conversational speech	1st grade: 125 wpm 5th grade: 142 wpm	Purcell & Runyan (1980)

Note: Discrepancies in speaking rates are due to variations in calculation methods (e.g., wpm versus sps) and task differences.

3. Modify speaking rate through manipulation of the number and duration of pauses rather than attempting to alter the articulatory movements required for speech sound production. This can be accomplished through the use of metronomes, pacing boards, DAF, or tapping. In each of these strategies, the client modifies habitual speech rate by producing each syllable or word in unison with the imposed beat or tempo. Speech rate also can be modified by requiring the client to write the initial letter of each word uttered.

Example Profiles

Following are three profiles that characterize the speech disturbances exhibited by individuals with different types of dysarthria (i.e., flaccid, hypokinetic, and ataxic). These examples have been designed to illustrate the selection of intervention targets as well as specific therapy activities and materials. Most of the chosen activities can be implemented in either individual or group therapy settings.

PROFILE 1

Mr. Patel, a 75-year-old male, suffered a brainstem stroke two weeks ago. He presents with mild paresis of all limbs, intact receptive and expressive language skills, and a moderate flaccid dysarthria. Assessment of the speech musculature indicates reduced strength and range of motion of the velum, tongue, and lips. Laryngeal movement is judged to be less affected. Respiratory support for speech appears to be within normal limits as measured by his ability to adequately sustain the vowel /a/. Mr. Patel's speech output is characterized by marked hypernasality; breathy voice quality; and slowed, labored articulation. The prosodic features of Mr. Patel's speech are unremarkable. Overall speech intelligibility is rated as 50% to 65% when the context is unknown to the listener.

Selection of therapy targets. The subsystems to be targeted for therapy are resonance, articulation, and prosody. The first two areas were selected because the degree of Mr. Patel's hypernasality and imprecise articulation contributes most significantly to a reduction in perceived speech intelligibility. In the area of prosody, Mr. Patel's habitual speech rate can be reduced in an attempt to improve intelligibility.

Sample Activities

1. Employ a Nasometer, which is a computerized instrument that calculates and visually displays the ratio of nasal versus nasal + oral acoustic energy. (Consult Nasometer Instruction Manual; Kay Elemetrics Corporation, Pine Brook, New Jersey). Develop a list of 80 stimuli that include 20 CV, VC, CVC, and VCV syllables containing low or mid vowels and liquid consonants (e.g., CV: *yo* and *ro*; VC: *all* and *air*; CVC: *war, roll*; VCV: *olo* and *airo*). Set the threshold line on the Nasometer to indicate an acceptable percentage of nasal resonance. Instruct the client to produce each syllable three times while closely watching the computer screen. Explain that the visual display of the client's valving behavior should consistently fall within the targeted range of resonance. The threshold line can be reduced in 5% steps as the client demonstrates increased mastery of velopharyngeal valving. If the client has difficulty achieving success at a particular percentage level, the threshold line can be raised 10%.

2. Instruct the client to elevate the tongue tip to the alveolar ridge and then raise the tongue tip outside the mouth beyond the upper lip. Provide a mirror for visual feedback. Repeat this elevation movement pattern three times and then pause. Continue the activity by gradually increasing the number of repetitions between each pause. To strengthen this lingual movement, use a tongue depressor to push against the tongue tip to provide resistance that the client must overcome during tongue elevation.

3. Make a list of 25 sentences, 7 to 10 words in length, and type them on a sheet of paper. Double space the sentences and leave large spaces between the words in each sentence. Sample sentences include the following:

   I really enjoyed my vacation last month.

   I don't know what you mean by that.

   The people are walking in the park.

Sometimes I watch TV in the evening.

Do you want spaghetti for dinner tonight?

My family visited the museum in London last year.

I saw your wife at the store yesterday.

What time do you usually get home from work?

I am sad to hear that you are not coming.

I heard that there is a big sale at the mall.

Cut a slit in the center of a piece of paper with the approximate dimensions of a 12-inch ruler. The size of the slit should correspond to the length and height of the longest word in the sentence set (e.g., spaghetti or yesterday). The clinician places the slit card over the first sentence and moves it slowly across the paper. Instruct the client to read each word aloud as it is revealed by the slit in the card. After each sentence is completed, remove the card and instruct the client to read the sentence again, maintaining the slowed speech rate of the first production.

PROFILE 2

Mrs. Fields, a 58-year-old female, presents with a moderate hypokinetic dysarthria secondary to Parkinson's disease. Her overall status (including speech musculature) is characterized by muscle rigidity, limited range of movement, and rest tremors (involuntary, rhythmic movements exhibited when muscles are at rest). Voice quality is breathy with monopitch and decreased loudness due to limited capacity and control of the respiratory musculature. Resonance is judged to be unaffected. Mrs. Fields's articulatory precision is mildly to moderately affected and is marked by short bursts of hurried speech separated by grammatically inappropriate and abrupt pauses. She demonstrates reduced prosody of speech. Her speech intelligibility is rated as moderately unintelligible, primarily as a result of vocal abnormalities with a more modest contribution from her articulation errors. Language abilities appear to be within normal limits.

Selection of therapy targets. The areas to be targeted are the respiratory, phonatory, and articulatory subsystems. These were selected according to the subsystem hierarchy. The first two were chosen based on Mrs. Fields's presenting vocal symptoms of breathiness and reduced pitch and loudness. The third was targeted in an effort to increase her intelligibility to its maximum level. Respiration was selected as the initial focus of therapy because it serves as the foundation for all other speech subsystems.

Sample Activities

1. Instruct the client to inhale deeply and hold the breath as the clinician slowly counts to three. Tell the client to exhale slowly while producing rhythmic patterns of a voiceless fricative (e.g., /s/). Sound productions of long and

short duration comprise the rhythmic patterns. Following are sample series
(_____ = long sound; __ = short sound):

__ ____ __ ____ __ ____

____ __ __ ____ __ __ ____

____ ____ __ ____ ____ __

__ __ __ ____ __ __ __ ____

____ __ ____ __ ____ __

Remind the client that each series must be produced on a single exhalation. This activity can be implemented with any rhythmic pattern and can be extended to gradually introduce additional voiceless fricatives such as /f/, /θ/ and /ʃ/.

2. Write the numbers 1 to 10 on 20 index cards. Highlight various combinations of numbers on each card by using bold print or type. Instruct the client to read the digit series on each card with increased loudness on the boldface numbers. Sit within five feet of the client and encourage her to project her voice without excessive muscular tension. Use the following series:

1 **2** 3 4 5 **6** 7 **8** 9 **10**

1 2 **3** 4 5 **6** 7 8 **9** 10

1 2 **3** **4** 5 6 **7** **8** 9 10

1 2 3 **4** **5** **6** 7 8 **9** **10**

1 **2** **3** 4 5 **6** **7** **8** 9 10

Increase the level of difficulty of this activity by gradually expanding the distance between the client and clinician.

3. Identify the client's articulation errors that result from limited range and strength of the oral musculature. Develop compensatory phonetic placements that effect acceptable approximations of the target sounds. Examples include the following:

Error Sound	Compensatory Placement
/p,b/	Place upper teeth on lower lip and abruptly drop the lower jaw to produce the desired plosive air burst.
/m/	Touch upper teeth to lower lip and produce sound with nasal resonance.
/t,d,l,s,z,n/	Elevate tongue blade to touch alveolar ridge while maintaining tongue tip in lower position.

PROFILE 3

Mr. Seymour, a 45-year-old male, presents with a mild to moderate ataxic dysarthria as a result of a tumor that caused localized damage to the cerebellum. His current condition is marked by hypotonia, slow and jerky voluntary movements, and inaccurate direction of movement. Mr. Seymour's breath support for speech appears to be adequate. His voice quality, although slightly harsh and monotone, is judged to be within normal limits. Resonance is unremarkable. In spontaneous speech, Mr. Seymour exhibits transient articulatory breakdown characterized by imprecise consonants and distorted vowels, prolongations of phonemes, and dysprosody of speech due to excess and equal stress of syllables and words. Overall speech intelligibility is rated at approximately 65% to 75% when the context is unknown to the listener.

Selection of therapy targets. The areas to be targeted are articulation and prosody. These were selected because Mr. Seymour's reduced speech intelligibility is caused primarily by deficits in these two subsystems.

Sample Activities

1. Develop three word lists for an intelligibility drill, each of which contains 10 CVC words that are similar except for a single phoneme. Sample word lists follow:

Paul	beer	ban
ball	dear	pan
call	fear	can
mall	near	man
small	cheer	ran
stall	tear	Dan
fall	gear	tan
tall	we're	span
hall	hear	fan
wall	mere	van

   Print each word on an index card and shuffle the cards so that the words are in random order. Instruct the client to select a card from the deck, keeping it out of the clinician's visual field, and read it aloud. The clinician is naive to the specific word being produced and must guess the identity of the utterance based solely on the client's intelligibility. The client indicates the accuracy of the clinician guess. If the clinician's first guess is incorrect, the client repeats the target word once. If the clinician's second guess is erroneous, the clinician reads the index card and models the correct production of the word. The client imitates this model five times, returns the index card to the pile, and draws another card.

2. Develop a set of 25 identical sentence pairs that contain at least a subject, verb, and object. Write each pair on a separate index card and underline or boldface a different word in each sentence. Explain that this activity focuses on the ways in which changes in prosody affect sentence meaning. Further explain that the clinician will ask a stimulus question that the client must answer by reading aloud the prosodically appropriate sentence from a corresponding index card. Instruct the client to choose one index card, listen to the

stimulus question, and read aloud the correct version using exaggerated intonation to highlight the bold word. Examples of stimulus questions and response sentences include the following:

Question	Response
What did you open?	I opened the **door**.
What did you do?	I **opened** the door.
Did she read the letter?	She **wrote** the letter.
Who wrote the letter?	**She** wrote the letter.
Whose car is John driving tomorrow?	John is driving **my** car tomorrow.
Is Phil driving your car tomorrow?	**John** is driving my car tomorrow.
What dance is Sadie doing?	Sadie is dancing the **tango** with Mel.
Who is she dancing with?	Sadie is dancing the tango with **Mel**.
Does Tom call Judy often?	Tom **always** calls Judy on her birthday.
When does Tom call Judy?	Tom always calls Judy on her **birthday**.

3. Gather several reading passages and highlight the syllables and words that receive primary stress. (**Note:** Stress patterns may vary according to regional dialect.) Instruct the client to read each passage aloud while concentrating on stress, rhythm, and intonation. Explain that this can be achieved by *strongly* emphasizing the highlighted portions. Examples of reading materials include the following:

The Little Girl and the Wolf
(From *The Thurber Carnival* by James Thurber, 1945)

One **after**noon a big **wolf wai**ted in a **dark for**est for a **li**ttle **girl** to come a**long carry**ing a **bas**ket of **food** to her **grand**mother. **Fin**ally a **li**ttle **girl did** come a**long** and **she** was **carry**ing a **bas**ket of **food**. "Are you **carry**ing that **bas**ket to your **grand**mother?" **asked** the **wolf**. The **li**ttle **girl** said **yes**, she **was**. So the **wolf asked** her **where** her **grand**mother **lived** and the **li**ttle **girl told** him and he **dis**appeared into the **wood**.

When the **li**ttle **girl o**pened the **door** of her **grand**mother's **house** she **saw** that there was **some**body in **bed** with a **night**cap and **night**-gown on. She had a**pproached** no **near**er than **twen**ty-five **feet** from the **bed** when she **saw** that it was **not** her **grand**mother but the **wolf**, for **e**ven in a **night**cap a **wolf** does **not** look any **more** like your **grand**mother than the **M-G-M li**on looks like **Cal**vin **Coo**lidge. So the **li**ttle **girl** took an auto**mat**ic out of her **bas**ket and **shot** the **wolf dead**.

Moral: It is **not** so **ea**sy to **fool li**ttle **girls now**adays as it **used** to be.

Oh When I Was . . .

(From *A Shropshire Lad* by A. E. Housman)

Oh when **I** was in **love** with **you**,
Then I was **clean** and **brave**,
And **miles around** the **won**der **grew**,
How **well** did I be**have**.
And **now** the **fan**cy **pass**es **by**,
And **noth**ing will re**main**,
And **miles around** they'll **say** that **I**
Am **quite** my**self again**.

Helpful Hints

1. It is important to avoid the tendency to simply instruct a client to slow down, speak up, or try harder. Explicit and intensive drills are required to successfully modify the prosodic features of a client's speech.

2. Verbal instructions for therapy activities may have to be simplified for clients who present with language deficits due to a concomitant aphasia.

3. Mirrors, audiotapes, and videotapes are useful adjuncts for developing a client's self-monitoring skills for speech production.

4. When working with adults, it is extremely important to explain why a given task is being implemented rather than merely describing how the task should be performed.

5. Clinicians should be aware that a client's reluctance to perform speech tasks may be related to fears about cosmetic changes (e.g., facial asymmetry, drooling) resulting from oral-facial sensory deficits.

6. Family education is an integral part of therapy programming for clients with dysarthria. For useful handouts about the nature of dysarthria and tips for effective communication strategies, see Yorkston, Miller, and Strand (2004) and Tanner (1999) in the recommended readings section at end of this chapter.

APRAXIA OF SPEECH

Apraxia is an inability to plan and execute volitional motor movements due to central nervous system damage despite intact muscle strength and coordination. This deficit can affect any system that requires purposeful sequences of muscle movement. In a **limb apraxia**, voluntary movements of the extremities are affected in gestures such as waving good-bye or making a fist on command. An **oral apraxia** involves difficulty with nonspeech movements of the oral mechanism such as tongue protrusion and lip pursing on command.

Apraxia of speech (or verbal apraxia) is a neurologically based articulation disorder characterized by difficulty in positioning speech muscles and sequencing muscle movements for the voluntary production of speech. This disorder is not associated with weakness, slowness, or incoordination of these muscles during automatic and reflexive acts (McNeil, Robin, & Schmidt, 1997). Verbal apraxia is a motor speech disorder; therefore, language comprehension and the grammatical system are not affected. However, it should be noted that apraxia frequently co-occurs with aphasia. Apraxia results from a lesion in the left frontal lobe near Broca's area. The main causes of apraxia are quite similar to those associated with aphasia and include CVA, trauma, tumors, and disease processes such as Alzheimer's.

Severity of apraxia ranges along a continuum from very subtle articulatory errors to completely unintelligible speech. At the most extreme level of impairment, an individual may be unable to initiate phonation volitionally. Following are the most significant characteristics of verbal apraxia (Croot, 2002; Wertz, LaPointe, & Rosenbek, 1991):

- Highly unpredictable and inconsistent errors are made, even on repeated attempts at the same word. For example, an individual with apraxia may produce the following sequence in an attempt to produce the word "escalator": elescat, lator, scalator, lescatator, lescator, elescator.

- Substitutions and transpositions are the most frequent type of speech production errors, but omissions and distortions are also common.

- Complex consonant blends are often substituted for simpler phonemes (e.g., "strondo" for "tornado").

- There is difficulty initiating speech as evidenced by frequent stops, restarts, long pauses and hesitations, and repetition of initial sounds and syllables.

- Articulatory accuracy deteriorates as word length increases.

- There are visible and audible groping behaviors in which the speaker struggles to achieve appropriate placement of the articulators through trial and error.

- Automatic speech generally contains fewer articulatory errors than purposeful productions. For example, rote recitation of the months of the year may be relatively error-free (i.e., January, February, March . . .), while meaningful production of any of these words is likely to include numerous articulation errors (e.g., In response to the clinician question, "When are you going to visit your daughter?" the client says, "Ferry . . . ferrary . . . fruary . . . befuary").

- Client may be aware of the articulation errors but is unable to correct them on subsequent attempts.

- Prosody of speech is atypical with respect to rhythm, word stress, and intonational contour.

- Speech rate is slowed.

As discussed in the aphasia section of this chapter, a period of spontaneous recovery follows the initial neurological insult. This period may continue for up to six months, with the most significant improvement occurring during the first eight weeks. The prognosis is determined by many of the same factors that affect recovery from aphasia, including size, location, and etiology of lesion, age at onset, and overall health of the client. However, there are certain apraxia-specific

TABLE 6-7
Differential Characteristics of Apraxia and Dysarthria

Apraxia	Dysarthria
Articulation is better in involuntary/automatic speech; periods of error-free speech may exist.	Automatic and voluntary speech are similarly impaired; there are no periods of error-free speech.
Errors are unpredictable and highly inconsistent.	Errors are predictable and highly consistent.
Substitution and transposition errors predominate.	Distortion and omission errors predominate.
There is significant difficulty with the initiation of speech, evidenced by hesitations, pauses, restarts, and repetitions.	Initiation of speech is usually not affected.
Visible and audible groping postures of the articulators are evident.	There are no visible or audible groping postures of the articulators, including respiration, prosody, and resonance.
Deficits occur primarily in articulation and prosody.	All speech processes are involved, including respiration, phonation, articulation, prosody, and resonance.

Sources: Adapted from Wertz, LaPointe, & Rosenbek (1991); LaPointe & Katz (2002); and Duffy (1995).

indicators that are associated with a less favorable prognosis. These include (1) presence of an accompanying oral apraxia, particularly lasting more than two months, and (2) the severity and duration of an accompanying aphasia.

Although apraxia and dysarthria are both motor speech disorders, their symptomologies are considerably different. Table 6-7 presents the differentiating characteristics of these disorders.

Treatment Efficacy

Few studies have been conducted that directly address either efficacy or outcome issues in apraxia of speech. Van Heugten, Dekker, Deelman, Stehmann-Saris, and Kinebanian (2000) investigated the effect of a functional treatment program with 33 stroke patients with apraxia and 36 stroke patients without apraxia. Their results suggest that traditional prognostic variables such as cognitive impairment, motor impairment, and advanced age were not related to treatment outcome. Ballard's (2001) critical review of the existing literature suggests that response generalization effects are slight, especially in the application of trained behaviors to novel situations.

Treatment for Apraxia of Speech

The ultimate aim of intervention for apraxia of speech (heretofore referred to simply as apraxia) is to increase a client's voluntary control over the articulatory movements necessary for accurate speech production to the limits imposed by the neurological impairment. For clients with severe to profound apraxia, intelligible speech may not be a realistic goal. Therapy for these individuals should focus on developing augmentative or alternative means of communication.

Structure. Intervention programs for apraxia can be structured in several different ways. The central feature of nearly all approaches is the use of drill; motor learning is dependent on repeated opportunities to practice desired movement patterns.

One well-known paradigm for structuring apraxia therapy is the eight-step task continuum developed by Wertz, LaPointe, and Rosenbek (1991). This continuum incorporates Milisen's (1954) concept of "integral stimulation," which emphasizes simultaneous input in multiple modalities, especially auditory and visual. This paradigm utilizes imitation as the primary teaching strategy and attempts to facilitate increased voluntary articulatory control through systematic, gradual fading of clinician cues. Following are the eight steps:

Step 1: Clinician presents integral stimulation (i.e., "Watch me; listen to me"); clinician and client then produce target utterance in unison.

Step 2: Clinician presents integral stimulation; then clinician offers visual cue only (i.e., mouths utterance without sound) while client simultaneously produces the target utterance aloud.

Step 3: Clinician presents integral stimulation; then client imitates target utterance independently.

Step 4: Repeat Step 3 but require the client to produce target utterance several times in a row without any intervening clinician model.

Step 5: Clinician presents written stimuli, which client reads aloud.

Step 6: Clinician presents and then removes written stimuli; client attempts target utterance.

Step 7: Clinician presents a question designed to elicit target utterance and client responds.

Step 8: Clinician engages client in role-play situations to elicit target utterance. (This step is most appropriate for target behaviors at the word level and beyond.)

Content. The hierarchy described above presents guidelines for "how to teach," or structure a therapy program. This section focuses on "what to teach," or the content of an intervention program for apraxia. In 1975, Darley, Aronson, and Brown recommended a basic treatment progression. This protocol was adapted for discussion in this chapter because of its simplicity and its suitability for almost any degree of apraxic impairment. The point in the progression at which therapy is initiated depends on an individual client's capabilities.

Phase I: Initiate Phonation. Instruct the client to:

• Produce a cough or sigh

• Prolong exhalation and shift from a cough or sigh to phonation

- Induce phonation through humming (or singing) in unison with clinician.
- Overlay a variety of mouth opening and tongue configurations to produce vowels and dipthongs.

Phase II: Increase Smoothness and Length of Speech.

- Use automatic speech such as TV jingles, Pledge of Allegiance, rotely memorized poems and songs, everyday expressions such as "How are you?" or "I feel fine" to experience the feel of easily produced speech.
- Use highly familiar or automatic speech patterns to provide a base for establishing propositional vocabulary, for example, "salt and _____" or "roses are _____."

Phase III: Phonemic Drill.
Individuals with apraxia exhibit the least amount of difficulty with vowels, glides, and nasal sounds; more difficulty with plosives; increased difficulty with fricatives and affricates; and the most difficulty with consonant clusters. This hierarchy of difficulty with respect to manner of production can guide the selection of therapy targets for drill work. Once a target phoneme has been identified, voluntary motor control can be increased using Darley et al.'s (1975) suggested 10-step therapy sequence.

Step 1: Hum the phoneme in isolation: /nnnnn/.

Step 2: Add a vowel to the consonant target and produce the syllable 20 times (e.g., /na/). Repeat this drill with other vowels.

Step 3: Produce a series of five or six different CV syllable combinations: nu, na, ny, now, naw.

Step 4: Produce reduplicative syllables first in isolation (nana, nana, nana; nini, nini, nini) and then in succession (nana, nini, nunu).

Step 5: Add the target phoneme as the final consonant to form a CVC syllable: nan, nin, nown. As in Step 4, first practice in isolation and then in succession.

Step 6: Produce the target phoneme in short words with simple phonetic environments: new, nine, nap, nag, nod, nail, bin, bone, run, loan, dune.

Step 7: Produce two-word phrases with the target phoneme in the initial position of both monosyllablic words: not now, no news, near noon, nice night, north Nile.

Step 8: Repeat Step 7 with target phoneme in the final position of words: down town, dine in, main man, one gown, lean on.

Step 9: Produce two-word utterances in which the target phoneme is in the initial position of the first word and the final position of the second word: knee pain, need ten, new phone, need loan.

Step 10: Produce multiword utterances with some polysyllabic words, gradually expanding them into sentences: Napoleon won the honor; Nan lives near Ned; John F. Kennedy; nutmeg and cinnamon; north of Jefferson County.

Once a client has mastered the production of several different target phonemes, introduce them in minimal word pairs to facilitate accurate articulatory transition from one target phoneme to another across word boundaries. Examples include name-game, run-rut, banner-backer.

Throughout phonemic drill training, encourage the client to anticipate upcoming phonemes in an utterance and plan or mentally rehearse appropriate articulatory postures. As the client's voluntary control over articulatory movements improves, foster more natural-sounding speech by increasing speech rate and highlighting other prosodic features.

Example Profiles

Following are two profiles that are representative of the speech characteristics of individuals with apraxia. These examples have been designed to illustrate the selection of intervention targets as well as specific therapy activities and materials. Most of the chosen activities can be implemented in either individual or group therapy settings.

PROFILE 1

Mrs. Elizondo, a 65-year-old female, exhibits a severe apraxia after surgery to remove a tumor localized in the left frontal lobe. She demonstrates no volitional speech but occasionally produces undifferentiated CV or VC syllables and some automatic utterances (e.g., "Oh my goodness"; "I don't know"). Mild to moderate oral and limb apraxia is present, with no evidence of an accompanying aphasia or hemiparesis. Currently, her sole means of communication is through writing.

Selection of therapy targets. Therapy will focus on ensuring the availability of an alternative mode of communication, the initiation of voluntary phonation, and the facilitation of propositional speech. An alternative system will be implemented to provide Mrs. Elizondo with an immediate means of communicating with others. The severity of her verbal apraxia dictates that treatment begin at the most basic level, which involves elicitation of volitional phonation. Because the only intelligible speech in her repertoire consists of sporadic automatic phrases, this type of utterance will be used to stimulate the production of propositional speech at the single-word level.

Sample Activities

1. The prognosis for significant improvement in speech production is difficult to determine so early in the recovery process. Therefore, the clinician should provide Mrs. Elizondo with a functional and reliable way of communicating. Many forms of alternative communication systems are available, including picture boards, alphabet boards, electronic devices, and computer-generated speech. It is the clinician's responsibility to review the available options and select the method within the client's linguistic and motoric capabilities that (a) is most

flexible, allowing for the expression of the broadest possible range of messages, and (b) generates messages that are most easily understood by listeners.

Given Mrs. Elizondo's current status, writing is judged to be the optimal choice for a nonvocal communication system. This selection was based on the fact that her language skills are essentially unimpaired and that the limb apraxia does not significantly impede her ability to write. At this stage in Mrs. Elizondo's recovery, it is not known whether writing will serve as an interim method of communication or eventually become a true alternative to speech as her permanent, primary mode of communication.

2. (Step 1 of Rosenbek's structural hierarchy and Phase I of the Darley et al., 1975, content hierarchy). Explain that the clinician will model a vocal behavior (i.e., a cough or sigh) two times. For the first trial, instruct the client to watch and listen carefully. On the second trial, instruct the client to attempt the cough or sigh in unison with the clinician's production. Repeat this sequence until the client can produce a cough on volition. Progress through the next three tasks in Phase I, using the same "integral stimulation-unison production" training paradigm. These tasks consist of (a) prolonging exhalation to transition from the cough or sigh to phonation, (b) extending phonation through humming, and (c) superimposing mouth opening and different tongue positions over the humming to produce vowels.

3. (Adaptation of Step 7 of Rosenbek's structural hierarchy and Phase II of the Darley et al., 1975 content hierarchy). Develop a set of 25 familiar or high-probability phrases. Examples include the following:

Salt and _____ (pepper)

Cup of _____ (coffee)

Knife and _____ (fork)

Look before you _____ (leap)

Birds of a _____ (feather)

Shoes and _____ (socks)

Turn over a new _____ (leaf)

Paper and _____ (pencil)

Peaches and _____ (cream)

Bacon and _____ (eggs)

Bread and _____ (butter)

The early bird catches the _____ (worm)

Gather pictures that represent the missing word in each fill-in-the-blank phrase. Explain that the clinician will say a phrase aloud while presenting the corresponding picture. Instruct the client to listen carefully, look at the picture, and produce the target word as quickly as possible. If the client is unsuccessful in the first attempt, the clinician can provide additional cues by demonstrating the appropriate placement of the first phoneme or by modeling the first phoneme aloud.

PROFILE 2

Mr. Collins, a 58-year-old male, sustained a left frontal lobe CVA one year ago, which resulted in a moderate apraxia with an accompanying mild to moderate nonfluent (Broca's) aphasia. He presents with a mild right-sided weakness with no significant oral or limb apraxia. Mr. Collins demonstrates good language comprehension for relatively simple oral and written material. With respect to expression, his utterances are pragmatically appropriate and consist of short effortful phrases marked by morphological and syntactic errors. Mr. Collins exhibits the ability to imitate verbal utterances; however, his performance deteriorates as utterance length and complexity increase. His speech is characterized by unpredictable articulation errors consisting mainly of sound substitutions and transpositions on plosives, fricatives, and affricates. These errors occur more frequently in multisyllabic utterances. Errors on nasal consonants are noted in connected speech. Speech melody is atypical with respect to stress and intonation; struggle behaviors to achieve accurate articulation placement were clearly visible. Overall, speech is rated as moderately unintelligible, particularly in unknown contexts. Mr. Collins recognizes the inadequacy of his communication skills and is frustrated by them.

Selection of therapy targets. The areas to be targeted are the /m/, /p/, and /s/ phonemes as well as the prosodic feature of stress. These sounds were selected according to the hierarchy of difficulty identified by Darley et al. (1975) based on their experience with apraxic individuals. Stress, particularly at the phrase level, was chosen as a means of increasing Mr. Collins's speech intelligibility.

Sample Activities

1. (Adapted from Steps 5 and 6 of Rosenbek's structural hierarchy and Step 9 of the Darley et al. [1975] phonemic drill sequence). Develop a list of 25 two-word phrases in which /m/ is in the initial position of the first word and the final position of the second word. Select short words with simple phonetic environments. Write each phrase on an index card and place the pile face-down on the table. Examples include the following:

make ti*m*e	*m*eet hi*m*
*m*y roo*m*	*m*iss To*m*
*m*ail the*m*	*m*ore gu*m*
*m*ade ha*m*	*m*eal ti*m*e
*m*en ca*m*e	*m*oon bea*m*

   Instruct the client to select the top card and read the phrase aloud. Remove the card and tell the client to repeat the same phrase three times. Following the last production, provide feedback such as "You did a nice job saying /m/ in 'make time'" to expose the client to a clearly articulated indirect model of the target sound. The difficulty of this activity can be increased by gradually incorporating polysyllabic words that contain the target sound into longer phrases and sentences.

2. (Step 4 of Rosenbek's structural hierarchy and Step 3 of the Darley et al. [1975] phonemic drill sequence). Write the target phoneme in the center of a large index card or sheet of paper and surround it with four vowels or dipthongs (e.g., ɑ, o, ɔ, ə). Arrange the vowels as follows, using traditional spelling rather than phonetic symbols.

ah

↑

aw ← p → o

↓

uh

Explain to the client that this activity is designed to improve his or her ability to transition quickly from one syllable to another. Instruct the client to watch and listen (integral stimulation) as the clinician models CV syllables at a relatively rapid rate. This is accomplished by pairing the target consonant with each of the four vowels in a clockwise progression from *ah* to *aw*. Client imitates the clinician's model of the syllable series 10 times. This activity also can be used to provide intense drill work on the other target phoneme: /s/.

3. Create a set of 20 pairs of phrases or short sentences in which manipulations of stress and pause time alter meaning. Examples include the following:

The sky is falling.	This guy is falling.
An ice man.	A nice man.
A man eating shark.	A man-eating shark.
Oranges have a peel.	Oranges have appeal.
He's a gentle man.	He's a gentleman.
What a dark room!	What a darkroom!
I don't like cross words.	I don't like crosswords.

Each phrase/sentence is written on separate index cards, which are then shuffled and placed in a pile facedown on the table. Instruct the client to select one card, keeping it out of the clinician's view, and read it aloud using the appropriate stress pattern. The clinician guesses the utterance based on the client's prosody and coarticulation cues and writes it down on a blank index card. The two cards are then compared to determine whether the client successfully communicated the intended message. If the cards do not match, the clinician models both stress patterns. The client is asked to identify the target pattern and imitate it.

Helpful Hints

1. To avoid or minimize client confusion during the initial stages of phonemic drill training, the clinician should select successive sound targets that are maximally different from one another.

2. A client's success on imitation tasks is sometimes facilitated by the clinician's use of an exaggerated stress or intonation when modeling stimuli.

3. A metronome is a particularly effective temporal cue for regulating the pace of a client's speech.

4. For some clients, a productive strategy for promoting speech initiation or output is to encourage them to pair a gesture with a word.

5. Melodic Intonation Therapy (MIT) (Helm-Estabrooks & Albert, 2004) can be used successfully to promote speech output; the rhythmic nature of intoning a melody serves to facilitate production for some clients with apraxia.

6. Counseling must frequently address the fact that other individuals may negatively judge a client's intellectual/language comprehension skills based on poor speech intelligibility.

7. Families may require considerable education regarding the nature of apraxia to ensure that the client's inconsistent speech errors are not misperceived as signs of laziness or lack of motivation.

INTRODUCTION TO DYSPHAGIA

Dysphagia is a swallowing disorder characterized by difficulty moving food from mouth to stomach including all the behavioral and physiological aspects of the process (Leopold & Kagel, 1996). Dysphagia occurs in all age groups and may result from a variety of structural or physiological abnormalities. The onset of dysphagia can be acute (e.g., resulting from a stroke) or characterized by gradual deterioration (e.g., resulting from a progressive disease process such amyotrophic lateral sclerosis). Difficulties can occur in any of the four stages of the normal swallow which correspond to the approximate location of the food bolus as it moves through the system: a) preparatory (chewing); b) oral (back of mouth); c) pharyngeal (throat); and d) esophageal (toward stomach). See Edgar (2003) for an extensive review of research on swallowing in normal adults. Intervention designed for preparatory and/or oral stage problems is generally referred to as "feeding" techniques while pharyngeal stage intervention is described as "swallowing" therapy. A speech-language pathologist's role in treatment is generally limited to difficulties in the first three stages of swallowing; problems in the esophageal stage are usually managed medically or surgically.

In 2002, the American Speech-Language-Hearing Association (ASHA) published a position statement on the roles of the SLP in swallowing and feeding disorders. Speech-language pathologists' education and clinical background in anatomy and physiology of respiration, swallowing, and speech prepares them to assume a variety of roles including:

- Developing and implementing treatment plans for individuals with dysphagia
- Providing education and counseling to patients and their families
- Serving as members of a multidisciplinary/interdisciplinary management team
- Advocating for services for individuals with dysphagia
- Advancing the knowledge base on swallowing and feeding disorders through research activities

Treatment

The two paramount goals of dysphagia management are: (1) prevention of aspiration, malnutrition, and dehydration; and (2) re-establishment of oral intake of food and liquid. These aims can be achieved through retraining muscle function, teaching new sequences of muscle activity, or stimulating increased sensory input (Logemann, 1998). Clinical decision-making is often carried out through a multidisciplinary team which may include a physician, dietitian, radiologist, or occupational therapist.

Intervention for feeding and swallowing disorders can be categorized into two main approaches: *compensatory strategies* or *therapy strategies*. The goal for compensatory strategies is to eliminate or reduce abnormal symptoms without changing the underlying physiology of the client's swallow. This approach requires minimal cognitive or physical effort from the client and largely involves manipulation of the following variables:

- Changing head and/or body posture (to redirect the flow of the bolus by changing the dimensions of the vocal tract)

- Increasing sensory input/awareness (heightening sensitivity of the CNS may result in improved initiation and timing of the swallow)

- Adjusting amount and rate of food presentation

- Modifying food consistency or texture (see McCullough, Pelletier, & Steele, 2003 for information on the National Dysphagia Diet published by the American Dietetic Associaton)

The goal of therapy strategies is to effect change in the client's swallow pattern. This approach generally focuses on range of motion and coordination/timing of movement. Clients must be able to follow instructions and have the capacity to practice exercises independently. Intervention may be implemented indirectly with just saliva or directly with food/liquid. This decision should be made solely on the basis of aspiration findings from radiographic studies (Logemann, 1998). Strategies utilized with this treatment approach include the following:

- Improving oral control and oral/pharyngeal range-of-motion

- Increasing sensory awareness prior to the swallow attempt

- Increasing voluntary control of pharyngeal movement through a variety of modified swallow maneuvers

- Improving self-monitoring of the swallow through biofeedback tools such as ultrasound, electromyography, video endoscopy, and video fluoroscopy

Intervention for feeding and swallowing disorders can have life-and-death consequences. Ethical issues in this area are complex and extremely serious (Sharp & Bryant, 2003). At this point, no universal guidelines exist for acceptable amounts of aspiration (i.e., entry of food/liquid into airway below level of the vocal folds). Radiographic evaluation is *absolutely* required to identify the existence, severity, and cause of aspiration. Logemann (1998) suggests oral intake of a given food consistency be prohibited if a client aspirates more than 10% of each bolus despite the use of optimal intervention techniques. However, clinicians should be aware that the wishes of clients and/or their families may run contrary to therapeutic recommendations. An instructive example involves a terminally ill client for whom the clinician has determined that oral intake be prohibited due to excessive aspiration under all conditions. Yet the client and family insist on continuing to eat by mouth. The clinician's ethical dilemma is whether to provide information/training on the least harmful way to swallow within a range of life-threatening alternatives.

Helpful Hints

1. If the client's progress plateaus for at least four weeks, active therapy can be terminated until/unless status changes.

2. Clinicians must carefully consider the eligibility question: "Will this client benefit from intervention?" Individuals with severe cognitive limitations or advanced motor neuron disease may not be considered good candidates for swallowing treatment.

CONCLUSION

The last three sections presented basic information, protocols, and procedures for intervention with dysarthria, apraxia of speech, and dysphagia at an **introductory** level. This information is intended only as a starting point in the reader's clinical education and training. For more in-depth coverage of these areas, the following readings are recommended:

Brookshire, R. H. (2003). *Introduction to neurogenic communication disorders.* St. Louis, MO: Mosby.

Duffy, J. R. (1995). *Motor speech disorders: Substrates, differential diagnosis, and management.* St. Louis, MO: Mosby.

Dworkin, J. D. (1991). *Motor speech disorders: A treatment guide.* St. Louis, MO: Mosby-Year Book.

Freed, D. (2000). *Motor speech disorders: Diagnosis and treatment.* San Diego, CA: Singular Thomson Learning.

Love, R. J., & Webb, W. G. (1996). *Neurology for the speech-language pathologist.* Woburn, MA: Butterworth-Heinemann.

McNeil, M. R. (1997). *Clinical management of sensorimotor speech disorders.* New York: Thieme.

Yorkston, K. M., Miller, R. M., & Strand, E. A. (2004). *Management of speech and swallowing in degenerative disorders.* Austin, TX: Pro-Ed.

Selected references for dysphagia, traumatic brain injury, and right hemisphere dysfunction include:

Dysphagia

Crary, M., & Groher, M. (2003). *Introduction to adult swallowing disorders.* Little Rock, AR: Elsevier.

Groher, M. E. (Ed.). (1997). *Dysphagia: Diagnosis and management.* Little Rock, AR: Elsevier.

Leonard, R., & Kendall, K. (1997). *Dysphagia assessment and treatment planning: A team approach.* San Diego, CA: Singular Thomson Learning.

Logemann, J. A. (1998). *Evaluation and treatment of swallowing disorders.* Austin, TX: Pro-Ed.

Traumatic Brain Injury

Blosser, J. L. (2003). *Pediatric traumatic brain injury: Proactive intervention.* Albany, NY: Singular Thomson Learning.

Hartley, L. L. (1995). *Cognitive-communicative abilities following brain injury: A functional approach.* San Diego, CA: Singular Publishing Group.

Murdoch, B. & Theodoros, D. G. (2001). *Traumatic brain injury: Associated speech, language, and swallowing disorders.* Albany, NY: Singular Thomson Learning.

Ylvisaker, M., & Feeney, T. (1998). *Collaborative brain injury intervention: Positive everyday routines.* San Diego, CA: Singular Thompson Learning.

Right Hemisphere Dysfunction

Myers, P. S. (1999). *Right hemisphere damage: Disorders of communication and cognition.* San Diego, CA: Singular Thomson Learning.

Myers, P. S. (2001). Communication disorders associated with right hemisphere damage. In R. Chapcy (Ed.), *Language intervention strategies in aphasia and related neurogenic communication disorders* (pp. 809–828). Baltimore: Lippincott Williams & Wilkins.

Tompkins, C. A. (1995). *Right hemisphere communication disorders: Theory and management.* San Diego, CA: Singular Publishing Group.

ADDITIONAL RESOURCES

Aphasia

The Speech Bin

1965 Twenty-Fifth Avenue
Vero Beach, FL 32960
Phone: 800-4-SPEECH
Fax: 888-FAX 2 BIN
Web site: www.speechbin.com

Workbook for Cognitive Skills
For adults and adolescents with moderate cognitive impairments or learning disabilities. Target areas include word formation, familiar phrases, definition usage, visual recognition, letter placement, and logical solutions.

Workbook for Aphasia
For adults with mild-to-moderate language and cognitive deficits. Target areas include word usage, development of syntax, use of factual information, and concrete and abstract reasoning.

Workbook for Language Skills
For adults with mild-to-severe language impairment. Target areas include spelling, sentence completion, sentence construction, sentence comprehension, figurative language, general knowledge, and word recall.

Workbook for Reasoning Skills

For adolescents and adults with mild-to-moderate impairment in problem solving, reasoning, and comprehension skills. Target areas include drawing conclusions, problem solving, following directions, visual/logical sequencing, humor, and numbers/systems.

Recall

Set includes 640 reproducible stimulus cards and a manual of activity worksheets all designed to improve word retrieval. The cards may be used in games or drills. Can be used from middle elementary school age through adults.

Potpourri

Set includes 100 cards, an instruction manual, and 10 worksheets for home reinforcement practice. Designed to increase skills in analogies, time, cause/effect, true/false, sentence types, categories, descriptive language, associations, rhyming, and cultural literacy.

Workbook for Verbal Expression

Hundreds of exercises including simple naming, automatic speech sequences, repetition, complex tasks using sentences, abstract reasoning, question formulation, word retrieval, restating factual information, and spontaneous speech drills. Functional real-life tasks range from high to low complexity; appropriate for both adult and child clients.

Cognitive Reorganization

4,200+ stimuli plus activities for functional applications help meet the diverse needs of clients who cannot use functional language skills in any organized, sequential, or pragmatic way. Responses may be written, verbal, or graphic.

Pro-Ed
8700 Shoal Creek Boulevard
Austin, TX 78757-6897
Phone: 800-897-3202
Fax: 800-397-7633
Web site: www.proedinc.com

Focus on Function: Retraining for the Communicatively Impaired Client
Targets independent living skills for adolescents and adults by having them practice a variety of daily tasks. Includes reproducible evaluation forms, task cards, picture cards, manipulatives, and practical activities that emphasize everyday verbal, phone, reading, writing, and numerical skills.

Language Activity Resource Kit (LARK)
A portable kit with objects (two of each), illustrated cards, color photographs, word and phrase cards, and line drawings of the objects in use. Designed especially for the itinerant SLP treating adults with aphasia and/or TBI. Optional LARK workbook with reproducible worksheets can be purchased.

Laureate
110 East Spring Street
Winooski, VT 05404-1898
Phone: 800-562-6801
Fax: 802-655-4757
Web site: www.laureatelearning.com

The Words and Concepts Series
Computer software designed to build vocabulary, strengthen language comprehension and word relationships, and develop important concepts. Consists of three instructional programs and three companion game programs, which use a core vocabulary of 40 referential nouns in six related language units: Vocabulary, Categorization, Word Identification by Function, Word Association, and Same and Different Concepts. Most activities contain three levels of difficulty, which can be set to branch among each other, following the progress of the individual.

The Following Directions Series
Computer software that includes eight activities to help clients learn to follow one-level, sequential, and two-level commands using spatial relations concepts and directional terms. Also includes 10 activities to improve clients' ability to follow directions and develop right/left discrimination concepts through activities such as simple left- and right-hand matching, practice crossing midline, and moving objects to left and right using hands in mirrored and nonmirrored positions.

The Language Activities of Daily Living Series: My House and My Town
Talking instructional computer software programs designed to help clients understand and express the language encountered during daily routines. Each program has four different activities designed to increase understanding of object names and their functions or descriptions: Discover Names, Identify Names, Discover Functions, and Identify Functions. In *My House*, the scenes represent typical rooms in a house: a bedroom, bathroom, dining room, kitchen, living room, and utility room. In *My Town*, a doctor's office, dentist's office, restaurant, park, city neighborhood, and suburban neighborhood are included.

Dysarthia and Apraxia of Speech

LinguiSystems
3100 Fourth Avenue
East Moline, IL 61244-9700
Phone: 800-776-4332
Fax: 800-577-4555
E-mail: linguisys@aol.com
Web site: www.linguisystems.com

The Source for Dysarthria
A comprehensive manual that includes information about dysarthria such as the different types, etiologies, evaluation and treatment planning options, and treatment objectives for respiration, phonation, resonance, articulation, and prosody. Also includes examples of documentation and sample reports.

The Source for Apraxia Therapy
A resource that combines a visual-auditory-kinesthetic approach to improve intelligibility in clients with mild, moderate, or severe apraxia. Divided into three sections, which focus on production of words and simple sentences, articulation, fluency, phrasing, and paralinguistic drills.

The Speech Bin
1965 Twenty-Fifth Avenue
Vero Beach, FL 32960
Phone: 800-4-SPEECH
Fax: 888-FAX 2 BIN
Web site: www.speechbin.com

The Apraxia of Speech Stimulus Library
Includes a research-based manual, four boxed sets of stimulus cards, and reproducible data collection sheets. Uses high-interest words (depicted graphically or by pictures) and practical phrases to improve production of phonemes and phoneme sequences.

Dysarthria Sourcebook
Activities for improving intelligibility, articulation, intonation, and stress. Clear, large, bold type is ideal for clients with visual impairments.

Dysarthria Treatment Manual
Imaginative treatment approach emphasizing self-monitoring and self-reliance. Its practical exercises target oral-motor, resonance, relaxation, respiration, prosody, and intelligibility. It offers client and family handouts, a simple communication board, and home practice activities.

Pro-Ed
8700 Shoal Creek Boulevard
Austin, TX 78757-6897
Phone: 800-897-3202
Fax: 800-397-7633
Web site: www.proedinc.com

Dysarthria Rehabilitation Program, second edition
For adolescents and adults. Exercises focus on improvement of speech intelligibility through exaggeration of articulatory movements, reduction of speech rate via vowel prolongation, and improvement of speech prosody. Includes 60 pictures, words, and reproducible data-collection and tracking forms for use with multiple clients.

Dysphagia

The Speech Bin
1965 Twenty-Fifth Avenue
Vero Beach, FL 32960
Phone: 800-4-SPEECH
Fax: 888-FAX 2 BIN
Web site: www.speechbin.com

Pre-Feeding Skills, second edition

This program for infants to adolescents discusses normal development, limitations, and management of tube feeding, cleft palate, drooling, prematurity, and feeding in autism. It covers evaluation, treatment, oral stimulation, positioning, oral-motor limitations, and nutritional factors. It features reproducibles, mealtime exercises, and Spanish translations of parent questionnaires.

PAIS: Program for the Assessment and Instruction of Swallowing

This program is easy and quick to use with forms for documentation required for third party reimbursement. PAIS includes a clinical protocol for evaluation of swallowing, modified barium swallow report, swallowing protocols, and warning stickers. Complete kit has a book, 25 copies of each form, and 25 stickers.

LinguiSystems

3100 Fourth Avenue
East Moline, IL 61244-9700
Phone: 800-776-4332
Fax: 800-577-4555
Web site: www.linguisystems.com

The Source for Dysphagia

This 305-page workbook includes Medicare changes related to swallowing treatment; detailed educational handouts for physicians, patients, and staff; information on fiberoptic endoscopic evaluation of swallowing (FEES); new information on how to perform and interpret a modified barium swallow; and descriptions of new therapy techniques and references to document efficacy.

The Source for Pediatric Dysphagia

For ages birth–18. It provides information on feeding, swallowing, and treatment goals for young patients. The techniques also can be applied to older children with cerebral palsy, neurological disorders, or any swallowing disorder. From diagnosis through treatment, chapters cover anatomy and physiology, diagnostic procedures, infant feeding techniques, behavioral feeding disorders, goals and treatment objectives, and tools for feeding.

Pro-Ed

8700 Shoal Creek Boulevard
Austin, TX 78757-6897
Phone: 800-897-3202
Fax: 800-397-7633
Web site: www.proedinc.com

Clinical Management of Dysphagia in Adults and Children, second edition

The new edition includes an overview of oral-motor and swallowing skills in the infant and child; clinical evaluation of dysphagia in adults and feeding/swallowing in infants and children; treatment of dysphagia in adults and children; developing quality assurance monitors for dysphagia; forms for bedside evaluation of dysphagia in adults and children; and discussion on videofluoroscopy and other diagnostic procedures.

Dysphagia: A Manual for Use by Families and Caregivers under the Direction of a Speech-Language Pathologist, third edition
An educational and instructional text for primary caregivers of dysphagic patients. This book provides the professional, family members, and the patient with a working understanding of swallowing problems and management approaches.

Swallowing Disorders Treatment Manual, second edition
Hands-on manual covering assessment and treatment with information on how to conduct a patient interview, bedside evaluation, and videofluoroscopy study. Intervention includes thermal-tactile stimulation, the Mendelsohn maneuver, supraglottic swallow, posture changes in feeding position, diet consistency, oral-motor exercises, compensatory strategies, as well as reproducible swallowing guidelines. A list of dysphagia products is also included.

AliMed
297 High Street
Dedham, MA 02026
Phone: 800-225-2610
Fax: 800-437-2966
Web site: www.alimed.com

Swallow Right
Comprehensive exercise manual for evaluation and treatment of oral myofunctional disorders. Suitable for individual, group, or carryover programming. Program covers theory, treatment, and tracking charts for the three main stages of swallowing.

Swallowing Disorders Treatment Videotape
High-quality videotape that covers treatment of oral and pharyngeal swallowing disorders in adults. Includes step-by-step demonstrations of various techniques and strategies. Information provided on compensatory strategies (e.g., posture, diet) and rehabilitation techniques (thermal-tactile stimulation, oral-motor exercises).

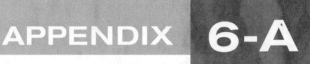

APPENDIX 6-A

GLOSSARY OF SELECTED MEDICAL TERMS

Acute care: Intense medical intervention to stabilize physical condition and ensure survival.

Alzheimer's disease: Progressive dementia caused by cerebral atrophy, resulting in memory loss, confusion, and speech disturbances beginning in late middle life with death occurring in 5 to 10 years.

Amyotrophic lateral sclerosis (ALS): Progressive disease of the spinal cord, resulting in degenerative muscular atrophy with accompanying mixed dysarthria.

Angular gyrus: Prominent rounded elevation (convolution) in the posterior portion of the parietal lobe.

Anoxia: Lack of oxygen in the blood supply to the brain.

Arcuate fasciculus: Nerve fiber bundle in the brain that transmits impulses from Wernicke's area to Broca's area.

Ataxia: Impairment in movement and balance resulting from cerebellar damage; a type of dysarthria characterized by articulation, rhythm, loudness, and stress disturbances.

Bolus: Rounded mass of food prepared by the mouth for swallowing.

Brainstem: Lower section of the brain that connects the spinal cord to the cerebrum; regulates functions such as breathing and blood pressure.

Broca's area: Motor speech area in the frontal lobe dominant for speech and language (usually left).

Bulbar palsy: Impairment and atrophy of the oral mechanism (lips, tongue, pharnyx, and so on) due to lesions in the medulla oblongata region of the brainstem.

Carotid artery: A major pathway of blood supply from the heart to the brain.

Catastrophic reaction: Sudden and extreme emotional/physical response to ordinary events or situations often exhibited by individuals with brain injury.

Central nervous system: The brain, brainstem, and spinal cord.

Chorea: Irregular, spasmodic, involuntary movements of the face and extremities.

Cortex: Convoluted outer layer of the brain responsible for higher-level sensory and motor functions.

CT scan: Computed tomography; sophisticated x-ray technique that provides cross-sectional images of the body.

Dementia: General deterioration of mental faculties characterized by disorientation, as well as impaired judgment, memory, and intellect.

Dyskinesia: Impairment in the ability to perform voluntary movements.

Dysphagia: Impairment in the ability to swallow normally.

Dystonia: A state of abnormal muscle tone (increased or decreased) associated with involuntary rhythmic twisting of the trunk or extremities.

Edema: Swelling resulting from an excessive amount of fluid retention in cells or tissues.

Extrapyramidal: Nerve fibers involved in regulation of automatic, subconscious aspects of motor coordination and posture.

Flaccid: Inability of a muscle to contract volitionally; relaxed, flabby, without tone; hypotonicity.

(continues)

Frontal lobe: Largest lobe of the brain located at the anterior portion of the cerebrum; responsible for primary motor control for all parts of the body.

Hematoma: A pooling of blood in an organ, tissue, or other area.

Hemorrhage: Escape of blood through ruptured blood vessels.

Huntington's chorea: Progressive neuromuscular disorder, usually beginning between the ages of 30 and 50 years, characterized by irregular and involuntary movements in the face and limbs; accompanied by gradual deterioration of mental status, resulting in dementia.

Hyperkinesia: Excessive, uncontrolled movement of any part of the body.

Infarct: An area of dead tissue resulting from an interruption of blood supply.

Ischemia: Decrease in blood supply due to mechanical obstruction (mainly narrowing of arteries). A cerebral ischemia involves a deficiency of the blood to the brain. Transient ischemic attacks (TIAs) generally last less than 24 hours.

MRI: Magnetic resonance imaging; computerized scan that utilizes nuclear magnetic resonance to produce cross-sectional images of the body.

Multiple sclerosis (MS): Progressive neuromuscular disorder resulting in paralysis, tremors, and speech disturbances; begins in early adulthood and is marked by periods of exacerbations and remissions.

Myasthenia gravis: Progressive muscular disorder resulting from impaired conduction of neural impulses to the muscles, beginning in the face and throat.

Myoclonus: Spasms in a muscle or group of muscles.

Nystagmus: Involuntary movement of the eyes often exhibited by individuals with brain injury.

Parietal lobe: The medial and upper lateral areas of the cerebrum responsible for reception and analysis of tactile and kinesthetic sensory impulses (touch and muscle movement awareness).

Parkinson's disease: Degenerative neurological syndrome characterized by rhythmic tremors, muscle rigidity, masklike face, general muscular weakness, and limp posture; often accompanied by a hypokinetic dysarthria.

Peripheral nervous system: Nerve bundles outside of the brain and spinal cord.

Premorbid: Preceding the occurrence of the disease or lesion.

Pseudobulbar palsy: Impairments in swallowing, chewing, and articulation due to bilateral upper motor neuron damage.

Pyramidal: Two nerve bundles originating in the sensorimotor area of the cortex inserting into the spinal cord, responsible for refined spatially oriented voluntary movements.

Rolandic fissure: A prominent groove on the lateral portion of each hemisphere forming the boundary between the frontal and parietal lobes.

Seizure: Episodes of excessive electrical activity in the brain.

Spastic: Muscle contractions that are involuntary and jerky; hypertonicity.

Subacute care: Rehabilitation program for individuals with stable medical conditions that provides daily nursing care and a range of other treatment services such as physical therapy, occupational therapy, and so on.

Supramarginal gyrus: Prominent rounded elevation (convolution) in the inferior half of the parietal lobe, surrounding the posterior part of the Sylvian fissure.

Temporal gyrus: Prominent rounded elevation (convolution) in the lateral surface of the temporal lobe.

(continues)

Appendix 6-A (continued)

Temporal lobe: Lower lateral portion of the cerebrum, responsible for sensation and interpretation of auditory impulses.

Tourette's syndrome: Neurological disorder characterized by verbal and facial tics, coprolalia (cursing), and motor incoordination; usually beginning in childhood.

Traumatic brain injury (TBI): Open or closed head injury resulting from impact or penetrating force.

Tremor: Repetitive and involuntary shaking or vibration of a body part or muscle group.

Wernicke's area: Large region of the temporal lobe responsible for auditory language comprehension.

Wilson's disease: Metabolic disorder associated with damage to the basal ganglia due to inadequate processing of the dietary intake of copper; often accompanied by mixed dysarthria.

APPENDIX 6-B

SUGGESTIONS FOR ENHANCING VERBAL INTERACTION WITH AN APHASIC FAMILY MEMBER

- Establish eye contact before you begin speaking.

- Speak slowly and with normal inflection at a natural loudness level.

- Keep messages relatively short and to the point.

- Combine speech with gestures, facial expressions, and other nonverbal communication to clarify the meaning of your messages.

- Pause frequently and check to make sure you are being understood (e.g., ask yes/no questions such as "Are you following me?"; "Is that clear?").

- Be sure that paper and pencil are readily accessible to communicate your message, if needed.

- Avoid abrupt or rapid changes in topic or speakers.

- Give ample time for the aphasic family member to respond to your message.

- Indicate when you do not understand a message rather than pretending you do.

Source: Adapted from Holland (1995).

APPENDIX 6-C

GUIDELINES FOR CONVERSATIONAL COACHING

I. Scriptwriting

- Scripts should be brief and written at the upper limits of a client's communicative range.

- Scripts should be written to highlight specific communicative behaviors that the clinician wishes to target. For example, if a client is learning to use synonyms as a compensatory strategy for word retrieval difficulties, the script should contain words that have many alternate lexical forms (e.g., car: automobile, sedan, convertible, vehicle, minivan).

- Scripts should be written in a conversational style.

- Scripts should be written in short utterances to promote successful expression and listener comprehension.

II. Levels of Difficulty

- Communication of shared information with a familiar listener

- Communication of new information with a familiar listener

- Communication of shared information with an unfamiliar listener

- Communication of new information with an unfamiliar listener

III. Advantages

- Simulates a conversational interaction in a highly structured setting

- Targets both speaker and listener communication behaviors in the same activity

- Permits the modification of both conversational content and communicative strategies

- Permits the observation of client in the role of conversational partner

Source: Adapted from Holland (1995).

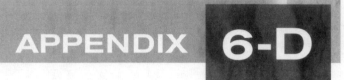

APPENDIX 6-D

NORMATIVE DATA FOR ADULT DIADOCHOKINETIC RATES
(Number of Syllables per Second)

pʌ	6.0–7.0
tʌ	6.0–7.0
kʌ	5.5–6.5
pʌtəkə	2.5

Source: From Kent, Kent, & Rosenbek (1987)

CHAPTER 7

Intervention
for
Fluency

The focus of this chapter is on **stuttering**, the major type of fluency disorder exhibited by children and adults. Cluttering, an associated fluency disorder, is beyond the scope of this chapter. Readers who are interested in this topic are referred to Daly & Burnett (1999); and St. Louis (1996).

Stuttering is characterized by an abnormally high frequency and/or duration of stoppages in the forward flow of speech (Andrews & Harris, 1964; Wingate, 1964; Yaruss, 1998). Prevalence studies indicate that stuttering occurs in approximately 1% to 1.5% of the population, with males outnumbering females by a ratio of 3:1. Many theories have been proposed regarding the cause of stuttering, ranging from genetic and other organic explanations to learned, environmental, or linguistic accounts. Certain theories emphasize differences in cerebral dominance (Travis, 1931), disruptions of speech motor timing (Kent, 1984; Van Riper, 1982), or anticipatory struggle to avoid communicative failure (Bloodstein, 1987). The covert repair hypothesis proposed by Kolk and colleagues (Kolk, 1991; Kolk & Postma, 1997) suggests that stutterers are prone to errors in phonological planning; their attempts to edit these errors prior to producing the utterance are manifested as disfluencies. In addition, several recent multifactorial theories have emphasized the interaction between stuttering and a variety of intrinsic/extrinsic factors. One account is the capacities and demands model, which posits that stuttering results from demands for performance that exceed the speaker's capacities in one or more domains (i.e., linguistic, motor, cognitive, or emotional) (Starkweather, 1987). The three-factor hypothesis (Wall & Myers, 1995) claims that a combination of psycholinguistic, psychosocial, and physiological factors are involved in the phenomenon of stuttering. In the multifactorial-dynamic model, Smith and colleagues (Smith, 1999; Smith & Kelly, 1997) argue that interaction among these factors occurs on multiple levels and that stuttered moments should be viewed as dynamic rather than static events. Similarly, De Nil's (1999) interpretation of the interactionist approach to stuttering stresses that all environmental and intrinsic factors are ultimately filtered through the stutterer's neurophysiological system. The specific interactions among linguistic, motor, cognitive, genetic, emotional, and social factors are yet to be determined, as well as their influence on the variable nature and complexity of stuttering. (See Manning, 2001, for a review of different theoretical positions.)

The onset of stuttering usually occurs between 2 and 5 years of age and may emerge in a sudden or severe manner (Yairi & Ambrose, 1992). Some researchers report that approximately 80% of children who stutter will spontaneously recover before the age of puberty (Andrews & Harris, 1964; Yairi & Ambrose, 1999). Some evidence suggests that spontaneous recovery is a gradual process that may begin within the first year of stuttering and not reach completion until three or four years post-onset (Yairi & Ambrose, 1999). Differences in terminology, methodology, and interpretation of data make it difficult to compare results (Ingham & Bothe, 2001; Onslow & Packman, 1999; Yairi & Ambrose, 1999, 2001). Many clinicians use a rule of thumb that 50% to 80% of children who stutter will recover with or without treatment (Guitar, 1998). For individuals who continue to stutter, the characteristics of the disorder may gradually change over time. Several viewpoints regarding the development of stuttering have been proposed. Bloodstein (1960) describes a four-phase model that progresses from mild episodic disfluencies to severe, chronic stuttering accompanied by fear and avoidance reactions. Van Riper (1982) suggests a three-stage progression that includes primary, transitional, and secondary phases. A third hypothesis, put forth by Starkweather (1987), indicates that the development of stuttering fluctuates as a result of an individual's changing capacity to accommodate environmental demands for communicative performance. Finally, recent longitudinal data on preschool stutterers suggests that severity of stuttering at onset may remain unchanged up to three years post-onset (Throneburg & Yairi, 2001).

CATEGORIES OF STUTTERING BEHAVIORS

Two main categories of characteristics are associated with stuttering: core behaviors and secondary behaviors.

Core Behaviors

Core behaviors are the basic manifestations that seem beyond the voluntary control of the stutterer and include the following:

- Repetitions of sounds, syllables, or whole words (e.g., c-c-cat; ba-ba-balloon; we-we-we are going)
- Prolongations of single sounds (e.g., ssssssoap; fffffishing)
- Blocks of airflow/voicing during speech (inappropriate stoppage of air or voice at any level of the vocal tract)

Secondary Behaviors

Secondary behaviors develop over time as learned reactions to the core behaviors and are categorized as escape or avoidance behaviors. Escape behaviors occur during a stuttering moment and are attempts to break out of the stutter. Common examples of escape behaviors include head nods, eye blinks, foot taps, and jaw tremors. In the more advanced stages of stuttering, these behaviors may be accompanied by visible struggle and muscular tension. Avoidance behaviors occur in anticipation of a stuttering moment and are attempts to refrain from stuttering at all. Typical avoidance behaviors are circumlocutions (substitutions of less feared vocabulary words), unfilled pauses without accompanying tension and struggle within or between words, and use of "um" or other interjections to postpone speaking.

Developmental Disfluencies versus Stuttering

Most typically developing children between 2 and 4 years of age display relatively effortless disfluencies during the normal course of language acquisition (Gregory & Hill, 1993; Pellowski & Conture, 2002; Zebrowski, 1994).

- Hesitations (silent pauses)
- Interjections of sounds, syllables, or words (e.g., "Um, I went to school"; "Did you *you know* find her?")

- Revisions/repetitions of words, phrases, or sentences (e.g., "You have to touch, *no, turn* it"; "I have some . . . *I want you to look at* these baseball cards")
- Normal rhythm and stress patterns
- No tension or tremors noted

It is important to differentiate between these normal disfluencies and the atypical disfluencies in the following list, which are often the early signs of stuttering:

- Three or more **within-word** disfluencies per 100 words (especially fragmentation of syllables)
- Disfluencies on more than 10% of syllables spoken
- Predominant use of prolongations, blocks, and part-word repetitions (as opposed to interjections and whole-word or phrase repetitions)
- Presence of secondary behaviors/increased tension
- Vowel neutralization (schwa) during repetitions (e.g., buh-buh-beat)
- Duration of single instance of disfluency that exceeds two seconds
- Uncontrolled or abrupt changes in pitch or loudness

Ambrose and Yairi's (1999) large-scale study of preschool children provides strong evidence that stuttering can be differentiated from normal disfluency on the basis of three main characteristics: (1) part-word repetition; (2) single-syllable word repetition; and (3) disrhythmic phonation (i.e., prolongations, blocks, and broken words). This differential pattern of disfluency types was significant even at the early stages of stuttering.

TREATMENT

Regardless of theoretical orientation, the ultimate aim of most stuttering therapy programs is spontaneous fluency. Fluency can be described as consisting of four primary components: rate, continuity, rhythm, and effort (Starkweather, 1985, 1987). Accordingly, spontaneous fluent speech is smooth, relatively rapid, melodic (as opposed to monotonous), and appears free of conscious physical or mental effort. For people who demonstrate severe stuttering behavior, spontaneous fluency may not be considered a realistic goal. Controlled fluency or acceptable levels of stuttering may be identified as the ultimate goal of treatment for these individuals, depending on the clinician's philosophy of the general nature of stuttering. The client's cultural and linguistic background also may influence the choice of general approach to intervention. In addition, it is important to recognize that, unlike most other speech and language disorders, relapse is a common phenomenon in stuttering. People who stutter frequently experience periods of increased disfluency after treatment has been terminated. For this reason, periodic follow-up sessions should be an integral part of an effective fluency treatment program. For example, Blood (1995) advocates a cognitive-behavioral relapse management program for adolescents that is instituted following the completion of a traditional course of fluency therapy. This program provides training in five basic areas, including problem solving, general communication skills, assertiveness, coping strategies, and establishment of realistic expectations.

Individuals who stutter have been shown to demonstrate performance differences in some language and phonological skills when compared with typical speakers (Cuadrado & Webber-Fox, 2003; Melnick, Conture, & Ohde, 2003). Stuttering can also occur concomitantly with other communication problems such as language or phonology disorders, particularly in preschool and school-age children (Gregory, 2003). There are at least four programming alternatives for treating coexisting impairments (Ratner, 1995):

Discrete: A certain amount of therapy time is allotted to treat each disorder in isolation. For example, in a one-hour therapy session, a clinician may devote 20 minutes to fluency goals and the remaining 40 minutes to articulation goals. Alternatively, a twice-weekly therapy schedule can be divided to spend one session on each disorder area.

Modified cycles: Treatment for one disorder is implemented for a specified block of time (e.g., six weeks) and then discontinued. An equivalent time period is then devoted to treatment of the other communicative impairment. This cycle is alternated until long-term goals are achieved for each disorder.

Blended: Therapy goals for one disorder are incorporated into the therapy activities for a second disorder. For example, during articulation activities, the clinician can encourage fluency-enhancing behaviors such as slower speaking rate and increased pause time between conversational turns.

Lagged: This is a modified form of the blended approach that incorporates an initial time delay. Specifically, a period of initial therapy focuses on attaining a predetermined level of mastery in the concomitant disorder area (e.g., phonological or linguistic). Once the child has reached this level of mastery, fluency therapy can begin using the recently mastered phonological/ linguistic forms as the basis for practice. Fluency therapy continues to be programmed at comfortable levels of phonological/linguistic demand as the child progressively masters new objectives in the concomitant disorder area.

Treatment Efficacy/Evidence-Based Practice

Efficacy in the area of stuttering therapy is particularly difficult to measure because its definition must incorporate three interrelated factors: (1) objective measures of frequency and duration of stuttered moments, (2) client emotions and attitudes, and (3) the client's amenability to participate in communicative interactions with a variety of partners. Recently, the importance of treatment outcomes has been increasingly addressed in the stuttering literature. Several authors have attempted to clarify general principles of evidence-based practice as they relate to stuttering. They have proposed definitional and operational guidelines that can facilitate clinicians' ability to critically evaluate different approaches to stuttering treatment of young children and adults (Blood & Conture, 1998; Cordes & Ingham, 1998; Finn, 2003; Ingham, 2003; Ingham & Riley, 1998; Langevin &

Kully, 2003). Conture (1996) reviewed available data on treatment efficacy of stuttering. His summary organized studies according to four age groups: preschoolers, school-aged children, adolescents, and adults. The overall conclusion is that treatment for fluency disorders is generally effective across age ranges. Following are additional conclusions:

- Preschool children benefit from initiation of therapy in the early stages of stuttering.

- Efficacy information for school-age children and adolescents is scant, although preliminary data are emerging regarding predicting and/or minimizing relapse after treatment.

- Studies of adults indicate that prolonged speech and gentle onsets are two of the most effective treatment strategies for remediating stuttering.

- Future efficacy research is needed to address several critical issues, including the relationship between reduced stuttering and naturalness of speech, attitudinal changes, and long-term outcomes (e.g., more than five years) of intervention.

Intervention Techniques

A myriad of techniques are used in the treatment of stuttering. These include Shames and Florance's (1980) stutter-free speech program, Ryan's (1974) graduated increase in length and complexity model, computer-aided fluency establishment training (Goebel, 1986), Bloodstein's (1975) anticipatory struggle program, and Shine's (1980) systematic fluency training, to name just a few. More recently, Onslow and colleagues (Onslow & Andrews, 1994; Onslow & Packman, 1999) developed the Lidcombe program, an operant conditioning approach to stuttering intervention. The central component of the program is presentation of verbal contingencies for stuttered versus stutterfree speech (i.e., praise versus corrective feedback). It incorporates a strong focus on parental participation as well as a structured maintenance phase. Frequently, the client's age is a critical factor in determining how intervention will be implemented. Many clinicians use an indirect method of intervention with young children and more direct procedures with older clients. Philosophically, all the different approaches can be divided into two primary schools of thought: fluency shaping and stuttering modification.

Fluency Shaping. Fluency shaping is based on the assumption that stuttering is a learned behavior. The primary goal of fluency shaping is to eliminate disfluencies and gradually change the speaker's habitual speaking pattern to one of fluent speech. This is accomplished through the use of several fluency enhancing techniques:

- **Easy onset/prevoice exhalation:** The speaker is taught to exhale slightly before beginning phonation and reach conversational loudness gradually.

- **Decreased speaking rate (prolonged speech):** The speaker is trained to stretch out the sounds (primarily vowels) in his speech and produce words at a slower-than-normal speaking rate while maintaining normal stress and intonation.

- **Light articulatory contacts:** The speaker is taught to move the articulators in a loose and relaxed manner.
- **Continuous phonation:** The speaker is trained to reduce all breaks between words by maintaining voicing continuously until he naturally needs to take a breath.

The ultimate aim of programs based on a fluency shaping philosophy is to completely change speech behavior by teaching clients to use these techniques at all times, not just during disfluent moments. These techniques are designed to interfere with the stuttering behaviors, thus reducing them. Overall, most fluency shaping programs can be categorized according to which parameter of communicative interaction is the focus of change: speech rate, length of utterance, or provision of contingent feedback. Therapy sessions focus solely on acquisition of fluency enhancing behaviors and generally do not address a client's secondary behaviors or the negative feelings and attitudes that may be associated with the stuttering.

Delayed auditory feedback (DAF) is a fluency shaping technique that has been widely used in the treatment of stuttering. It is a system in which a speaker's own words are returned to her through headphones after an imposed electronic delay of a few milliseconds. For normal speakers, the use of DAF disrupts the smooth flow of speech and results in a significant breakdown in fluency. DAF has the opposite effect on the speech of many individuals who stutter; it decreases their speech rate and reduces the number of notable disfluencies. As a general rule, therapy is initiated at a delay time of approximately 250 ms. The time delay is then reduced in 50-ms intervals (i.e., 200 ms, 150 ms, 100 ms, and so on) as the client stabilizes her fluency skills at each level. (See Ham, 1999, for detailed information on the implementation of DAF as a clinical procedure.)

Use of DAF in stuttering therapy has been recommended by many authors, including Van Riper (1973); Webster, Schumacher, and Lubker (1970); and Shames & Florance (1980). Proponents of this technique suggest that it tends to generate increased fluency in the early stages of therapy. DAF is also believed to enhance the speaker's ability to monitor oral-sensory feedback cues from his own speech mechanism. Finally, it facilitates a slower speaking rate by increasing a client's syllable duration and phonation time. However, other writers have cautioned about the possible drawbacks of DAF (Sheehan, 1968; Wingate, 1976). Among the most commonly cited disadvantages are difficulty in weaning clients from the DAF equipment and the development of a "DAF voice" (slow, labored, lacking in inflection and stress variation). For a detailed review of the literature on the effects of DAF, see Bloodstein (1995).

Stuttering Modification. Stuttering modification is based on the premise that stuttering may involve a physiological predisposition. The primary goals of stuttering modification are to modify each disfluent moment by stuttering more easily and to eliminate struggle and avoidance behaviors (Van Riper, 1973). Gregory

(1979) called this the "stutter more fluently" approach. These goals are accomplished through the use of a combination of the following techniques:

- **Self-analysis:** Increase the client's awareness of the type, severity, and loci of disfluencies as well as any accompanying secondary behaviors (see Activity 1 in Profile 3 for stuttering modification approach). Attention also may be given to increasing the client's self-awareness of the characteristics of his nonstuttered speech and monitoring his proprioceptive awareness of the oral musculature.

- **Relaxation:** Reduce the client's anxiety and muscle tension through relaxation training (see Table 7-1 for specific steps).

- **Desensitization:** Reduce negative emotions associated with stuttering (e.g., fear, frustration, embarrassment) by decreasing sensitivity to core behaviors and listener reactions through activities such as voluntary stuttering or freezing (see Activities 2 and 3, respectively, in Profile 4 for stuttering modification approach).

In this philosophy, therapy outcomes are not defined strictly by decreases in stuttering frequency counts. Rather, progress is measured along a qualitative continuum as the nature of stuttering shifts from high-struggle with syllable fragmentations to less effortful, forward-moving speech.

TABLE 7-1
Progressive Relaxation Training

Step 1:	Ensure that the client is seated comfortably.
Step 2:	Explain that this procedure involves the deliberate contracting and relaxing of various muscles to help the client recognize and discriminate between muscular tension and relaxation.
Step 3:	Starting at the level of the abdomen, instruct the client to tightly contract his stomach muscles for at least five seconds and then relax them. Encourage the client to concentrate on how his muscles feel when they are in a tensed versus relaxed state. Require the client to perform this activity three to five times.
Step 4:	Repeat the contraction-relaxation sequence with other muscle groups moving progressively toward the head (i.e., arms, shoulders, neck, face). The clinician should periodically check the client's level of relaxation during the release phase by placing one hand on the target muscle group and pushing slightly to determine the degree of muscle resistance. Noticeable resistance indicates an insufficient degree of relaxation.
Step 5:	At the level of the face, instruct the client to perform each of the following movement sequences three to five times: clench the mandible against the upper molars and release; pucker and release the lips; push the blade of the tongue strongly against the hard palate and release; tightly close both eyes and then open; frown in an exaggerated manner and relax.

Note: The aim of teaching progressive relaxation is to enable the stutterer to consistently identify instances of excessive muscular tension during speech and to immediately transition into a relaxed state without having to work through the entire stepwise progression.
Sources: Adapted from Jacobson (1938) and Ham (1986).

Clinicians who employ a stuttering modification approach work with clients to identify hierarchies of feared speaking situations. These hierarchies are valuable tools for a variety of therapeutic purposes: a) developing clients' self-awareness and ability to analyze their behavior; b) recognizing variations in clients' stuttering patterns across different settings; and c) facilitating development of sequential behavioral objectives and collection of data. (See Figure 7-1 for sample hierarchies.)

The following techniques are generally intended to be used as a three-part sequence in the following order:

- **Cancellations:** When experiencing a disfluency, the speaker is encouraged to *complete* the intended word without attempting to break out of the disfluency. After the disfluency has been produced, the speaker is instructed to pause and mentally rehearse a technique for producing the word more fluently (or with an easier stutter) and then repeat the word.

- **Pull-outs:** When experiencing a disfluency, the speaker is taught to stop in the *middle* of the stuttering moment, mentally rehearse the intended word using a fluency enhancing technique (or easier stuttering pattern) and then reproduce it.

- **Preparatory sets:** The speaker is encouraged to anticipate an imminent disfluency and pause briefly to mentally rehearse fluent (or gentle stuttering) production *before* the word is attempted.

The ultimate aim of programs based on a stuttering modification philosophy is to modify stuttering behaviors to an acceptable level rather than eliminate them entirely. The client's negative attitudes and feelings toward his or her stuttering

FIGURE 7-1
Climbing the fear hierarchy.

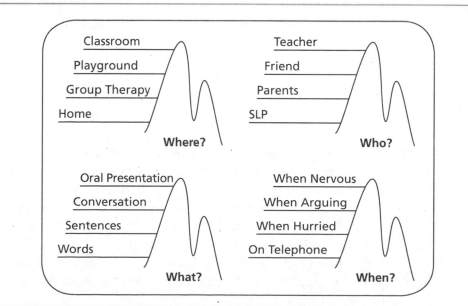

(Reprinted by permission Sisskin, 2002.)

are typically identified and monitored over time through the administration of attitudinal scales. Therapy sessions also give considerable attention to the reduction of speech fears and secondary behaviors as a means of minimizing stuttering. Elementary school-aged children and adolescents are particularly vulnerable to teasing and negative self-image. Effective therapy programs incorporate activities such as role playing and brainstorming to proactively address these issues. Detailed information on counseling techniques can be found in Chapter 9.

Guitar (1998) suggests that long-term fluency goals and clinical methods are two important treatment issues that differentiate fluency shaping and stuttering modification approaches. With regard to fluency goals, the three possible outcomes of therapy are spontaneous fluency, controlled fluency, and acceptable stuttering. The outcome of choice for both therapy approaches is spontaneous fluency with a secondary goal of controlled fluency.

Guitar (1998) and others advocate the integration of fluency shaping and stuttering modification techniques in the treatment of stuttering. They believe that stuttering results from an interaction of physiologic factors and learned behaviors. Therefore, facets of each approach are viewed as essential components of an effective treatment paradigm.

Example Profiles

Four profiles representative of fluency problems exhibited by clients of different age ranges (i.e., preschool, school-age, and adult) are presented in this section. These examples have been designed to illustrate the selection of intervention targets, specific therapy activities, and materials. Implementation of both fluency shaping and stuttering modification approaches is demonstrated for each profile.

PROFILE 1

Eli is 3 years old and his speech is characterized by hesitations, whole-word/phrase repetitions, and interjections of syllables/words (e.g., "um," "well") with no accompanying struggle behaviors. Analysis of a 200-syllable spontaneous speech sample indicated that 20% of the syllables uttered were disfluent. By parental report, Eli appears to exhibit no awareness of his communication difficulties. Receptive and expressive language abilities, as well as other developmental skills, appear age appropriate.

Selection of therapy targets. The overall communicative profile demonstrated by Eli is consistent with that of a child experiencing normal disfluencies, except for the relatively high frequency of the disfluencies. Based on Eli's disfluency rate and his young chronological age, an indirect approach to treatment is selected for use. An indirect approach focuses on the modification of the communicative environment rather than on treating the disfluencies themselves. The child's family is taught strategies for adapting its communicative behaviors in ways that create an environment conducive to the production of fluent speech. This is particularly important since survey evidence indicates that parents may unknowingly exacerbate children's disfluencies by correcting and/or finishing their utterances (ASHA Leader, 2003). Families are encouraged to do the following:

- Listen attentively to the child's message rather than to his speech pattern.
- Avoid speaking for the child; do not fill in or complete the child's message.
- Avoid communicative stresses such as time pressures.
- Decrease demands for verbal performance (e.g., "Tell Aunt Suzie what you did in school today.").
- Avoid interrupting the child or allowing siblings or friends to interrupt (emphasize the rules for turn-taking in conversation).
- Avoid the predominant use of questions that demand lengthy or complex responses in favor of those that require simple one- or two-word answers.
- Avoid using an excessively rapid speech pattern; be sure to model smooth, relaxed speech when talking with the child (Guitar & Marchinkoski, 2001).
- Avoid labeling disfluencies as stuttering.
- Maintain natural eye contact while the child speaks, even during disfluencies.
- Avoid correcting the child's mispronunciations of speech sounds.

An important aspect of the indirect approach is to facilitate parental awareness of the child's fluency status in the home environment. This can be accomplished through use of a fluency observation chart (Form 7-1) in which parents keep a record of each disfluency exhibited by the child at home and the factors that surround it.

It is essential to maintain regular contact with the family to monitor the effectiveness of these strategies in ameliorating the child's disfluencies. A more direct treatment approach should be considered when no significant improvement is reported after a predetermined time period (e.g., 3–4 months), or more immediately if the child's communication performance deteriorates (i.e., demonstrates a higher frequency or longer duration of disfluencies, emergence of struggle behaviors).

Helpful Hints

1. Videotapes of natural family interactions (e.g., birthday party, family vacation, family reunion) can be helpful in identifying the communication patterns used by different family members with the child.
2. The effectiveness of an indirect treatment approach can be enhanced by preparing simple, clear materials that outline the desired communication strategies listed previously. These materials can be given to individuals with whom the child has regular contact (i.e., daycare providers, preschool teachers, babysitters, grandparents, and so on).
3. For families that seem overly sensitive to their child's disfluencies, it may be helpful to have them chart the type and number of disfluencies that occur naturally in everyday conversations among normally fluent speakers.

FORM 7-1 HOME FLUENCY OBSERVATION CHART

Child's Name: _____   Informant: _____

Instructions: Over the next week, write down at least five situations in which your child experiences disfluency. Please indicate the circumstances in which the disfluency occurs by recording the information below. It is recommended that a separate recording chart be maintained by each observer.

Date/Time	Situation/ Topic	Type of Disfluency	Child's Reaction to Disfluency	Listener Name/ Reaction to Disfluency	What Triggered the Disfluency

4. Parents often express feelings of guilt regarding a child's disfluencies. It is important to assure parents that they did not cause the fluency problem and that their consistent use of the recommended communication strategies can be the most powerful, positive facilitator of fluent speech for their child. (Refer to Chapter 9 for additional information on counseling strategies.)

5. Clinicians may need to make parents aware that the severity of their child's stuttering can vary considerably from one day to the next. This inconsistent behavior is typical of stuttering and should not to be interpreted as voluntary in nature or indicative of permanent change in fluency status.

6. In their attempts to minimize disfluent moments, families may inadvertently reduce or alter the amount/variety of verbal exchanges with their children. Clinicians should encourage family members to maintain natural levels of communicative interactions that typically occur in the home environment.

For each of the remaining profiles, two sets of therapy targets will be presented, one based on a fluency shaping approach and the other on stuttering modification. The sample activities that are included were designed to illustrate how each of these treatment paradigms can be implemented.

PROFILE 2

Kate is 3 years old and her speech is characterized by hesitations, whole-word/phrase repetitions, and interjections of syllables/words. Unlike Eli in Profile 1, Kate also demonstrates occasional word-initial syllable repetitions, accompanied by the incipient secondary behaviors of eye blinks and head nods. Analysis of a 200-syllable spontaneous speech sample indicated that 23% of the syllables uttered were disfluent. According to her parents, Kate is extremely frustrated by her disfluencies and often states, "I can't say that word." Her receptive and expressive language abilities, as well as other developmental milestones, appear age appropriate.

Selection of therapy targets using a fluency shaping approach. The behaviors to be targeted are decreased speech rate and easy onset of phonation. These techniques were chosen because they are relatively easy for a young child to conceptualize and generally yield a marked decrease in disfluencies. In addition, the use of easy onset is particularly appropriate because it tends to inhibit the production of word-initial disfluencies.

Sample Activities

1. Fill a large bag or pillowcase with 25 to 30 small toys and objects. Collect pictures of one slow-moving and one fast-moving animal (e.g., whale and rabbit). Point to each picture while modeling the animals' special voices. Demonstrate the whale's voice by producing simple sentences using an exaggerated slow speech rate (approximately three to four syllables per second) and easy onset of phonation. Repeat the same sentences to demonstrate the rabbit's voice with an extremely rapid speech rate and abrupt onset of phonation.

Select a carrier phrase that begins with a vowel, such as "I have a
_____." Tell the child that she should close her eyes and pick one object
from the bag. Have the child say the carrier phrase five times, including the
name of the chosen object, using the preferred "whale voice" (e.g., "I have a
ball"). As each utterance is produced, the clinician identifies the child's
speech pattern by pointing to one of the animal pictures. Whenever the
child's utterance is more like the rabbit's voice, the clinician provides another
model of the whale's smooth, easy speaking voice and asks the child to imitate it. The child is then given a brief opportunity to play with the selected
toy before repeating the sequence with another toy.

2. Obtain an empty coffee can and punch 20 holes (approximately the width of
a pencil) in the plastic lid. Place a small toy or other prize inside the can.
Gather 20 lengths of colored yarn (each approximately 12 inches long) and tie
a large knot at one end of each piece. Put the knotted ends of the strings at
the bottom of the can and replace the lid on the can with unknotted ends of
each piece protruding slightly from the top of the lid. Select a book that contains pictures of common objects and activities with which the child is familiar. The clinician shows the child the first picture in the book and models
simple three- to five-word sentences (e.g., There's a doggie; I see a baby; The
man is running; The house is red) using a very slow, easy speaking voice. The
child is required to imitate the sentence using the same speech pattern while
pulling one string of yarn through the coffee can lid in a correspondingly
slow and gentle manner (until the yarn is stopped by the knot). Model a different sentence for each successive picture until all the yarn pieces are
"sprouting" from the can. After the last string has been pulled, the child may
remove the lid to find the prize hidden inside.

Selection of therapy targets using a stuttering modification approach.
Stuttering modification may be of limited usefulness with a child of this age
because many of the techniques employed in this approach require relatively
advanced cognitive skills and are beyond the grasp of a 3-year-old child (e.g., self-
analysis, cancellations, pull-outs). However, parents can be encouraged to minimize their child's anxiety by using appropriate vocabulary for casual reference to
disfluencies (e.g., bumpy speech) and modeling expressions that mirror their child's
feelings (e.g., That one was really tough to say). One aspect of this approach that
can be extremely effective with very young disfluent children is desensitization.
Therefore, the goal is to lessen the child's sensitivity to her own disfluencies.

Sample Activities

1. Obtain two Colorform sets (or two simple puzzles) and a deck of 25 cards
depicting different agent + action relationships. Give one set (puzzle) to each
player and place the card deck facedown on the table. Introduce a "Catch Me
if You Can" game by explaining that each person will take a turn picking a
card from the deck, placing it faceup on the table, and describing it. The clinician should be prepared to pseudo-stutter (pretend to be disfluent) using

the child's habitual pattern on about half of her turns. The child is instructed to listen carefully for any instances of "bumpy" (disfluent) speech during the clinician's or her own turn and to immediately slap the picture as soon as she hears it. The clinician provides feedback regarding the smoothness or bumpiness of every production. The player who slaps the picture first earns a chance to put a piece on the Colorform set. Repeat this sequence until the card deck is depleted.

2. Gather three puppets with movable mouths. One is for the clinician; the others are given to the child. Select a storybook that has a repetitive refrain or story line (e.g., *Green Eggs and Ham, The Little Red Hen*, and so on). Explain to the child that her puppets both have "bumpy" voices, but that "Snappy" has more trouble with his words and gets stuck more often than "Max." The clinician uses her puppet to model both voices. The bumpier voice should reflect the child's habitual disfluency pattern in a slightly exaggerated manner and be accompanied by the child's secondary behaviors. The other voice is produced with just a few easy whole-word repetitions. Tell the child that the clinician's puppet is going to read a story out loud alternately using one or the other of her puppets' voices. The child's puppets will supply the refrain or repetitive line. The child must identify which voice the clinician's puppet is producing by making either Snappy or Max say the refrain in the same voice as the clinician's model. The clinician should gradually increase the frequency with which Max's less bumpy voice is presented as a model for imitation.

PROFILE 3

Susan is 9 years old and her speech is characterized by part word repetitions, whole-word repetitions, prolongations of initial sounds (approximately two to three seconds), and phrase revisions. She was noted to demonstrate several secondary behaviors, of which she did not seem consistently aware. These included excessive leg movements, lip tremors, and eye gaze aversion. Analysis of a 200-syllable spontaneous speech sample indicated that 29% of the syllables uttered were disfluent. According to parental report, Susan is extremely anxious about her speech difficulties. Developmental history is unremarkable and her academic performance is appropriate for her grade level.

Selection of therapy targets using a fluency shaping approach. The behaviors to be targeted are easy onset of phonation, light articulatory contacts, and decreased speaking rate. An analysis of Susan's disfluency profile indicates that her most severe stuttering characteristics are initial sound prolongations and part-word repetitions. Easy onset and light articulatory contacts were chosen because they are effective in addressing these types of disfluencies, especially when they occur in the word-initial position. Decreased speaking rate is considered a basic intervention technique that generally results in an immediate observable decrease in frequency of stuttering and thus provides the child with success in the very early stages of therapy.

Sample Activities

1. Play a modified version of an "I Spy" game in which the clinician is "it." Before beginning the game, teach the fluency enhancing techniques of easy onset of phonation and light articulatory contacts. Instruct the child to release a little bit of air before starting her voice and to move her tongue and lips gently during speech. The clinician models each of the target techniques in single words. As soon as the child demonstrates some mastery of these behaviors (e.g., five consecutive correct responses), the "I Spy" game can be initiated. The clinician thinks of an object in the room and gives the child clues to its identity by describing its attributes one at a time (e.g., "I spy something black"; "I spy something heavy"; and so on), employing a slightly exaggerated rendition of both techniques. After each clue, the child takes one guess at identifying the object (at the single-word level) using both fluency techniques. Continue to present clues until the object is named. In the early phases of therapy, a slight modification of the game is recommended when the child takes his turn to be "it." Following the child's selection of an object, the clinician supplies the carrier phrase, "I spy something . . . ," for the child to complete with a single word clue using the target fluency techniques.

2. Obtain a book of Mad Libs. Mad Libs are stories or vignettes in which specific parts of speech (e.g., noun, proper noun, adverb, adjective, and so on) have been omitted. When the missing parts are filled in, the result is a semantically absurd and funny text. The clinician selects one of the stories and says, "Give me an example of a _____" for each of the omitted parts of speech. These utterances should be produced with a slightly decreased speaking rate to highlight the target behavior. The child provides a word or phrase, which the clinician inserts into the written story. When all the blanks have been filled in, the child is instructed to read the whole story aloud using a predetermined slow rate of speech. The child then takes a turn choosing a Mad Lib and asks the clinician to supply the missing parts, remembering to use her slow speech rate. Instruct the child to read the completed story aloud to give her maximal opportunities to practice the target behavior. (This task is best used with children who have already demonstrated initial mastery of decreased speaking rate at the level of imitation.)

Selection of therapy targets using a stuttering modification approach. Based on Susan's fluency profile, the therapy targets are her secondary behaviors, prolongation of initial sounds, and part-word repetitions. The secondary behaviors were selected because Susan shows little awareness of them and because these behaviors are highly distracting to conversational partners. The prolongations and part-word repetitions were identified as therapy targets because they represent Susan's most severe disfluency types.

Sample Activities

1. Obtain a 20- to 30-minute videotaped sample of the child's connected speech that represents her typical pattern and level of disfluencies. Explain to the

child that when she stutters, she often exhibits some extra body movements and tends to look away from the listener. Tell her that she and the clinician will review the videotape to increase her awareness of the occurrence of these accompanying behaviors (i.e., leg movements, lip tremors, and eye gaze aversion). Select one of the secondary characteristics and tell the child that she and the clinician will watch the tape carefully for instances of that behavior. The first person to notice an occurrence of the target should signal by raising her hand. The person who signals correct identifications most frequently is declared the winner. Particularly clear examples of the behaviors may be played again to reinforce the child's understanding of the nature of the secondary characteristic. The initial stages of this activity should entail the use of brief segments of videotape (i.e., one minute), which can be gradually increased as the child demonstrates greater facility with the task.

2. Compile a list of 25 animal riddles (e.g., Q: Why do chimpanzees like bananas? A: Because they have a-peel). Underline one word in the question part of each riddle, being sure to vary location of the underlined word in the sentence. Tell the child that she is going to read the riddles to the clinician using cancellations.

   Before beginning this activity, review this stuttering modification technique with the child. Remind the child that, whenever she gets stuck on a word, she should complete the stutter without trying to start the word or sentence again. Once the word is finished, the child should pause to think about what went wrong, using the self-analysis skills learned in previous stages of therapy. The child should plan how to correct it by silently rehearsing how it would feel to say the word fluently. Then, have the child repeat the word in a smooth, prolonged manner. Provide the child with several opportunities to practice the technique by modeling some disfluencies and cancellations for her to imitate.

   Instruct the child to read the first part of each riddle and to deliberately stutter on the underlined word in the question. Each disfluency should be modified using cancellation. Once the cancellation has been successfully completed, the child can finish reading the whole riddle. Any spontaneous disfluencies that occur on words other than the underlined target should also be cancelled.

PROFILE 4

Patrick is 29 years old and his speech is characterized by laryngeal blocks and prolongations of initial sounds. Duration of blocks ranges between 2 to 20 seconds, while prolongations tend to last 3 to 5 seconds. Patrick was observed to demonstrate numerous secondary behaviors, including head jerks, jaw tremors, eye blinks, and audible inhalation. Analysis of a 200-syllable spontaneous speech sample indicated that 35% of syllables uttered were disfluent. During the case history interview, Patrick stated that stuttering has been a problem since childhood and that he is currently seeking treatment because his disfluencies are interfering with career advancement as well as interpersonal relationships.

Selection of therapy targets using a fluency shaping approach. The behaviors to be targeted are easy onset of phonation and continuous phonation. These techniques were chosen because they require an open vocal fold posture and, therefore, inhibit the production of laryngeal blocks, Patrick's most severe type of disfluency.

Sample Activities

1. Draw a graphic representation of two breath curves, like the ones shown in Figure 7-2. Explain that the first drawing represents the usual pattern of speaking in which voicing (the dotted line) is initiated at the same time as the onset of exhalation (the solid line). Explain to the client that his attempts to use this pattern often result in complete involuntary closure of the vocal folds (i.e., laryngeal blocks). Introduce the second drawing and tell him that it illustrates an alternative phonation pattern that will help prevent these blocks. Explain that the solid line again represents the point at which inhalation ends and exhalation begins and that the dotted line has been moved to indicate that his voice should start *after* exhalation has begun. Using the easy onset graph, instruct the client to place his finger at the beginning of the breath curve. Tell him to move his finger slowly along the curve as he inhales. When his finger reaches the solid line, he should begin to exhale slowly and continuously. As his finger reaches the dotted line, the client should *maintain* his open vocal fold posture and smoothly produce an isolated vowel such as /o, a, uh/. Once the client can easily initiate phonation without blocking, the task can progress hierarchically from isolated vowels to h-initial words, and then to more complex units of speech. (See Appendix 7-A for sample materials including phrases, questions, and monologue topics.)

2. Prepare a list of 50 simple three-word phrases (see Appendix 7-A). Introduce the technique of continuous phonation by explaining to the client that he should keep his voice turned on even between words, but without increasing his habitual speech rate. Model use of the technique by first producing an

FIGURE 7-2
Breath curves.

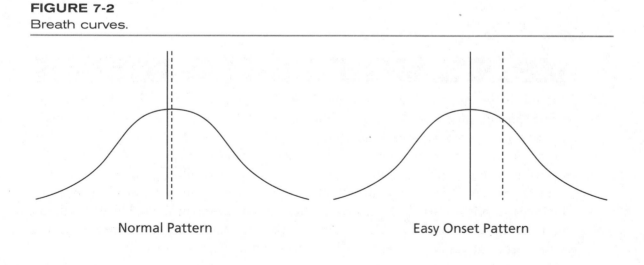

Normal Pattern   Easy Onset Pattern

audible yawn, which is characterized by continuous voicing. Produce the yawn a second time, and overlay a four-word utterance that lasts throughout its duration. Stress the idea that speaking over the yawn results in a smooth, unbroken utterance stream. Instruct the client to produce several audible yawns to heighten his awareness of how it feels to produce smooth, flowing streams of phonation. Read phrases from the prepared list and have the client imitate each stimulus phrase using the yawn technique to emphasize the production of continuous phonation.

Selection of therapy targets using a stuttering modification approach. Based on Patrick's fluency profile, the therapy targets are his secondary behaviors, laryngeal blocks, and prolongations of initial sounds. The secondary behaviors were chosen because their bizarre nature tends to invoke severe listener penalty. Patrick's two main disfluency types were selected because both blocks and prolongations interfere significantly with his ability to communicate.

Sample Activities

1. Help the client to generate a list of anxiety-producing speaking situations and arrange them hierarchically from least to most feared. Teach the client a tension reduction procedure such as progressive relaxation (Jacobson, 1938). This technique can be modified specifically for stutterers by using the steps outlined in Table 7-1. Once the client demonstrates the ability to consciously achieve a relaxed state, explain that relaxation will be used to desensitize him to the previously identified feared speaking situations. Beginning with the least feared situation in the hierarchy, instruct the client to use visual imagery to imagine himself in that situation. Tell him to monitor his overall level of muscle tone for any significant increase in tension. Whenever the client identifies an occurrence of excessive tension, he is instructed to employ the relaxation skills learned in progressive relaxation training. Continue to have the client focus on the same speaking situation until he demonstrates the ability to remain relaxed throughout the entire visualization. Once the client can maintain a relaxed state at this level with minimal discernible effort, move to the next situation in the hierarchy. Repeat the visualization-relaxation sequence for each successive entry until the client is effectively desensitized to the thought of all the feared speaking situations in the hierarchy. Once the client can consciously induce a relaxed state, progress to more difficult environments such as including strangers in the therapy session and going outside the clinic setting (e.g., a store or library).

2. Introduce the technique of voluntary stuttering and the rationale for its use in the treatment process. Explain that this technique requires clients to stutter on purpose and then analyze their own feelings as well as listener reactions. The goal of voluntary stuttering is to reduce/minimize the stutterer's feelings of fear or embarrassment associated with disfluent moments. Model easy repetitions and prolongations for the client during a short conversational

interaction. Then instruct the client to produce at least five of these voluntary stutters on nonfeared words during another three-minute conversation. Provide visual cues (e.g., hand gestures), as necessary, to prompt the client's use of easy repetitions and prolongations. Following the conversation, the client should rank feelings of anxiety on a five-point scale. Once the client is comfortable with this technique in the clinical setting, the task can be implemented gradually in real-world situations with other conversational partners. In addition, the rating scale can be expanded to rank degrees of negative listener reactions.

3. Introduce the concept of freezing, which involves purposefully extending the moment of stuttering to increase the client's tolerance for and control over core stuttering behaviors. Instruct the client to read aloud lists of short phrases (e.g., Appendix 7-A). Explain that when a disfluency occurs, the clinician will signal the client to continue the stutter. The client should maintain the same disfluency pattern (prolongation, repetition, or block) until the clinician signals to release it.

4. Obtain a board game suitable for adults that generally requires the production of multiword responses, such as Jeopardy. Explain the rules of the game and inform the client that he will assume the role of contestant. Tell him that each of his responses must contain at least one pseudo or real disfluency, which he will modify using pull-outs. Review this stuttering modification technique by reminding the client that whenever he gets stuck on a word, he should (a) stop in the middle of the disfluency; (b) pause to mentally rehearse how it would feel to produce that word fluently; (c) say the word a second time in a smooth, prolonged manner; and (d) complete the rest of the intended utterance without going back to the beginning of the sentence. Provide several opportunities to practice this technique by modeling some disfluencies and pull-outs for him to imitate. Begin the game by instructing the client to choose a topic category and a difficulty level. Read the designated "answer" to which the client must respond in the form of a question that contains a pull-out. Provide the opportunity for the client to produce at least 50 "questions" during the game.

Helpful Hints

1. For each of the activities listed, the difficulty of the task can be manipulated systematically with regard to utterance length using the traditional hierarchy of single words, carrier phrase + word, sentence, two- to four-word sentences, conversation. Provision of consistent clinician models should be faded gradually until all client responses are spontaneously generated without any model.

2. As therapy progresses, introduce activities that simulate natural speaking situations. For young children, these might include asking for a turn to play with a toy, asking for assistance in completing a puzzle, describing pictures in a book, playing house or tea party, telling stories, and negotiating the rules

of a game. For older children and adults, activities may involve talking on the telephone, ordering food at a restaurant, asking for directions, interviewing for a job, and giving presentations in class or at work.

3. Fluency shaping and stuttering modification techniques can be combined within the same therapy session. It is best to begin the session with stuttering modification techniques and then move on to fluency shaping. If implemented in the reverse order, carryover from fluency shaping practice may significantly decrease the number of disfluencies the client produces during the treatment visit. The reduced frequency of stuttering may not provide the client with adequate opportunities to learn and practice stuttering modification techniques later in the session.

4. Once the target concepts and techniques have been established in individual sessions, group therapy can be particularly effective for strengthening and refining clients' fluency skills.

5. It is essential for the clinician to monitor her or his reactions to client disfluencies. Even subtle indications of discomfort (e.g., averted eye gaze) may adversely affect the therapeutic relationship between client and clinician.

6. A client's feelings about his stuttering can be monitored over the course of therapy by periodic readministration of a stuttering attitude checklist (see Form 7-2). Such scales are not intended to be scored quantitatively along a continuum of severity, but rather to provide descriptive information about changes in the client's emotions and attitudes.

7. Families should be encouraged to avoid a conspiracy of silence regarding stuttering. Open acknowledgment and discussion can minimize feelings of isolation and shame often experienced by individuals who stutter. (Refer to Chapter 9 for additional information on counseling strategies.)

8. Stuttering modification therapy frequently results in a noticeable increase in observable disfluencies as the client begins to relinquish habitual avoidance strategies. The focus of counseling at this point is twofold: (a) to help the client understand that this stage of therapy is temporary and (b) to provide consistent and direct support as the client confronts feared speaking situations during this phase.

9. Clinicians should be aware that older children and adolescents (i.e., between approximately 10 and 17 years of age) frequently demonstrate extreme resistance to any type of fluency therapy. Parents may require considerable counseling support to accept the fact that their child may not be emotionally ready to benefit from direct intervention during this period. Clinicians should also reassure parents that willingness to participate in therapy reemerges with increased maturity.

10. Individuals with a long-standing history of severe stuttering often limit their participation in social interactions, resulting in a relative lack of practice with conversational skills in both speaker and listener roles. Clinicians can incorporate pragmatic language goals into the fluency treatment plan in order to facilitate maximal communicative effectiveness.

FORM 7-2 STUTTERING ATTITUDE CHECKLIST

Instructions: Respond to the following by circling "Y" to indicate that "Yes, I agree" or "N" to indicate "No, I do not agree" with each statement. Record your initial reaction rather than analyzing or deliberating over each statement.

1.   Y   N   I often feel that stuttering is my own fault.

2.   Y   N   I find it easy to talk to people in authority such as my teacher or my employer.

3.   Y   N   Sometimes I wonder if I stutter on purpose to get attention.

4.   Y   N   I have more trouble saying some words/sounds than others.

5.   Y   N   Most people think that stutterers are not quite as smart as people who do not stutter.

6.   Y   N   People always seem comfortable when I am talking to them.

7.   Y   N   I think that stuttering is caused by some kind of mental or emotional problem.

8.   Y   N   My stuttering keeps me from doing the kind of work that I would really like to do.

9.   Y   N   I sometimes think that other people are responsible for having caused my stuttering.

10.   Y   N   The way I talk does not embarrass me.

11.   Y   N   Stuttering is my biggest problem.

12.   Y   N   Even when I know the right answer to a question, I often keep silent because of my stuttering.

13.   Y   N   I think speech therapy can help me a great deal.

14.   Y   N   My stuttering would go away if I stopped worrying about it all the time.

15.   Y   N   I feel that I should be able to stop my stuttering without help from anyone else.

Sources: Adapted from Cooper & Cooper (1985) and Andrews & Cutler (1974).

CONCLUSION

This chapter presented basic information, protocols, and procedures for intervention with fluency disorders at an **introductory** level. This information is intended only as a starting point in the reader's clinical education and training. For more in-depth coverage of this area, the following readings are recommended:

Guitar, B. (1998). *Stuttering: An integrated approach to its nature and treatment.* Baltimore: Williams & Wilkins.

Ham, R. E. (1990). *Therapy of stuttering: Preschool through adolescence.* Englewood Cliffs, NJ: Prentice Hall.

Ham, R. E. (1999). *Clinical management of stuttering in older children and adults.* Austin, TX: Pro-Ed.

Manning, W.H. (2001). *Clinical decision making in fluency disorders.* Albany, NY: Singular Thomson Learning.

Shapiro, D. (1999). *Stuttering intervention: A collaborative journey to fluency freedom.* Austin, TX: Pro-Ed.

Van Riper, C. (1982). *The nature of stuttering.* Englewood Cliffs, NJ: Prentice Hall.

ADDITIONAL RESOURCES

The Speech Bin
1965 Twenty-Fifth Avenue
Vero Beach, FL 32960
Phone: 800-4-SPEECH
Fax: 888-FAX 2 BIN
Web site: www.speechbin.com

Systematic Fluency Training for Young Children
Highly structured program that addresses phonatory, articulatory, and respiratory aspects of speech; includes cards, therapy objects, storybooks, and audiocassettes.

Successful Stuttering Management Program
Step-by-step approach for adolescent and adult stutterers. Includes reproducible handouts, home assignments, an audiotape, and an e-mail component for the maintenance phase. Ideal for use in group or individual sessions and to guide clients in self-help.

Stepping Up to Fluency
Systematic program for clients ages 5 years to adult. Presents strategies and materials in two levels, K–3 (Level I) and grade 4 to adult (Level II), in a series of four stages: identification, target training, evaluation, and carryover. Includes reproducible activities and suggestions for fluency maintenance.

Winning in Speech: A Workbook for Fluency
For children ages 7 to 14. Explores factors that interfere with the ability to speak fluently, including struggle reactions, self-concepts, fears about speaking, and perceptions about listeners. Provides reproducible worksheets to facilitate carryover as well as to show parents how to help their child.

Easy Talker: A Fluency Workbook for School-Age Children
For children in grades 3 to 12. Uses a three-step approach for working on and coping with stuttering by focusing on cognition, emotion, and behavior. Incorporates these issues into real-life situations and solutions.

Coping for Kids Who Stutter
A helpful resource to teach children, their families, and teachers about the nature of stuttering. This matter-of-fact book presents a multitude of facts about stuttering and gives good advice about what to do in a nonthreatening, convincing manner. It also helps children who stutter rid themselves of feelings of diminished self-esteem.

Pro-Ed
8700 Shoal Creek Boulevard
Austin, TX 78757-6897
Phone: 800-897-3202
Fax: 800-397-7633
Web site: www.proedinc.com

Cooper Personalized Fluency Control Therapy, third edition
Separate children and adult/adolescent programs that include comprehensive fluency assessment and treatment processes addressing the affective, behavioral, and cognitive components of fluency disorders. A list of references is included and appendices include stuttering information and support sources.

The Lidcombe Program of Early Stuttering Intervention: A Clinician's Guide
This text is written for clinicians to provide detailed information on the method and implementation of the Lidcombe Program, a parent-conducted, behavioral treatment for stuttering that is designed for children younger than age 6.

LinguiSystems
3100 Fourth Avenue
East Moline, IL 61244-9700
Phone: 800-776-4332
Fax: 800-577-4555
E-mail: linguisys@aol.com
Web site: www.linguisystems.com

Easy Does It for Fluency
Two separate programs for preschool/primary children aged 2 to 6 years and intermediate children aged 6 to 11 years. The preschool/primary program focuses on the use of slow, easy speech to maintain fluency presented through five steps; the intermediate program presents a six-step curriculum for obtaining fluency. Each program includes therapy manuals and materials books that provide all the reproducible activities needed for each lesson.

The Source for School-Age Stuttering
This comprehensive resource for ages 7 to 18 includes all phases of the therapeutic process from assessment through diagnosis and treatment. Tool, tips, activities, and strategies to help develop skills including planning and implementing

therapy, providing "real world" practice, working effectively with parents and teachers, and much more.

Stuttering Foundation of America

3100 Walnut Grove Road, Suite 603
P.O. Box 11749
Memphis, TN 38111-0749
Phone: 800-992-9392
Fax: 901-452-3931
Web site: www.stutteringhelp.org

Stuttering and Your Child: A Videotape for Parents
Appropriate for viewing in any home, daycare, clinical, or educational setting. This 30-minute video provides parents with up-to-date information about what stuttering is, what is thought to cause and worsen childhood stuttering, and what parents can do to help their child.

Counseling Stutterers
This book helps the clinician have a better understanding of the counseling aspect of therapy and suggests ways to use it effectively.

The School-Age Child Who Stutters: Working Effectively with Attitudes and Emotions
Focuses on assessing and treating feelings/beliefs in school-age children who stutter. Contains practical, concrete ideas for documentation and strategies to achieve change.

The Power R Game!
Uses a gameboard format to change attitudes and feelings about stuttering. Contains 94 game cards with 564 statements for directing discussions about stuttering and an additional 50 cards containing diversion scenarios. Second edition provides an updated manual with additional resources and references.

APPENDIX 7-A

SAMPLE PHRASES, QUESTIONS, AND MONOLOGUES

PHRASES

LIST 1

Two adjacent alveolar phonemes in linking positions

1. on his doorstep
2. those turnip greens
3. broom and dustpan
4. brand new bicycle
5. a price tag
6. an August day
7. an afternoon snack
8. gas station pump
9. cloak and dagger
10. be on time
11. in a sand trap
12. that steamy pot
13. in a candy store
14. cats and dogs
15. old spark plug
16. a Cuban cigar

LIST 2

With "the" in linking position

1. over the rainbow
2. behind the tree
3. in the hall
4. over the bridge
5. beside the pool
6. in the meadow
7. ring the doorbell
8. tour the museum
9. melt the butter
10. in the birdhouse
11. up the hill
12. close the lid
13. climb the ladder
14. dial the phone
15. ride the subway
16. near the table

LIST 3

Two adjacent alveolar phonemes in linking positions

1. in a slump
2. smell an aroma
3. this smeary ink
4. smaller and smaller
5. give a speech
6. stay a while
7. swear under oath
8. all eyes and ears
9. smoke a cigar
10. a joyous smile
11. be a small fry
12. spin around
13. sugar and spice
14. clean a stain
15. swam in a race
16. sweltering weather

(continues)

Appendix 7-A (continued)

QUESTIONS

What country is shaped like a boot?	(Italy)
What Chinese medical procedure uses needles?	(acupuncture)
Who won the Civil War?	(Union Army)
What are the ditches around castles called?	(moats)
What bird is the emblem of the United States?	(bald eagle)
Who is said to have shot Abraham Lincoln?	(John W. Booth)
In the United States, who takes command if the president dies or leaves office?	(vice president)
What were the last two states admitted to the United States?	(Hawaii and Alaska)
Why did the Pilgrims come to North America?	(freedom of religion)
What book gives synonyms?	(thesaurus)
Who fought in the Gulf War?	(U.S. and Iraq)
What kind of war is fought between people who live in the same country?	(civil war)
Which president was involved in the Watergate scandal?	(Nixon)
Who wrote Hamlet and Macbeth?	(Shakespeare)
Name one of O. J. Simpson's lawyers.	(Shapiro, Cochran, Bailey, and so on)
Ringo Starr was the drummer for what famous rock group?	(Beatles)

MONOLOGUE TOPICS

Tell me about your summer vacation.

Tell me about the last movie you saw.

What do you like most about your job?

What do you like least about your job?

Tell me about your brothers and sisters.

If you won $10 million in the lottery, what would you do with it?

How would you change things if you had your boss's job?

If you could go anywhere in the world this afternoon, where would it be?

What foreign language would you most like to learn and why?

If you could relive any year in your life, which would it be and why?

If you could redesign an automobile, what things would you change?

If you were able to read another person's mind, would you do it?

If you could have three wishes come true, what would they be?

If you were president of the United States, what is the first law you would make?

If you had to choose between being blind or deaf, which would you choose and why?

CHAPTER 8

Intervention for Voice and Alaryngeal Speech

This chapter will address impairments in phonation (traditionally referred to as voice disorders) as well as alaryngeal speech resulting from surgical removal of the larynx. To competently diagnose and treat phonatory disorders, clinicians must be well acquainted with the mechanisms involved in normal voice production. The reader is referred to Aronson (1990), Boone and McFarlane (2000), Seikel and Drumright (2004), and Zemlin (1998) for detailed discussions of laryngeal anatomy and physiology.

VOICE DISORDERS

A voice disorder is a disturbance of pitch, loudness, or quality in relation to an individual's age, gender, and cultural background. Voice disorders are identified on the basis of a listener's judgment rather than by any absolute or standardized criteria for normal voice production. The term **dysphonia** refers to any deviation in phonation, whereas **aphonia** is a term used to indicate the absence of audible phonation.

In the normal production of voice, the airstream is generated by the lungs. As the air passes through the larynx, the vocal folds are set into vibratory motion, which results in the production of sound (i.e., phonation). The sound continues to travel through the upper vocal tract and is modified by the resonating characteristics of the pharynx and oral and nasal cavities. Loudness and pitch are controlled by different physiologic mechanisms. Loudness is the perceptual counterpart to amplitude (the height of a sound wave). It is determined primarily by the amount and speed of subglottal air pressure. A voice becomes louder when there is an increase in the volume and velocity of the airstream as it passes through the glottis. Pitch is the perceptual correlate of frequency (number of vibratory closing and opening cycles per second). The relative length and thickness of the vocal folds determine voice pitch. The voice becomes higher in pitch when the vocal folds are elongated with a concurrent decrease in mass and an increase in elasticity of the vocal folds. The pitch most frequently used by an individual speaker during spontaneous speech production is known as **fundamental frequency** or **habitual pitch**. The fundamental frequencies used by normal speakers of different ages and genders are shown in Table 8-1.

Normal voices function in at least three pitch ranges, or **voice registers**. These are the pulse (the lower range of fundamental frequencies), modal (the range of fundamental frequencies used in normal speech), and loft (the highest range of fundamental frequencies) registers. Each register is characterized by a distinct pattern of vocal fold approximation. The vocal folds vibrate in the same manner throughout a given pitch range; the pattern of vibration changes as the maximum limit for the range is exceeded and a new voice register is entered.

Voice quality is difficult to define but can be described as the aspects of a voice that differentiate it from another voice at identical pitch and loudness levels. It is regulated, at least in part, by the manner and force with which the vocal folds approximate one another. For example, if the folds are loosely approximated during phonation, the resulting voice quality is generally labeled as breathy,

TABLE 8-1
Normal Fundamental Frequencies for Males and Females

Fundamental Frequency (Hz)		
Age	Male	Female
1–2	400	400
3	300	300
4	285	285
5–7	265	265
8	250	255
9–13	235	240
14	175	225
15	165	220
16	150	215
17	135	210
18	125	205
20–29	120	227
30–39	112	214
40–49	107	214
50–59	118	214
60–69	112	209
70–79	132	206
80–89	146	197

Sources: Adapted from Aronson (1990), Hollien & Shipp (1972), Kelley (1977), and Wilson (1987).

whereas overly tense vocal fold approximation is generally associated with a harsh, strained voice quality.

Resonance is another factor that affects voice production. The sound generated at the laryngeal level is amplified or filtered as it passes through the resonating cavities of the upper vocal tract (i.e., pharynx, oral and nasal cavities). Vocal resonance can be affected by a variety of neurological and structural factors. Information regarding voice symptoms and resonance problems associated with various kinds of dysarthrias is discussed in Chapter 7; resonance problems that accompany cleft palate are described in Chapter 3.

The incidence of voice disorders is not well documented. However, studies suggest that they occur in approximately 3%–9% of the general population including children and adults (Senturia & Wilson, 1968; Silverman & Zimmer, 1975; Verdolini, 1998, 2000; Yairi, Currin, Bulian, & Yairi, 1974).

Classification of Voice Disorders

Traditionally, voice disorders have been classified as either **organic** or **functional** (Aronson, 1990; Boone & McFarlane, 2000). Organic voice disorders result from pathology or disease that affects the anatomy or physiology of the larynx and other regions of the vocal tract. Functional voice disorders are dysphonias related to vocal abuse/misuse or psychogenic factors in the absence of an identifiable physical etiology. The distinction between these two diagnostic categories is not always clear. For example, a pattern of long-term vocal abuse may eventually lead to organic pathology of the vocal folds. The most common voice disorders are functional in nature and involve faulty habits of vocal usage (Boone & McFarlane, 2000). However, several organic etiologies have significant impact on voice production.

The speech-language pathologist should be familiar with the range of possible organic and functional etiologies and their implications for treatment planning. Table 8-2 lists the most common organic and functional voice problems.

Organic. Many organic factors alter the mass of vocal folds and result in lowered pitch; decreased loudness; and a breathy, hoarse voice quality. These alterations affect the shape, the mobility, and/or the muscular tension of the vocal folds. Lower pitch is a result of the inability of the vocal folds to be lengthened and thinned. Reduced loudness and the breathy, hoarse voice quality will occur if the folds cannot achieve adequate closure (adduction). Examples of these organic factors include the following:

- **Edema** (swelling) related to **laryngitis** (inflammation of the folds and other regions of the larynx usually caused by bacterial infection)
- Mass lesions such as **tumors**, large **granulomas**, and **papillomas**
- **Neurologic or endocrine disorders** (e.g., degenerative diseases such as Parkinsonism and hypothyroidism)
- **Laryngeal webs** (membranes that extend from one vocal fold to the other and partially occlude the airway)
- **Vocal fold paralysis** due to impairment in the recurrent or superior laryngeal nerves that innervate the larynx

Functional. Functional voice disorders arise from faulty voice usage or psychogenic factors. Symptoms range from a breathy whispered voice to a strained tight voice with inappropriate loudness and pitch.

TABLE 8-2
Organic and Functional Voice Problems

Organic	Functional
Vocal fold paralysis	Abuse/misuse
Laryngeal webs	Vocal nodules
Papilloma	Contact ulcers
Edema	Ventricular dysphonia
Tumor	Psychogenic
Granuloma	Conversion dysphonia
Neurologic/endocrine disease	Mutational falsetto
Spasmodic dysphonia*	

*Several varieties have been described; etiology is not known.

Vocal abuse/misuse is directly related to excessive muscle tension (i.e., laryngeal hyperfunction). In laryngeal hyperfunction, the pattern of vocal fold closure is abrupt and forceful. The most common types of abuse/misuse include shouting, screaming, and excessive talking as well excessive coughing or throat clearing. Initiation of phonation is accomplished by **hard glottal attack**, which is characterized by tight glottal closure, increased subglottal air pressure, and explosive abduction (opening) of the folds. Consistent use of faulty patterns can result in pathology (i.e., chronic laryngitis, **vocal nodules**, or **contact ulcers**). Vocal nodules are benign whitish protuberances that occur at the junction of the anterior and middle thirds of the vocal folds, the area of maximum impact during vocal fold closure. These calluslike formations prevent complete adduction of the folds and result in a lower pitch and breathy, hoarse voice quality. Contact ulcers are benign bilateral sorelike lesions on the posterior third of the vocal folds caused by habitual use of hard glottal attacks and excessively low pitch. Symptoms include hoarseness and laryngeal pain. Another example of vocal misuse is **ventricular dysphonia**. This disorder involves the use of the ventricular (false vocal folds) as the primary source of phonation, while the true folds are held in an abducted position.

Psychogenic voice disorders arise from emotional or mental factors such as anxiety, depression, or personality disturbance that interfere with voluntary control over voice production (Aronson, 1990). These disorders may develop subsequent to an occurrence of physiologic changes in the larynx, such as laryngitis, and persist long after the physical symptoms have disappeared. Two primary examples of psychogenic voice disorders are **conversion dysphonias** and **mutational falsetto**. Conversion dysphonias are the physical manifestations of psychological conflict and range in severity from mild hoarseness to whispering to complete absence of voice (i.e., dysphonia → aphonia → mutism). A mutational falsetto is characterized by the continued use of a higher-pitched childhood voice into adolescence and adulthood in the presence of a normal laryngeal system. This condition is seen mainly in males and results in a voice that is high-pitched, breathy, hoarse, and gives the overall impression of immaturity.

Spasmodic dysphonia is a voice disorder that resists easy classification. Several different types of these dysphonias have been described, some of which are considered organic and others functional in origin (Aronson, 1990; Stemple, Glaze, & Klaben, 2000). However, there is mounting evidence of an underlying neurologic etiology for all types. This growing consensus suggests that SD is a focal dystonia, a condition characterized by involuntary movement in an isolated body part. These abnormal movement patterns occur predominantly during purposeful tasks such as speech and may not affect reflexive functions such as coughing, laughing, or sneezing. This disorder involves severe spasmodic movements of the vocal folds that interrupt the normal adduction-abduction cycle of phonation. The disorder is traditionally divided into two main categories: **adductor spasmodic dysphonia** and **abductor spasmodic dysphonia** depending on when the vocal fold spasms occur. In the more common adductor type, glottal closure is so tight that the vocal folds cannot vibrate in the usual sustained fashion. This overadduction results in a voice that can be described as hoarse, strained, and staccato. It is accompanied by periodic cessation in phonation (phonation breaks) and sudden, unpredictable changes in pitch (pitch breaks). Abductor spasmodic dysphonia is less common than the adductor type and is characterized by excessive and spasmodic opening of the vocal folds during phonation. This uncontrolled abduction allows a great deal of unphonated air to pass through the larynx, causing a breathy voice quality.

There is a distinct lack of research data regarding prognostic indicators related to voice disorders. The same factors generally associated with improvement of any communication disorder also can be applied to individuals with vocal abnormalities. A favorable outcome is generally associated with structural adequacy of the speech production mechanism with little or no organic impairment, a high degree of client motivation and cooperation, and a client's ability to discriminate and self-monitor target behavior.

TREATMENT EFFICACY/EVIDENCE-BASED PRACTICE

Ramig and Verdolini (1998) provided a comprehensive summary of available data on treatment efficacy for voice disorders. They reviewed group and single-subject experimental designs, retrospective analyses, case studies, and program evaluation data. Their overall conclusion was that voice treatment is effective for both functional and organic voice disorders. Their analysis also resulted in several additional conclusions:

- Disorders of vocal misuse and hyperfunction can be effectively treated with a variety of intervention techniques, including biofeedback of laryngeal muscle activity, progressive relaxation, yawn-sigh procedure, and vocal intensity reduction.

- Voice therapy significantly reduces the recurrence of vocal nodules after surgical removal. (See also McCrory, 2001; Speyer et al., 2002.)

- Voice therapy is effective in reducing/eliminating contact ulcers for most individuals.

- Lee Silverman Voice Treatment (LSVT) successfully increases vocal fold adduction in individuals with Parkinson's disease. (See also Ramig et al., 2001.)

- A combination of voice therapy and botulinum toxin injection significantly improves laryngeal function for clients with spasmodic dysphonia. (See also Boutsen, Cannito, Taylor, & Bender, 2002.)

- Future treatment efficacy research should expand the current focus on single-subject studies to include more large group experimental designs.

TREATMENT

The goal of treatment for voice disorders is to help a client produce a voice of the best possible pitch, loudness, and quality in relation to the individual's age and gender within the context of cultural and linguistic background. There are three main approaches to voice treatment: (1) medical, (2) environmental, and (3) behavioral. Medical interventions include surgery, medication, and radiation (e.g., removal of vocal fold polyps). Environmental strategies involve modifying a client's daily surroundings or helping a client adjust to the vocal demands of his or her environment (e.g., suggesting the use of a microphone or visual communication system for a client employed in a noisy workplace). Behavioral strategies (also referred to as symptomatic voice therapy) consist of intervention techniques designed to modify specific vocal symptoms such as hoarseness, breathiness, and monoloudness (Casper & Murray, 2000; Stemple, Glaze, & Klaben, 2000).

The approach to intervention for some organic voice disorders is strictly medical. For example, papillomas (wartlike growths on the inner margin of the vocal folds) are effectively treated only through surgical removal. Other organic disorders are best treated through a combination of medical and behavioral therapies. For instance, treatment for a neurological disorder such as Parkinson's disease generally consists of medications as well as symptomatic voice therapy. Functional voice disorders are usually treated effectively with voice therapy alone.

Numerous intervention techniques for voice disorders have been described in the literature. Certain approaches are applicable to any voice disorder regardless of symptomatology or etiology. These include the following:

- *Listening skills:* These techniques are used to increase client awareness of his or her vocal behaviors. The clinician demonstrates and contrasts appropriate and inappropriate vocal behaviors. The client is asked to identify and discriminate between the two in live and tape-recorded samples.

- *Respiratory control:* These strategies are used to optimize respiratory support for voice production. Attention is given to posture, breathing patterns, and expiratory control for phonation. The client may be asked to prolong phonation for as long as possible at a variety of different pitch and intensity levels.

- *Vocal rest:* Reduction or elimination of phonation is sometimes recommended to limit laryngeal irritation and to permit the vocal folds to recover from surgery or misuse. A client may be asked to modify or totally refrain from talking for a specified amount of time (usually four days to two weeks). Individuals most likely to be placed on vocal rest have (1) fluid-filled lesions that may rupture (e.g., cysts), (2) vascular conditions such as hematoma, and (3) just undergone laryngeal surgery. The strategy of complete voice rest is highly controversial with regard to its value and practicality.

Intervention Techniques

The remainder of the chapter is devoted to a discussion of therapy techniques associated with specific voice abnormalities. Although the organic versus functional paradigm was appropriate for a description of voice disorder classification, we find it clinically more useful to organize treatment information according to the following four categories: vocal hyperfunction, vocal hypofunction, psychogenic disorders, and spastic dysphonias.

Vocal Hyperfunction. This category includes any voice disorder characterized by excessive laryngeal tension or overly forceful closure of the vocal folds. It consists primarily of dysphonias related to vocal abuse or misuse. The majority of voice problems encountered by speech-language pathologists are related to vocal hyperfunction caused by vocal abuse or misuse. The following techniques are useful in treating symptoms associated with laryngeal hyperfunction (Boone & McFarlane, 2000; Deem & Miller, 2000). The overall aims of these techniques are to (1) reduce muscular tension and (2) eliminate abusive vocal behaviors.

Relaxing Muscles. Techniques can be directed specifically to the vocal tract musculature or toward relaxation of the whole body. One method of tension reduction for the muscles of the larynx is the adoption of an open-mouth posture during speech because muscular tension in the jaw area is usually related to tension in the laryngeal musculature. The client visualizes the contrasting mouth postures of a ventriloquist and an opera singer. The client then practices speaking alternately with a closed-mouth and open-mouth posture in front of a mirror. Other vocal relaxation techniques include laryngeal massage and head and neck rolls. (For step-by-step instructions, see Deem & Miller, 2000.) One of the most common approaches to tension reduction for the whole body is progressive relaxation, which is described in detail in Chapter 7. Muscle relaxation typically is used in conjunction with one or more of the following techniques.

Reducing Loudness. The client reads short phrases or sentences aloud, using a different intensity level for each one. A lower intensity level that is optimal for the client is identified (described by Boone and McFarlane [2000] as the voice to use when not wanting to waken a sleeping person). This quieter voice is practiced in drills that require reading utterances of increasing length (i.e., single sentences → multiple sentences → short paragraphs).

Softening Glottal Attacks. Several techniques can be used to soften hard glottal attacks.

- *Yawn-sigh:* The client yawns in a natural manner and phonates a gentle sigh on exhalation. Once relaxed phonation is mastered, the client produces words on the exhalation. Begin with single words that begin with /h/ or a vowel and progress to four to five words per exhalation. The eventual goal is for the client to induce easy phonation by imagining the relaxed oral feeling associated with the yawn-sigh approach.

- *Chewing:* The client chews in a natural but exaggerated manner while simultaneously producing phonation (Froeschels, 1952). Start with vowels and gradually increase the length of the utterance on successive exhalations. The client practices variations in pitch and loudness levels while chewing/phonating. Relaxation of laryngeal musculature should be maintained.

- *Easy onset:* The client produces syllable combinations of /h/ + vowel to practice relaxed initiation of phonation. This phoneme sequence establishes airflow through the glottis prior to phonation. Gradually lengthen utterances to polysyllabic words and short sentences. Expand the drills to include other voiceless fricatives and other sound classes.

- *Chant talk:* The client listens to and imitates a tape of chanting, a speaking pattern characterized by the production of words in a continuous unbroken monotone, prolongation of vowels, and lack of syllable stress (i.e., Gregorian chant). Once this speaking style can be reliably produced, the client reads aloud for 20-second periods, alternating between habitual voice and chant talk.

Adjusting Pitch. A habitual pitch that requires the least amount of physical effort and tension results in the most pleasant sounding voice. The client produces a "um-hum" with a closed-mouth posture using a rising inflection. This vocalization should simulate the conversational device that is commonly used to signal agreement with a partner's statement. Once identified, a pitch pipe can be used to provide a model for the client to imitate. Begin with isolated vowels and progress to single words, sentences, and paragraphs. Instrumentation (e.g., Visi-Pitch from Kay Elemetrics Corporation) can be used to provide visual feedback, which helps the client maintain appropriate pitch use for longer periods of time.

Phonating on Inhalation. The client inhales slowly while attempting to phonate a hum as modeled by the clinician. Once this behavior is reliably established, the client attempts to phonate on exhalation and match the pitch produced during the previous inhalation. Gradually, phonation is produced only on exhalation and at a wide variety of pitch levels. This technique is often used with cases of ventricular phonation because phonating on inhalation requires the use of the true vocal folds rather than the false folds.

Vocal Hypofunction. This category refers to voice disorders characterized by incomplete closure of the vocal folds. It involves dysphonias resulting from neurologic disorders such as unilateral vocal fold paralysis, myasthenia gravis, and muscular dystrophy. The techniques described next are useful in treating symptoms associated with laryngeal hypofunction (Boone & McFarlane, 2000). The main purposes of these techniques are to achieve firmer closure of the vocal folds and/or compensatory movements (e.g., one fold moves across the midline to compensate for the other in unilateral paralysis).

Pushing/Pulling. The client engages in forceful muscular activity that elicits reflexive glottal closure (Froeschels, Kastein, & Weiss, 1955). These activities should be used for short periods of time and discontinued as soon as the client demonstrates an awareness of the "feel" of tighter vocal fold closure. Care must be taken to ensure that an overly hyperfunctional behavior does not occur. In one method, the client is seated in a chair, firmly grasps each side of the seat, and pushes downward with both arms while producing a vowel such as /a/. A variation of this activity requires the client to raise both fists to the level of the chest with elbows extended outward. The client then pushes both fists downward forcefully while producing a vowel sound as loudly as possible. A third method requires the client to link the fingers of both hands together at the level of the chest and to pull in opposite directions while producing a vowel such as /a/. Length of phonation should be gradually increased while continuing to maintain the improved loudness and voice quality.

Increasing Loudness. In some cases, loudness can be improved by establishing a more efficient respiratory pattern (i.e., abdominal-diaphragmatic breathing). The client lies on his or her back and places one hand on the chest and the other on the abdomen. The client inhales though the nose and closely monitors movement of the abdomen (not the chest) while exhaling through the mouth. During subsequent respiratory cycles, the client deliberately relaxes the abdominal muscles during inhalation and tenses the same muscles during exhalation. Once this respiratory pattern has been established, the client begins to produce prolonged vowels on exhalation at an increased level of loudness. Progress occurs from vowels to syllables to words to phrases to sentences. Vocal loudness also can be addressed through the use of the pushing/pulling techniques described in the previous section.

A programmed approach to remediating reduced vocal loudness in clients with Parkinson's disease is the Lee Silverman Voice Treatment (Ramig, 1998; Ramig, Pawlas, & Countryman, 1995). This approach utilizes high phonatory effort tasks to increase vocal fold adduction and respiratory support. The goal of this program is to improve functional speech intelligibility to a realistic level. A minimum of 16 intensive individual sessions within a four-week period is required regardless of a client's severity of impairment. The program also provides specific guidelines for posttreatment maintenance and reevaluation.

Psychogenic. This category involves voice disorders that arise from psychological or emotional factors. Symptoms associated with psychogenic voice disorders range from mild dysphonia to complete loss of voice and can involve pitch, loudness, or voice quality. The overall purpose of treatment is to reestablish a client's access to his or her own normal voice. This purpose is generally achieved through three sequential stages of intervention (Aronson, 1990).

Client Education. The clinician discusses available medical reports with the client and emphasizes that the client's laryngeal anatomy and physiology are intact and, more important, that the client is capable of producing normal voice.

Symptomatic Therapy. The clinician attempts to elicit normal phonation through vegetative vocal functions. The client produces a variety of these sounds (i.e., coughing, throat clearing, laughing, gargling, humming). When normal phonation occurs during one of the vegetative behaviors, it should be brought to the client's attention immediately. The client then extends this normal voice into vowels, single words, and sentences. For clients with mutational falsetto, inhalation phonation (as described in the section on hyperfunction) also may be an effective technique for eliciting normal phonation.

Referral. The clinician considers the possibility that voice intervention alone is insufficient to resolve a client's underlying emotional problems and may counsel the client to seek psychological or psychiatric services as needed.

Spasmodic Dysphonia. This category encompasses two distinct types of voice disorders characterized by spasms that result in abnormalities of vocal fold approximation. Adductor spasmodic dysphonia has been treated with a variety of surgical and medical interventions. In general, the surgical approach focuses on removal of a small segment (resection) of the recurrent laryngeal nerve to improve vocal fold function (Berke et al., 1999; Dedo & Izdebski, 1983). More recently, injection of botulinum toxin (Botox) into the vocal folds has become the treatment of first choice for this type of dysphonia (Blitzer, Brin, Fahn, & Lovelace, 1988; Sulica, Brin, Blitzer, & Stewart, 2003; Langeveld et al., 2001). Botox injections are also used to treat the abductor type of SD, although with somewhat less effectiveness. According to Blitzer, Brin, and Stewart's (1998) retrospective analysis, adductor SD patients demonstrated approximately 90% normal vocal function over an average of 15 weeks while adductor SD patients had an average benefit of almost 67% normal function over an average of 10.5 weeks.

Spasmodic dysphonias are also treated with symptomatic voice techniques, although voice therapy alone usually does not result in significantly improved voice production. These techniques are similar to those employed for treating laryngeal hyperfunction/hypofunction and are generally on a trial basis before and after medical intervention. The overall goal of symptomatic voice therapy is to help the client achieve the best possible voice, with the recognition that normal voice quality may never be regained.

Premedical Therapy Techniques. Techniques aimed at reducing laryngeal muscle tension are employed, including chewing, chant talk, yawn-sigh, and easy onset. (See section on vocal hyperfunction for a description of these techniques.)

Postmedical Therapy Techniques. Techniques aimed at decreasing breathiness, increasing loudness, and establishing a new pitch are employed, including pushing/pulling and abdominal-diaphragmatic breathing. (See section on vocal hypofunction for a description of these techniques.)

Example Profiles

The following three profiles represent typical dysphonias of children and adults with different types of voice disorders. These examples have been designed to illustrate the selection of intervention targets as well as specific therapy activities and materials. Most of the chosen activities are easily implemented in either individual or group therapy settings.

PROFILE 1

Brian, an 8-year-old male, presents with a hoarse, low-pitched voice. Otolaryngological findings reveal prominent bilateral vocal nodules approximately 2 mm in size. Both vocal folds are swollen and irritated. Case history information obtained from his parents indicates that Brian is an extremely active child whose play activities are frequently accompanied by shouting and screaming. According to his mom, "Brian talks incessantly, from the moment he wakes up until it's time for bed." She also reported that Brian likes to make "sound effects," including car noises and monster voices. Brian shows no awareness of the dysphonic nature of his voice. Both Brian's parents and his classroom teacher noted that his voice quality deteriorates as the day progresses.

Selection of therapy targets. The overall communicative profile demonstrated by Brian is consistent with a dysphonia caused by vocal abuse/misuse. Based on his age and the pattern of hyperfunctional vocal behaviors, therapy will focus on the following areas: (1) identification of vocally abusive situations, (2) establishment of the target voice, and (3) elimination of the abusive behaviors. Most children with voice disorders do not recognize that a problem exists. Therefore, an important aspect of this approach is to facilitate an awareness in Brian, his parents, and his teacher of what constitutes abusive vocal behaviors, as well as the situations in which these behaviors most frequently occur.

Sample Activities

1. Observe Brian in home, play, and school settings for specified units of time (e.g., 15 minutes, recess period, and so on) to identify instances of hyperfunctional vocal behavior. Use this information to establish baselines regarding the type, context, and frequency of vocal abuse/misuse. These observations should be conducted on at least three occasions to ensure gathering of a representative sample of Brian's communicative behavior. Interviews with family members and others also can yield useful information regarding Brian's habitual vocal patterns. Develop a list of his most common types of vocal abuse/misuse and the situations in which they most frequently occur. Review this list with Brian and discuss how these behaviors have "bothered his voice."

2. Help Brian generate a list of 25 of his "likes" and "dislikes". Likes might include soccer, chocolate shakes, video games, ping-pong, and playing with his best friend, Ian. Dislikes might include homework, broccoli, brushing his teeth, going shopping, and cleaning his room. Gather pictures or photographs depicting each item and tack the positive and negative items to separate walls. Model an excessively loud voice and a more desirable quiet voice until Brian can easily imitate each pattern. Explain to Brian that he will talk about the pictured items, alternately using his old loud voice and the new quieter voice. Instruct Brian to select one picture from the negative set and produce it along with the carrier phrase, "I don't like _____," using his old voice pattern. Then ask him to choose an item from the positive group and say the carrier phrase, "I do like _____," using the target voice. Encourage Brian to pay attention to the differences in how these voices sound and feel. Continue to compare and contrast the desirable and undesirable loudness levels by repeating this alternating sequence until all items have been named.

3. Provide Brian with a tally card or a simple behavioral response counter. Instruct Brian to record each time he catches himself yelling during a given time period. The clinician should specify time periods in which there will likely be at least 10 instances of the abusive behavior (e.g., recess). Have Brian tally the number of recorded behaviors at the end of each day and plot the number on a simple graph like the one shown in Form 8-1. As Brian's ability to accurately identify instances of vocal abuses improves, the specified time frame for self-monitoring can be progressively increased.

FORM 8-1 VOCAL ABUSE CHART

Client's Name:_____ Setting: _____

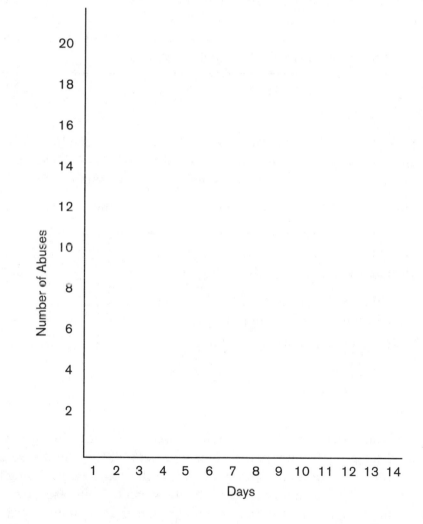

PROFILE 2

Mr. Abdul, a 48-year-old professor of political science, reports a two-year history of hoarseness and throat pain associated with teaching. He states that these symptoms are more severe during summer school because lecture periods are substantially longer than during the fall and spring semesters. A videotape of a typical lecture indicates that Mr. Abdul's speaking style in the classroom can be described as loud, forceful, and low pitched. In addition, Mr. Abdul is a member of a local repertory theater company and frequently performs in plays and musicals. A recent laryngoscopic examination reveals the presence of bilateral contact ulcers.

Selection of therapy targets. The aspects of voice production to be targeted are inappropriately low pitch, abrupt initiation of phonation, and excessive loudness. These features were selected because they constitute the primary symptoms of laryngeal hyperfunction in Mr. Abdul's profile.

Sample Activities

1. Determine the client's optimal pitch through the procedure described in the section on treatment techniques for vocal hyperfunction. Devise a list 25 sentences for a cloze task. Examples include the following:

   I'm going to the store and I'm going to buy some _____.

   I'm going on a trip and I'm packing _____.

   I'm going on a picnic and I'm taking _____.

   My favorite chili is made with _____.

   On our last vacation, we visited _____.

   If I win the lottery, I would buy _____.

   I'm sending a Christmas card to _____.

   My favorite baseball player is _____.

   Last night for dinner I had _____.

   This old car needs new _____.

   Explain that the clinician will read each sentence and present a cue or prompt (e.g., pitch pipe, piano note) representing the client's optimum pitch. Then the client completes the statement with a single word using the targeted pitch level. The difficulty level of this task can be increased by requiring the client to answer with a series of items rather than a single word.

2. The clinician models a soft glottal attack by yawning and producing single words that begin with /h/ or a vowel during the exhalation. Once the client can easily imitate this relaxed initiation of phonation, utterances can be progressively lengthened and may include initial phonemes other than /h/.

   Explain to the client that the game of "20 Questions" will be used to practice the yawn-sign approach to phonation at the carrier phrase level. Instruct the client to think of a person, place, or thing. The clinician then asks yes/no questions to determine the correct answer. Emphasize that the client should employ the yawn-sigh approach at the beginning of each response to the clinician's queries. For example:

Clinician: Are you thinking of a person?

Client: Yes, I'm thinking of a person.

Clinician: Is the person a female?

Client: No, the person is not a female.

Clinician: Is the person alive?

Client: Yes, the person is alive.

Task difficulty can be increased by reversing roles and instructing the client to spontaneously formulate the questions.

3. Identify the optimal loudness level for the client as described in the section on vocal hyperfunction. Select listlike reading materials that can be easily divided into segments corresponding to single breath groups (e.g., directions to a destination such as a restaurant or movie theater, a recipe, instructions for assembling or operating a VCR, and so on). Write each topic on an index card or sheet of paper and clearly delineate the utterance to be produced on each exhalation. Sample formats may include the following:

Turn left at the second traffic light/Pass the Shell station on the right/Go two blocks and make your first left/The restaurant will be on your right

1. Combine flour and sugar in a bowl.
2. Add melted butter and one egg.
3. Mix thoroughly until batter is stiff.
4. Drop by the spoonful onto cookie sheet.
5. Bake at 350 degrees for 20 minutes.

Model reading each utterance aloud on a single exhalation. Instruct the client to imitate each production using the optimal loudness level identified previously.

PROFILE 3

Mrs. Simon, a 39-year-old female, was diagnosed with right unilateral adductor vocal fold paralysis two months ago. She sustained damage to the vagus nerve as a result of intubation during surgery. Mrs. Simon presents with an extremely quiet, weak, and breathy voice. Also evident are a hoarse vocal quality and low pitch with occasional pitch breaks. Decisions regarding surgical interventions such as phonosurgery are deferred for six months to allow for any spontaneous recovery of laryngeal function.

Selection of therapy targets. The vocal symptoms to be targeted are breathy, hoarse voice quality and reduced loudness level. These areas were chosen because they represent the primary characteristics of laryngeal hypofunction in Mrs. Simon's profile.

Sample Activities

1. Instruct the client to use one of the pushing/pulling techniques described in the section on laryngeal hypofunction to achieve firmer vocal fold approximation during phonation. Once closure has been achieved, emphasize the importance of an easy, relaxed pattern. Begin with prolongation of single vowels and progress hierarchically to the level of connected speech. At the connected speech level, the clinician poses simple questions and the client responds while employing the pushing/pulling technique. Sample questions include the following:

    Where do you live?

    How long have you lived there?

    Do you have any brothers or sisters?

    What are their names?

    When is your birthday?

    Where do you work?

    What was your first job?

    What has been your favorite vacation?

    What did you do last weekend?

    What kind of car do you drive?

    What kind of car would you like to drive?

    What are your hobbies?

    What is your favorite movie?

    What do you like most about your job?

    What is your favorite holiday?

2. Instruct the client to use the abdominal-diaphragmatic breathing pattern with phonation as discussed in the section on vocal hypofunction to achieve increased loudness. Stimuli may begin at the level of isolated vowels and advance systematically to the discourse level. At the discourse level, the clinician creates several written dialogues and provides two copies of each scenario. Assign the client one of the roles. Instruct her to place one hand on her abdomen to monitor the use of the target breathing pattern while reading her lines in the script. Following are sample scripts; additional dialogues can be found in Appendix 8-A.

    Calling Information

    Operator: Hello. What city please?

    Caller: College Park.

    O: Yes?

    C: I'd like the number for Kinko's on Route 1.

    O: Thank you. That number is 555-2200.

Ordering a Pizza

Operator: Thank you for calling Domino's. Can you hold please?

Caller: Yes.

O: Thanks for holding. Can I take your order?

C: Yes, I'd like a large pepperoni pizza with extra cheese.

O: Any sodas with that?

C: I'll take two large Diet Cokes.

O: What's your address?

C: 1600 Pennsylvania Avenue.

O: And the phone number?

C: 203-4000.

O: OK. We'll be there in 30 minutes or less.

C: What's the total?

O: $14.50.

C: Thanks.

Helpful Hints

1. Clients with voice disorders that result from psychogenic factors, such as conversion dysphonias, may regain a completely normal voice within a single session.

2. Puppets can be very useful in negative practice activities for children who demonstrate dysphonias related to hyperfunction. For example, large or ugly puppets can adopt the abusive vocal pattern, while small or attractive puppets speak in the target voice.

3. With respect to the treatment of conversion disorders, the clinician must recognize that, although the voice is not actually lost, the loss of voice control is very real to the client.

4. Relatively loud masking or ambient noise can be useful for increasing loudness in some clients with weak, ineffective voices.

5. Irritating substances such as tobacco or alcohol can exacerbate the symptoms of an existing dysphonia.

6. Clinicians should be able to translate anatomical, physiological, and medical terminology used by other professionals (e.g., otolaryngologists) into clear and understandable explanations of a client's voice disorder.

7. Some aspects of voice production are difficult to explain verbally; use of visual imagery such as a Nasometer or computer display often helps clients grasp these concepts in a more concrete manner.

8. Despite the effectiveness of botox injections, clients with long-standing SD may persist in their tendency to "push out" their voice. These individuals may benefit from direct counseling/education to realize that their habit of effortful phonation is now unnecessary.

ALARYNGEAL SPEECH

Alaryngeal speech refers to voice that emanates from a sound source other than the larynx. The surgical procedure known as **total laryngectomy** involves complete removal of the larynx due to malignant tumor or severe trauma. During total laryngectomy surgery, the larynx and its intrinsic muscles as well as the hyoid bone are removed. The trachea is then surgically attached to an opening (stoma) created in the neck just above the notch of the sternum. As a result, air from the lungs can no longer enter the vocal tract, and the voicing source has been removed, making normal phonation impossible. In addition to surgery, some individuals with laryngeal cancer may receive pre- or postoperative radiation and/or chemotherapy. In fact, a recent study (Weber et al., 2003) indicates that patients who receive simultaneous chemotherapy and radiation therapy are less likely to require surgical removal of the larynx.

A preoperative visit by the speech-language pathologist plays an important role. The clinician can clearly explain the consequences of the surgical procedure on voice production and describe various methods of alaryngeal speech production. The visit also provides an ideal opportunity for assessment of the individual's habitual speaking patterns prior to surgery. Deem and Miller (2000) suggest that the following factors be noted during the preoperative visit: (1) articulatory proficiency, (2) conversational speech rate, (3) dialectal patterns, and (4) degree of mouth opening used in conversation. Client and family counseling forms a major part of this preoperative visit and continues throughout the therapeutic process. Overall personal adjustment can facilitate successful long-term rehabilitation efforts (Renner, 1995).

The goal of therapy with individuals with laryngectomies is to establish an alternative mode of sound production that can be used for communication. Many factors may affect the prognosis for successful intervention:

- Extent of surgery (especially if significant portions of the tongue are also removed)

- Presence of significant hearing impairment (greatly reduces an individual's ability to acquire alaryngeal speech)

- Presence of excessive esophageal muscle tone

- Lengthy course of concurrent radiation treatment (may produce side effects that interfere with easy acquisition of alaryngeal speech)

- Limitations in cognitive, linguistic, or emotional status (may negatively affect an individual's ability to learn alaryngeal speech)

TREATMENT

The search for an alternative method of sound production subsequent to laryngectomy is based on three general sources: external mechanical devices, functional use of the sphincterlike tissue at the junction of the pharynx and esophagus (PE segment) to produce esophageal speech, or the use of a prosthetic voice device inserted into a surgically created opening. The clinician should consult with the physician prior to and after surgery regarding the most appropriate form of alaryngeal speech for a given individual.

Mechanical Devices

Pneumatic aids. These devices consist of a plastic housing that is held over the stoma connected to a small unit with a reed, and tubing that is placed in the mouth. Air exhaled from the lungs through the stoma vibrates the reed, and the sound is carried to the oral cavity through the tubing. The speaker articulates this sound to produce speech.

Electronic aids. There are several types of electronic artificial larynges that provide a battery-powered sound source.

- *Neck devices:* A handheld sound source is placed against the neck. Sound is transmitted through the skin into the vocal tract. The clinician locates the most supple area on the client's neck and the aid is placed there, with the head of the aid in full contact with the skin. Typically, the best location is approximately one to two inches below the mandible near the midline of the neck. The client is instructed to hold the electrolarynx in his nondominant hand and turn it on while simultaneously shaping monosyllabic words containing bilabial consonants as clearly as possible. The client should be cautioned against the instinct to forcefully exhale because this results in stoma noise that distracts the listener. As longer utterances are produced, the client must learn to turn the electrolarynx off during natural speech pauses and coordinate initiation of articulatory movement with finger movement for the "on" switch. The intelligibility of speech produced with an electrolarynx is greatly enhanced by the use of precise articulatory movements and reduced speaking rate.

- *Oral devices:* These devices are similar to the pneumatic aid described previously, except the sound source is battery driven rather than arising from air exhaled through the stoma. Tubing should be placed in a corner of the mouth and angled up toward the hard palate to ensure that it is not occluded by the tongue or cheek. The client learns to articulate the sound carried to the oral cavity by the tubing. This type of aid is often used immediately after surgery because it does not interfere with sutures or swollen tissues. As with the neck version, training in the use of this device generally begins with monosyllabic words that contain bilabial consonants.

There are some disadvantages to the use of artificial larynges. The quality of the sound source is often judged as "unnatural," and these devices severely restrict the individual's ability to vary the pitch and loudness of his or her speech. However, there are also many positive aspects to the use of an artificial larynx. The device can be demonstrated prior to surgery and can be employed in the immediate postoperative period. The device also provides a means of communication that can be learned rapidly by most clients. Some laryngectomees will continue to use an electrolarynx as the primary method of communication; others will employ it as a temporary alternative until they master other forms of alaryngeal communication.

Esophageal Speech

This method of communication consists of using air passing through a narrow constriction in the esophagus as an alternative source of sound for speech. The quality of sound produced is perceived as more natural than that generated by an electrolarynx. The client's ability to rapidly intake and expel air from the esophagus and perform precise articulatory movements is the most critical aspect of effective esophageal speech. According to Casper and Colton (1998), at least one-third of laryngectomees will be unable to produce esophageal speech that is intelligible for daily communication purposes. Esophageal speech production operates on the principle that air of greater pressure in one location (mouth) will flow to a location of lesser pressure (esophagus) if the locations are connected (PE segment). The six main goals of intervention with esophageal speech as originally identified by Aronson in 1980 remain unchanged (Deem & Miller, 2000):

1. Easily and rapidly phonate on demand
2. Use a rapid method of air intake
3. Short latency period between air intake and phonation
4. Production of four to nine syllables per air charge
5. Speaking rate of 85–129 words per minute
6. Adequate intelligibility

The basic sequence of training for esophageal speech includes the following steps:

Step 1: Establishing esophageal voice

Step 2: Gaining and maintaining control over production

Step 3: Increasing intelligibility of esophageal speech

Step 4: Increasing length of utterance production

Step 5: Mastering conversational nuances of pitch, loudness, and stress patterns

Esophageal speech training should begin as soon as possible after the client's discharge from the hospital. One rule of thumb states that an individual is ready to start learning esophageal speech when oral ingestion of food can be tolerated. A moderate pace of therapy is recommended. Although many clients are extremely eager to master this procedure, therapy that proceeds too rapidly may result in unintelligible, forced speech with excessive stoma noise. (See Table 8-3 for basic guidelines for home practice of esophageal speech techniques.)

There are four main techniques for obtaining an esophageal air supply. From most to least efficient, they are consonant-injection, glossopharyngeal press, inhalation, and swallowing. Therefore, it is generally recommended that the clinician begin with the consonant-injection method. If the client is unsuccessful,

TABLE 8-3
Homework Guidelines for Esophageal Speakers

1. Have reasonable expectations, especially during the initial period of treatment. It takes time to establish effective patterns of muscle control over esophageal speech production.

2. Practice for short, consistent periods (e.g., 10 minutes per hour) rather than for lengthy periods of time.

3. Exaggerated breathing patterns (either on inhalation or exhalation) do not make esophageal speech clearer or easier to understand.

4. Use of excessive muscular force does not make esophageal speech more intelligible; it only wears you out.

proceed sequentially through the other methods until the client can consistently initiate phonation. At that point, the clinician may want to retry one of the more efficient methods.

Consonant-Injection Method. This method uses the intraoral air pressure that normally builds during production of high-pressure consonants, such as stops and fricatives, to inflate the esophagus. It has been described as the most efficient technique of esophageal air intake because air can be injected *simultaneously* with the production of a consonant rather than only during a pause or phrase interval. This results in minimal or no interruption in communication unlike the other three methods.

Step 1: Client forces air into the esophagus by producing a whispered plosive bilabial consonant, such as /p/, repetitively four to five times. This repeated compression of air in the oral cavity should force some air into the esophagus.

Step 2: Client expels the air from the esophagus and attempts to phonate /pə/.

Step 3: Gradually introduce other voiceless plosives, fricatives, and affricates paired with /ə/ at the syllable level.

Step 4: Introduce monosyllabic words containing high-pressure consonants such as "pay," "tap," "toy," "skate," "stop," "scotch."

Step 5: Extend phonation to phrases that contain a preponderance of both voiced and voiceless high-pressure consonants such as "make it dark," "stop that cab," "cut the cake," and "take that skate."

For some clients, this method may be less effective with stimulus items that consist mainly of vowels and low-pressure consonants. The relatively open-mouth articulatory configurations of these sounds may not allow the buildup of sufficient air pressure to insufflate the esophagus.

Glossopharyngeal Press Method. This method achieves esophageal air intake through tongue movements and is a useful alternative to consonant-injection for utterances loaded with low-pressure phonemes.

Step 1: Client closes lips and anchors the tongue tip against the alveolar ridge.

Step 2: The posterior portion of the tongue is moved backward along the hard and soft palates to pump air into the esophagus.

Step 3: The client expels air from esophagus and attempts to phonate vowels or monosyllables. Extend length of utterance as the client's mastery of voluntary phonation improves.

Remind the client to refrain from actually completing a swallow when employing this technique.

Inhalation Method. In this method, air is supplied to the esophagus through relaxation of the PE segment during pulmonary inhalation. The expansion and contraction of chest muscles are used to direct air into the esophagus.

Step 1: The client inhales rapidly through the nose or covers stoma midway through a quick inhalation.

Step 2: The client immediately expels the air and attempts production of /a/.

Step 3: CV syllables that contain stops are gradually introduced and content progresses to monosyllabic words.

Swallow Method. This method utilizes a controlled swallowing pattern to inject air into the esophagus. It is based on the fact that the PE segment tends to open spontaneously during a swallow because air is forced backward by the posterior movement of the tongue. This is the least efficient method of air injection and should be used only as a last resort. Primary disadvantages include (1) the extended latency between initiation of a swallow and the production of phonation; (2) the accumulation of air in the stomach as a result of repeated attempts at rapid swallowing; and (3) the inability to produce rapid, repetitive dry swallows as required for speech.

Step 1: The client swallows in a normal fashion by moving the tongue backward toward the pharynx.

Step 2: The client releases air and attempts to produce a CV syllable with an alveolar stop consonant such as "ta" and "da."

Tracheoesophageal (TE) Speech

This method is an alternative to esophageal speech (Blom, Singer, & Hamaker, 1998). A small device made of silicone is inserted into a surgically created opening between the trachea and esophagus to allow air from the lungs to reach the PE segment. This procedure can be performed during the primary laryngectomy surgery or at a later date. This technique, called tracheoesophageal puncture (TEP), may be the quickest way for a client to regain near-normal speech after the larynx has been removed. Compared to users of artificial larynges, TE speakers report more positive long-term outcomes with regard to their communication abilities and their overall sense of well-being (Ward, Koh, Frisby, & Hodge, 2003).

Patient selection for this procedure is often made by the surgeon. However, the clinician should be aware of some guidelines that are relevant to the selection of candidates for TEP. First, the client's overall health should be stable in all areas other than the laryngectomy. For example, an individual with poor respiratory function due to emphysema might not be able to generate enough pressure to move pulmonary air through the prosthesis to the PE segment.

Second, the client should possess the manual dexterity and cognitive skills required to use and care for the prosthesis on a daily basis. Ideally, the clinician should be involved in evaluating the suitability of a client for the TEP procedure; sizing the prosthesis; and training the client to insert, remove, and clean the prosthesis.

Once the fistula (punctured area) has healed sufficiently and the prosthesis has been inserted, the clinician may begin intervention according to this basic sequence of steps:

Step 1: Ask the client to inhale and then phonate on exhalation while the clinician uses a finger to occlude the stoma. It is important that the stoma be covered completely, but with gentle pressure.

Step 2: The client digitally occludes the stoma during exhalation and attempts to phonate sustained sounds or words. Utterances should become longer and more effortless at a fairly rapid rate. (Note: Use of a tracheostoma valve can eliminate the need for manual occlusion of the stoma during speech production.)

(**Note:** For more information regarding this topic, consult the most recent technical report published by the American Speech-Language-Hearing Association in 2004).

Example Profile

The following profile illustrates characteristics typical of individuals who have undergone surgical removal of the larynx. Unlike other profiles throughout the book, the activities presented in this section are designed to illustrate a progression of intervention strategies that would be implemented over time with a single individual.

PROFILE

Mr. Evans, a 62-year-old male, underwent a total laryngectomy three months ago as a result of squamous cell carcinoma. Sutures have been removed, and he is currently able to take food by mouth. He received a postsurgical regimen of radiation treatment for eight weeks. Currently, Mr. Evans communicates with an electrolarynx and by writing.

Selection of therapy targets. The targets selected based on this profile illustrate the typical progression of esophageal speech programming and include (1) establishing phonation, (2) increasing duration of phonation, and (3) refining vocal pitch and intensity. One activity will address each of the target areas.

Sample Activities

1. Instruct the client in the consonant-injection method of esophageal sound production as described in the section on esophageal speech. Once Mr. Evans can produce /pə/ rapidly in 10 consecutive trials, introduce CV syllables containing other voiceless plosives, fricatives, and affricates and then progress to monosyllabic words containing high-pressure consonants. Example stimuli include the following:

CV Syllables	CVC Words
/tə/	cup
/tɔ/	tub
/ti/	pat
/to/	cut
/kæ/	bag
/kɛ/	cheese
/kɑ/	church
/kʊ/	bit
/sə/	punch
/so/	cash
/sʊ/	bed
/si/	cat
/tʃʌ/	day
/tʃo/	date
/tʃə/	ghost

2. Once esophageal speech has been reliably established at the level of monosyllabic CVC words, focus on increasing the duration of phonation. Write a list of three- to five-word phrases that are loaded with voiced and voiceless high-pressure consonants. Instruct the client to read these longer stimuli aloud while maintaining a consistent pattern of phonation. Sample stimuli include the following:

Stop that cab

Get the cup

Go to church

Buy the boot

Touch the cat

Pull the tag

Call the cop

Go to bed

The time of day

Put it in the bank

A day at the beach

Teach the kids

Shut the door

Make it good

Coach the team

Get in the tub

Put on the cap

A lot of cash

Cash in the chips

Cut the tape

As the client progresses, the difficulty of this task can be increased. Write each phrase on a separate index card, shuffle the cards, and place the deck facedown on the table. The client draws the top card from the pile without exposing its contents, reads it aloud, and the clinician attempts to imitate it. Emphasize that the clinician will be relying solely on the intelligibility of the client's esophageal speech to identify the entire phrase.

3. The next phase of therapy focuses on refining communicative effectiveness by improving the client's ability to manipulate the pitch and loudness characteristics of esophageal speech (to the extent possible). Develop 10 groups of three-sentence sets. Each set should contain declarative, interrogative, and tag question versions of the same sentence (three to five words in length). Write each set on a single index card. Instruct the client to select a card and read each of the three sentences aloud using the appropriate alterations of pitch and increased loudness on the second and third versions. Encourage the client to try a variety of different head postures, which may facilitate increased pitch and loudness (e.g., slight head turning, chin lowering, head and chin extension). Examples include the following:

They know she's gone.
They know she's gone?
They know she's gone, don't they?

There's no hot water.
There's no hot water?
There's no hot water, is there?

The office opens at 9 A.M.
The office opens at 9 A.M.?
The office opens at 9 A.M., doesn't it?

Mr. Smith is her dentist.
Mr. Smith is her dentist?
Mr. Smith is her dentist, isn't he?

They're going to the mall.
They're going to the mall?
They're going to the mall, aren't they?

The weather has improved.
The weather has improved?
The weather has improved, hasn't it?

It won't work for me.
It won't work for me?
It won't work for me, will it?

They shoot horses.
They shoot horses?
They shoot horses, don't they?

The budget was vetoed.
The budget was vetoed?
The budget was vetoed, wasn't it?

This is delicious soup.
This is delicious soup?
This is delicious soup, isn't it?

Helpful Hints

1. It is important for the client to avoid the use of excessive muscular tension during the production of esophageal speech. Overly rapid and effortful phonation is often accompanied by undesirable and distracting behaviors such as stoma noise, grimacing, and audible "klunking" during air injection.

2. A client can learn to self-monitor stoma noise using a microphone, stethoscope, or hand held in front of the stoma.

3. The clinician may want to avoid the use of velar plosives such as /k/ in the early stages of esophageal speech training to prevent inadvertent production of pharyngeal speech (i.e., a Donald Duck voice).

4. The clinician needs to remember that esophageal speakers have much smaller reservoirs of air available for speech (i.e., less than 5 cc) than normal speakers (i.e., greater than 5 L). Therefore, they have a reduced capacity to generate lengthy utterances on a single injection of air.

5. Whenever possible, the clinician should arrange for the client to meet with a successful esophageal speaker either immediately prior to or following surgery. This visit can accomplish several goals at once. It serves as a motivator for the client; it demonstrates the communicative effectiveness of esophageal speech; and it allows the client and family to ask specific questions about the entire rehabilitation process.

6. A nonspeech communication system may need to be provided on an interim basis while the client is learning one of the alternative sound production methods.

7. Clinicians should be aware that clients may experience difficulty focusing on therapy goals due to preoccupation with global issues such as physical survival, economic pressures, and self-identity.

CONCLUSION

This chapter has presented basic information, protocols, and procedures for intervention with voice disorders at an **introductory** level. This information is intended only as a starting point in the reader's clinical education and training. For in-depth coverage of these areas, the following readings are recommended:

Andrews, M., & Summers, A., (2002). *Voice treatment for children and adolescents.* Clifton Park, NY: Thomson Delmar Learning.

Aronson, A. E. (1990). *Clinical voice disorders.* New York: Thieme Medical Publishers.

Boone, D. R., & McFarlane, S. C. (2000). *The voice and voice therapy.* Englewood Cliffs, NJ: Prentice Hall.

Casper, J. K., & Colton, R. H. (1998). *Clinical manual for laryngectomy and head/neck cancer rehabilitation.* San Diego, CA: Singular Publishing Group.

Deem, J. F., & Miller, L. (1999). *Manual of voice therapy.* Austin, TX: Pro-Ed.

Salmon, S. J. (Ed.). (1999). *Alaryngeal speech rehabilitation.* Austin, TX: Pro-Ed.

Stemple, J. C., Glaze, L. E., & Klaben, B. G. (2000). *Clinical voice pathology: Theory and management.* Clifton Park, NY: Singular Thomson Learning.

ADDITIONAL RESOURCES

The Speech Bin
1965 Twenty-Fifth Avenue
Vero Beach, FL 32960
Phone: 800 4 SPEECH
FAX: 888-FAX 2 BIN

The Boone Voice Program for Children, revised
A cognitive approach to diagnosing and treating children's voice disorders. Kit includes an assessment manual, a remediation manual, and an audiocassette tape.

The Boone Voice Program for Adults, second edition
Program includes stimulus and practice materials, explanations of normal voice and vocal pathologies, and 15 approaches for achieving better voice quality. Kit includes evaluation and remediation manuals, an audiotape, and practice sheets.

Voice Choice
Teaches children in kindergarten through fifth grade the importance of rate, volume, pitch, and inflection through eight classroom lessons. Also includes follow-up activities to treat children with vocal nodules through reproducible charts, parent letters, reminder pages, anatomy illustrations, and activity assignments.

What Is Vocal Hoarseness?
For clients, families, and teachers. Gives clear and comprehensive explanations for the importance of accurate diagnosis; roles of laryngologist and speech-language pathologist; guidelines for appropriate treatment; and information on vocal nodules, polyps, and contact ulcers. Includes reproducible checklists that serve as valuable counseling tools.

Treatment of Vocal Hoarseness in Children, second edition
Step-by-step techniques and reproducibles to remediate vocal abuse using efficient vocal production methods. Includes anatomical drawings of a larynx with and without nodules, word cut-outs, lists of suggested vocal behaviors to replace abusive ones, and worksheets of activities for the "Voice Scrapbook" to ensure carryover of vocal behaviors.

Using Your Best Voice: Production Activities for Children
Worksheets and activities to teach 3–11 year olds important vocal concepts—how to demonstrate appropriate voice patterns, interpret meaning and feelings in vocal and nonverbal behaviors, and practice effective nonverbal behaviors. Activities in three sections—finding, practicing, and showing others your best voice—for voice disorders including hyperfunction, hypofunction, resonance, pitch, loudness, and rate/timing.

Using Your Voice Wisely and Well, second edition
Eight sequential lessons for elementary and middle-school students on how to prevent and deal with harmful voice problems. Activities explain how their vocalizations impact listeners' reactions and feelings. Includes discussion ideas, reproducible worksheets, reproducible board game, question cards, posters, and pre-/posttests.

LinguiSystems
3100 Fourth Avenue
East Moline, IL 61244
Phone: 800-776-4332
Fax: 800-577-4555
E-mail: linguisys@aol.com
Web site: www.linguisystems.com

Easy Does It for Voice
Vocal abuse detection and reduction program for children ages 6 to 12. Can be used with individuals or groups. Includes reproducible tracking charts, parent and medical letters, and a voice evaluation form.

Pro-Ed
8700 Shoal Creek Boulevard
Austin, TX 78757-6897
Phone: 800-897-3202
Fax: 800-397-7633
Web site: www.proedinc.com

Remediation of Vocal Hoarseness
Step-by-step techniques, reproducibles, and progress tracking forms to help remediate vocal abuse through relaxation and more efficient vocal production methods. Targeted for kindergarten through grade 6.

Manual of Voice Therapy
Comprehensive reference that includes information for pediatric through adult clients. It includes information about the various conditions that lead to voice

disorders, the most recent developments in treatment methods and approaches, instrumentation, related medico-surgical management, counseling, and the challenges in management of voice disorders. This resource also contains a set of reproducible informational handouts for clients and families.

Hypernasality Modification Program: A Systematic Approach
Carefully organized treatment protocol and stimulus materials to help clients, age 6 through adult, correct inappropriate resonance patterns—either hypernasality or denasality. The resonance evaluation is used to analyze each client's resonance pattern and there are 63 cards, word lists, and activities covering the 16 phonetic contexts for drill practice.

Alaryngeal Speech Rehabilitation: For Clinicians by Clinicians
A resource textbook that provides basic knowledge about the production of alaryngeal speech and information about solving treatment problems. Chapters include instructions for helping a patient select an artificial larynx, guidelines for terminating treatment, suggestions for the management of terminal patients and their families, and treatment and troubleshooting techniques for all methods of alaryngeal speech

Micro Video
210 Collingwood, Suite 100
P.O. Box 7357
Ann Arbor, MI 48103
Phone: 800-537-2182
Fax: 734-996-3838
Web site: www.videovoice.com

Videovoice
For use with clients aged preschool to adult. Computer software that covers 15 areas of vocal function, including volume awareness and control, intonation and stress, pitch training, and voice quality. Activities are conducted in a game format in which the model voice can be replaced with the clinician's or client's voice to facilitate responses across different speakers. Correct/incorrect productions are visually displayed for client; the program records the data.

APPENDIX 8-A

ADDITIONAL DIALOGUE SCRIPTS FOR VOICE THERAPY ACTIVITIES

MAKING A DENTAL APPOINTMENT

Secretary: Hello, can I help you?

Customer: Yes, I need to make an appointment with Dr. Brown.

S: Have you ever been here before?

C: No.

S: OK. What are you coming in for?

C: I need my teeth cleaned and checked.

S: OK. What day would you like to come in?

C: Are there any openings next Thursday?

S: Morning or afternoon?

C: I'd prefer the morning, and after 11 o'clock if possible.

S: I have an opening at 1 o'clock. Is that OK?

C: Yes, that's fine.

S: OK. Then we'll see you next Thursday at 1 o'clock.

C: What should I do if I have to cancel?

S: You need to call us and cancel at least 24 hours in advance.

C: OK. How much will this cost?

S: The initial visit is $50 and every visit after that is $45.

C: And will my insurance cover it? I have Blue Cross Blue Shield.

S: Yes. We are a preferred provider for Blue Cross Blue Shield. Just bring in your card on the day of the appointment.

C: OK. Thank you very much. See you next Thursday.

GOING TO A RESTAURANT

Hostess: Would you like smoking or nonsmoking?

Customer: I'd like nonsmoking please.

H: Right this way. Your waitress will be right with you.

C: Thank you very much.

Waitress: Can I take your order?

C: I'll take a hamburger and a large order of fries.

W: Would you like anything to drink with that?

C: I'd like a large Coke.

W: OK. I'll be right back with your drink.

Waitress brings the soda.

(continues)

Appendix 8-A (continued)

C: Excuse me—can I also get a salad?

W: Sure. What type of dressing would you like?

C: The house dressing would be fine.

Waitress comes to clean the table.

W: How was everything?

C: The food was really great.

W: I'm glad to hear that. Would you care for any dessert?

C: I don't think so.

W: What about some coffee?

C: I'll just take the check.

W: OK. I'll be right back.

BUYING A CAR

Salesperson: Good afternoon. Can I help you with something?

Buyer: Yes, I'm interested in buying a used car.

S: Did you have a particular car in mind?

B: Well, I was looking at this Honda yesterday, but I have a few questions about it.

S: OK. What are they?

B: What year car is it?

S: A 2000.

B: And how many miles does it have on it?

S: 35,000.

B: Oh, that's not very many.

S: No, and it's in really good condition.

B: What other features does it have?

S: It has an automatic transmission, air conditioning, cruise control, and a CD player.

B: Would it be possible for me to take it for a test drive?

S: Sure—let me get the keys.

After the test drive

S: So, what did you think?

B: It drives great. What kind of deal can you give me on it?

S: Well, with your first-time buyer discount I can give it to you for $11,500.

B: Would I be able to pay it off by paying $350 a month?

S: Yes, that's no problem. Should I go draw up the paperwork?

B: Not today—I'll get back to you.

OPENING A BANK ACCOUNT

Teller: Good afternoon. What can I do for you today?

Customer: I'd like to open an account.

T: Checking or savings?

C: Both types of accounts.

(continues)

Appendix 8-A (continued)

T: Do you want a MOST card with the account also?

C: Is there a charge when I use the card?

T: Only if you use it at a bank other than this one.

C: I'll take one then. Is there a monthly charge on the account?

T: Do you write more than 10 checks a month?

C: I usually write fewer than that.

T: We have an account that's free if you write fewer than 10 checks a month.

C: What if I write more than 10 checks a month?

T: You'll be charged 25 cents for each check over 10.

C: Are there any other free accounts?

T: We have another type of account that requires a minimum monthly balance of $100.

C: I'd like to go with the first type of account.

T: How much money will you be initially depositing?

C: I have a check for $300.

T: Here is your account number and some starter checks. You will receive your new checks in about two weeks.

C: Will they be delivered in the mail?

T: They will be delivered to your home address.

C: OK. Thanks for all your help.

BUYING A PLANE TICKET

Travel Agent: Hi. Can I help you?

Customer: Yes. I'm interested in getting a plane ticket from Baltimore to Florida.

TA: Where in Florida do you want to go?

C: Miami.

TA: OK. When do you want to leave?

C: Sometime between May 5 and May 10.

TA: And how long do you want to stay?

C: About two weeks.

TA: Did you have a particular airline in mind?

C: No, but I want to find the cheapest rate possible.

TA: OK, let's see. I have a discount fare on Delta leaving on May 6 and returning on May 20.

C: That sounds perfect.

TA: OK. Do you want to leave in the morning or afternoon?

C: Morning if possible.

TA: How's 9 A.M.?

C: What time would I land in Miami?

TA: 11:25 A.M.

C: That's good. And on the 20th, I'd like an evening flight.

TA: I have a flight leaving Miami at 8 P.M. and arriving in Baltimore at 10:30 P.M.—how's that?

C: Great.

(continues)

Appendix 8-A (continued)

TA: OK. I'll print these out. How will you be paying for them?

C: My credit card.

You pay and the agent returns with the tickets.

TA: Here are your tickets. Enjoy your trip.

C: I will and thanks for your help.

TA: You're welcome.

GETTING WORK DONE ON YOUR CAR

Mechanic: Hi, can I help you?

Customer: Yes, I need to have some work done on my car.

M: What's wrong with it?

C: Well, it needs an oil change, the brakes are squealing really badly, and the tires need to be rotated.

M: Can you leave it here today?

C: Yes, but I need to have it back by 6 P.M. tonight.

M: That's fine. We'll take a look at it and give you a call within the next two hours to let you know what's wrong.

C: OK—thanks.

MAKING A VETERINARY APPOINTMENT

Vet: Hello, can I help you?

Caller: Yes, I'd like to make an appointment for my dog.

V: What is your last name?

C: (Client states his/her last name.)

V: What's the dog's name?

C: Scruffy.

V: OK. What's he coming in for?

C: He just needs his shots updated.

V: We have a spot open Saturday at noon. How's that?

C: Saturday at noon is fine.

V: OK. We'll see you then.

CHAPTER 9

Client and Family Counseling

Counseling can be defined as an interpersonal relationship that is intended to alleviate emotional stress arising from or contributing to the primary communicative disorder. There are several theoretical schools of thought regarding the counseling process. Some of the most common include behavioral (Skinner, 1953), humanistic (Rogers, 1951), cognitive (Ellis, 1977), existential (Yalom, 1980), and interpersonal (Sullivan, 1953) orientations. This chapter takes an eclectic approach to counseling and integrates the underlying assumptions of several theoretical models (Flasher & Fogel, 2004):

1. Human behavior can change or be changed.

2. Some behaviors (e.g., inadequate, dysfunctional, undesirable) warrant change.

3. Particular counseling techniques/interventions will effect change in client behavior.

4. Clients generally acknowledge the possibility that change will occur.

5. Clinicians expect clients to be actively involved in the therapeutic counseling process.

In speech-language intervention, counseling is an essential aspect of the therapeutic process and fulfills several important functions:

- It allows the clinician to impart basic information to clients and their families.

- It provides opportunities for clients to verbalize feelings, fears, and uncertainties.

- It serves as an emotionally supportive milieu in which clients are comfortable making attitudinal and behavioral changes.

Although counseling is recognized as an integral part of treatment, clinicians typically do not receive formal education or training in basic counseling skills. Many clinicians feel uncomfortable with this aspect of their professional role and are uncertain about the differences between psychotherapy and counseling. Psychotherapy involves the identification of unconscious patterns of behavior in a client in order to effect major personality changes. In contrast, counseling focuses on helping a client acknowledge feelings and engage in problem solving to make personal adjustments.

Counseling is the aspect of speech-language therapy that focuses on the person rather than the disorder. An effective therapeutic relationship must be built on mutual confidence, trust, respect, and consideration (Biggs & Blocher, 1987; Brammer & McDonald, 1999; Rollin, 2000). Several variables can influence the counseling process. Both client and clinician bring their own needs, values, feelings, experiences, and expectations to the therapeutic relationship (Brammer & McDonald, 1999). Both participants must recognize that the client's welfare is the central concern of the relationship and work together to improve the client's communicative status. It is important to understand that individual clients require varying amounts of time to form a bond of trust with another person. Therefore, clinicians need to be patient with clients who are slower to risk self-disclosure. In addition, clinicians must realize that, in most cases, a communicative disorder is a family problem rather than a problem of a single individual. Thus, counseling must address clients in the context of their overall life situations.

Counseling is an ongoing process and should not be viewed as a one-time event. It is incorporated into diagnostic as well as treatment sessions. In some cases, counseling may constitute the treatment process itself. For example, an intervention program for a person who stutters may consist entirely of counseling sessions that focus on reducing anxiety, boosting self-confidence, and modifying the environment to eliminate communicative stress.

Counseling is a relationship, and for any relationship to be successful, boundaries must be established (Stone & Olswang, 1989; Stone, Shapiro, & Pasino, 1990). This is a necessary first step because boundaries define the function and role of each participant and clarify what will or will not be part of the therapeutic relationship. Setting specific parameters serves to reduce anxiety for clients whose expectations about therapy may be confused or unclear. In the initial stage of intervention, the clinician is responsible for ensuring that boundaries are established and understood.

Clinicians also need to recognize the limits of their training and experience and realize when referrals need to be made to professionals with specialized counseling expertise. Situations that are clearly beyond the scope of practice for a speech-language pathologist may involve either the content or the style of the interaction. Content refers to the topic areas discussed within the therapeutic relationship. Topics that are generally considered inappropriate for discussion within the domain of speech-language pathology may include a client's marital problems, chronic depression, or unrelated health problems. Style involves the manner in which the clinician and client interact. Examples of inappropriate style include a client's unhealthy dependency on the clinician, unpredictable and repeated fluctuations of mood and temper, or undue anxiety on the part of the clinician before and after each therapy session.

STAGES OF COUNSELING

Counseling is a dynamic process that continues throughout the course of a treatment program. As therapy progresses, the nature of counseling evolves through three main phases.

Establishing the Therapeutic Relationship

To initiate an effective counseling relationship, a clinician must demonstrate certain qualities. These qualities are fundamental to the establishment of good rapport between the client and clinician:

- Sensitivity to a client's feelings and perceptions
- Respect for client as an individual
- Empathy or identification with the client's feelings and circumstances
- Objectivity regarding personal feelings toward the client (e.g., "being friendly" rather than "being a friend") (Shipley, 1997)
- Honesty in the ability to communicate potentially unpleasant information in an undiluted yet tactful manner
- Ability to motivate the client to actively participate in the therapy process
- Effective listening in order to understand the content of a client's message or to allow the client to "vent" feelings

In this first phase, one of the clinician's primary responsibilities is to provide clients and their families with information. This information may pertain to the nature of the communicative disorder, possible treatment options, specific therapy techniques, the prognosis for improvement, and the level of commitment that therapy will require from the client and family. Clinicians must be sensitive to the amount of information that a client or family can handle at a given time. For example, the impact of an initial diagnosis of a communicative disorder may be devastating and preclude the processing of any other information presented at that time. When establishing a therapeutic relationship, the clinician functions in a directive role and assumes primary responsibility for setting the therapeutic agenda. The clinician determines the topics to be discussed, the activities to be performed, and the parameters of the client-clinician interpersonal relationship.

Implementing Counseling Intervention

This is the "work" stage of the client-clinician relationship. The focus of the counseling process shifts from an educational/informative mode to a problem-solving orientation. Therapy activities begin to focus directly on the client's deficits, and demands for behavioral change become more intense. Individual clients may demonstrate a variety of coping strategies or defense mechanisms such as avoidance, escape, humor, rationalization/intellectualization, and passive-aggression (Tanner, 2003). The client may begin to experience feelings of vulnerability and frustration, which may give rise to behaviors that are disruptive to the therapy process. Commonly seen manifestations may include (1) consistently arriving late for sessions, (2) chronically failing to complete homework assignments, (3) resisting therapy activities perceived as "too difficult," or (4) refusing/"forgetting" to attempt new communicative behaviors outside the therapy setting. The clinician needs to recognize the feelings that motivate these behaviors in the client and focus counseling efforts on resolving these issues. In this phase, the clinician begins to function in a more nondirective mode. The client is encouraged to assume more active responsibility for self-motivation and for determining the therapeutic agenda.

Terminating the Therapeutic Relationship

At this final stage, the clinician lays the groundwork for the closure of the relationship by preparing the client to become his or her own therapist. Counseling efforts focus on encouraging the client to assume full responsibility for maintaining the behavioral changes that have been accomplished in therapy. Counseling also should be directed toward ensuring that the client leaves therapy with a genuine conceptual understanding and healthy perspective regarding the nature of the communicative disorder.

CLIENT AND FAMILY EMOTIONAL REACTIONS TO COMMUNICATIVE DISORDERS

Clients and their families often receive the diagnosis of a communicative impairment with a great sense of loss. This sense of loss can be manifested through a variety of strong emotional responses. Clinicians need to be aware of the range of possible emotions that clients or families may experience at different stages in the therapy process. The most common reactions that clinicians must recognize and be prepared to handle include the following:

- *Grief* is deep sorrow in response to a significant loss. There have been numerous attempts to identify the stages of the grieving process. For example, Kubler-Ross (1969) discussed five stages, which include initial denial that a disorder exists, a bargaining phase in which "deals" are offered to ameliorate the severity or existence of the disorder (e.g., "If Billy stops stuttering, I'll never criticize him again"), and an acceptance stage in which the client and family adjust to the loss as a fact of life and begin focusing efforts toward rehabilitation. See Tanner (1999) for a sample discussion of the acceptance of unwanted change following stroke.

- *Anger* is a strong feeling of displeasure characterized by resentment, hostility, or rage. With respect to a communicative disorder, anger is often an instinctive attempt at self-protection resulting from fear, powerlessness, and frustration. Sometimes spouses or parents experience feelings of anger toward the family member with the communicative impairment. However, they perceive this reaction as socially unacceptable, and therefore may transfer their angry feelings toward the clinician.

- *Depression* is anger turned inward that results in passivity and feelings of helplessness. The client realizes that previous stages of anger and bargaining were ineffective and the fact of the communication disorder must be faced. Depression is a relatively common emotion encountered in the counseling process. The clinician should be aware that this emotional state can become self-perpetuating and seriously impede a client's therapy progress.

- *Guilt* refers to self-blame and is frequently demonstrated by a client's immediate family members. These feelings tend to center around two types of issues: "Did I do something to cause (or contribute to) John's communicative disorder?" and "Am I getting the right type and amount of therapy for John?" Parents and family members may not necessarily verbalize these feelings but may act them out in the form of behavioral extremes, such as withdrawal from or overinvolvement in the therapeutic process. Clinicians need to be aware that some questions or comments routinely addressed to family members may inadvertently trigger feelings of guilt (e.g., "When did you first seek therapy for John's problem?" or "How do you deal with John's behavior at home?").

- *Shame* is an emotional state characterized by a negative evaluation of one's entire self and is accompanied by feelings of worthlessness and failure. It generates strong avoidance behaviors that may have a significant impact on a client's ability to participate effectively in counseling. Shame can be difficult to detect because there is no easily recognized facial expression or other overt manifestation, as in anger or depression.

- *Anxiety* refers to feelings of apprehension or distress that are generally not directly related to an immediate situation. This reaction may be present throughout the therapeutic process. During the initial stages of intervention, clients and their families are often uncertain about what to expect and also may question whether the clinician can truly help them. As therapy progresses, the focus of client anxiety may shift to the educational, vocational, or social repercussions of the communicative disorder.

- *Inadequacy* encompasses feelings of insufficiency or incompetence. Clients and their families frequently are overwhelmed by the diagnosis and implications of a communicative disorder. As a result, they rely heavily on the information and support provided by the clinician, especially in the initial stages of intervention. If feelings of confidence and self-esteem are not cultivated, this dependent relationship is likely to continue, and the clinician can become cast in the role of "rescuer" rather than a facilitator of change (Luterman, 2001).

- *Isolation* is a sense of personal detachment and remoteness from society. It can be self-imposed or result from others' rejection of the client. Isolation may arise from feelings such as inadequacy and low self-esteem, or from the perception that no one else can truly understand the client's situation. Strong feelings of isolation may exacerbate the intensity or duration of all the emotional reactions just discussed. The client's isolation from social interactions may severely impede the clinician's ability to establish an effective counseling relationship.

Clients rarely verbalize these emotions directly. Therefore, the clinician must be a keen observer of nonverbal and vocal behaviors that may be indicative of client distress (see Form 9-1 on page 332, which is a behavioral checklist).

COUNSELING TECHNIQUES FOR COMMUNICATIVE DISORDERS

One of the primary goals of counseling is to help clients and their families cope with the reality of the communicative disorder and foster the perspective that it constitutes only one aspect of the client's overall identity. The clinician's role is to assist clients in assuming responsibility for their own behavior and decisions. This goal is generally achieved through implementation of a variety of counseling techniques. Selection of specific procedures will depend on the personalities of the client and clinician as well as the constraints imposed by the communicative disorder. The following section briefly describes several of the counseling techniques most commonly used by speech-language pathologists.

- *Desensitization:* The client is guided through a hierarchy of situations from least to most anxiety provoking within the context of a safe and relaxed counseling environment. For example, a college student with a severe lisp can be gradually exposed to feared speaking situations that range from (1) an informal conversation with the clinician, (2) a formal presentation to the clinician, and (3) the same formal presentation to unfamiliar listeners in a classroom setting.

- *Relaxation:* Tension is reduced in muscle groups to alleviate a client's feelings of anxiety. For example, a client with a hyperfunctional voice disorder can be instructed to (1) alternately contract and release laryngeal muscles, (2) mentally visualize a peaceful setting, and (3) engage in deep diaphragmatic breathing.

- *Counterquestion:* A client may ask questions that appear to be requests for technical information but are actually intended to gain the clinician's confirmation or validation of a decision that has already been made. The clinician can respond to these types of remarks by posing a counterquestion that encourages the client to reveal the true intent of the original query. For example, a clinician may recognize that a mother who repeatedly inquires about the interpretation of her child's cognitive and language test scores may not truly be seeking technical information. The clinician can pose a counterquestion such as "Is there something in particular about these test scores that bothers you?" At this point, the mother may acknowledge that she recently refused to allow an IEP team to label her child as mentally retarded, and she is actually seeking support for this decision from the clinician.

- *Reframing:* A client or family is encouraged to modify views or attitudes toward a negative situation that cannot be changed. For example, a clinician may point out that family members have analyzed and improved their interpersonal relationships as a result of the client's stroke and subsequent aphasia. This technique should be introduced in the later stages of the therapeutic relationship only after the client or family has demonstrated a genuine acceptance of the communicative disorder.

- *Open-ended and indirect questions:* Questions are formulated in a manner that does not restrict the client or family's response to a simple one- or two-word utterance. This technique is used to elicit spontaneous and detailed responses that provide insight into the client's attitudes, knowledge, and feelings. One common example of an open-ended question is: "What are your major concerns about wearing a hearing aid?" A typical indirect question is: "I'd be interested in knowing your opinion of the new hearing aid."

- *Role playing:* Problematic situations associated with the communicative disorder are identified, and structured opportunities are provided for a client to act out more appropriate behaviors in hypothetical contexts. For example, an adolescent who frequently misunderstands conversational messages may refuse to request clarification because "people will think I am stupid." Scripted scenarios can be developed and used to rehearse specific repair strategies for obtaining needed information without embarrassment.

- *Empathetic listening:* The clinician reflects back the content or emotions expressed by a client's message in a nonjudgmental manner. This is generally accomplished by merely repeating or rephrasing the client's comments in an objective fashion. Effective listening is characterized by consistent eye contact, attentive body language, and behaviors that encourage continued communication such as head nods and "um hmm."

- *Silence:* The clinician refrains from speaking in order to shift the conversational floor to a client. A purposeful silence can provide the client with a communicative disorder with the time needed to formulate responses. Also, clinicians who meet a client utterance with purposeful silence rather than an immediate rejoinder may encourage the client to share additional information that would not otherwise have been expressed. Beginning clinicians typically are uncomfortable with even brief silences during their interactions with clients. Counseling skills can be greatly enhanced by learning the judicious use of purposeful silences in the clinical setting.

(See Form 9-2 on page 333, which is a checklist clinicians can use to monitor their own verbal and nonverbal behaviors during counseling sessions.)

FORM 9-1 CLIENT NONVERBAL AND VOCAL BEHAVIOR CHECKLIST

Instructions: Observe a live or videotaped counseling session. Answer each of the following items by circling the letter in each set of three that corresponds to the most appropriate description of the client's nonverbal behaviors.

1. How is the client sitting?

   a. Rigidly   a. Very near the clinician   a. In constant motion
   b. Relaxed   b. At an average distance   b. In typical motion
   c. Slouched   c. Very far from the clinician   c. Motionless

2. How does the client look?

   a. Nervous   a. Happy   a. Well-dressed
   b. At ease   b. Concerned   b. Appropriately dressed
   c. Passive   c. Upset   c. Disheveled

   a. Markedly overweight   a. Friendly
   b. Average weight   b. Businesslike
   c. Markedly underweight   c. Belligerent

3. How does the client communicate?

   a. Very quickly   a. Loudly   a. High-pitched voice
   b. At a normal rate   b. At normal intensity   b. Average voice
   c. Very slowly   c. Quietly   c. Low-pitched voice

   a. With appropriate affect and intonation   a. With many gestures
   b. With inappropriate affect and intonation   b. With some gestures
   c. With no affect or intonation   c. With no gestures

Source: Adapted from McDonald & Haney (1997).

FORM 9-2 CLINICIAN/COUNSELOR BEHAVIOR CHECKLIST

Instructions: Observe a live or videotaped counseling session. Respond to each statement with "Yes," "No," or "Not applicable" to describe the clinician's counseling behaviors.

(Note: Y = Yes; N = No; NA = Not applicable)

Nonverbal

_____ 1. The clinician maintained appropriate eye contact with the client.

_____ 2. The clinician was alert and responded with animated facial expression.

_____ 3. The clinician refrained from nonverbally reinforcing the client's off-task or irrelevant remarks (i.e., head nods).

_____ 4. The clinician demonstrated relaxed body posture.

_____ 5. The clinician leaned forward as the client spoke.

_____ 6. The clinician used a variety of vocal intonation patterns.

_____ 7. The clinician's voice was sufficiently loud to be heard by the client.

_____ 8. The clinician used intermittent vocalization (i.e., mm-hmm) during the client's on-task, relevant remarks.

Verbal

_____ 1. The clinician's remarks usually addressed the most important aspects of each of the client's utterances.

_____ 2. The clinician encouraged the client to express feelings about the communicative disorder.

_____ 3. The clinician verbally identified and responded to the client's feelings.

_____ 4. Most of the clinician's questions were open-ended in nature and required more than a one- or two-word response from the client.

_____ 5. The clinician did not monopolize the available talk time in the session.

_____ 6. The clinician used purposeful silences to encourage the client to elaborate on responses.

_____ 7. The clinician made verbal responses that supported or reinforced some of the client's statements.

_____ 8. The clinician occasionally restated or clarified the client's remarks.

_____ 9. The clinician expressed a desire to understand the client's feelings and attitudes about the communication problem.

_____ 10. The clinician answered directly when the client asked for information and/or opinion.

_____ 11. The clinician occasionally used counterquestions to respond to certain client queries.

_____ 12. The clinician occasionally offered an alternative and more positive perspective of some situation that the client has identified as distressing.

_____ 13. The clinician summarized key points of the session at appropriate junctures.

Source: Adapted from Cormier & Hackney (1999).

GROUP COUNSELING

Some speech-language pathologists coordinate sessions that function as emotional support groups for clients and their families. Clinicians need to be knowledgeable about group dynamics and be aware of the issues that tend to arise in this setting. Effective counseling skills enable the clinician to do the following:

- Determine appropriate composition and size of a group
- Set the procedures and norms for group interactions
- Promote an atmosphere of trust and unity among the group members
- Assume a less directive leadership role as the group matures
- Encourage a particular group member to risk self-disclosure
- Manage a dominant member who is monopolizing the group's time
- Manage confrontational interactions between or among group members
- Determine the hidden agendas of individual group members
- Extinguish comments and behavior that tend to detract from therapy goals
- Reinforce group members who make constructive comments to other group members
- Recognize an individual group member's need for more specialized counseling services and broach the topic skillfully
- Determine the appropriate juncture for terminating a group

(See Chapter 1 for a detailed discussion of the advantages and disadvantages of group sessions.)

FAMILY SYSTEMS COUNSELING

Based on family systems theory, this approach acknowledges the central role that the family plays in a client's development and progress. Key concepts of this theory are: (a) change in one family member affects the entire family system; (b) the family unit is greater than the sum of its parts; and (c) families exist within the context of the larger society. In this view, families are dynamic units with specific communication and interaction patterns (Begun, 1996). Effective clinicians incorporate this family-centered perspective into their counseling efforts. It is noteworthy that such consideration is actually required by federal law under the provisions of the Individuals with Disabilities Education Act (IDEA).

An increasing variety of family structures are represented in clinical caseloads. Several societal factors contribute to this diversity and include differing cultural/ethnic backgrounds, poverty, and single-parent households, among a host of others. Accordingly, clinicians can expect a wide range of family involvement/participation in the intervention process. Therefore, the clinician's counseling efforts should be designed on a case-by-case basis to accommodate the needs of each family.

MULTICULTURAL ISSUES IN COUNSELING

The changing demographics of the United States have important implications for speech-language pathologists to consider as they engage in the counseling process. Currently, minorities represent approximately 25% of the United States population, and this number is projected to increase to over 30% between 2000 and 2015 (U.S. Bureau of the Census, 2000). If communication disorders occur at the same prevalence rate as in the general United States population, then approximately 6.2 million culturally/linguistically diverse Americans currently have a communication disorder (Battle, 2002). Further, at least 13% of individuals living in the United States speak a primary language other than English. When individuals in this group demonstrate communication disorders, they often experience difficulty using English to express abstract feelings and concerns about their communication problems. As a result, they may not be able to effectively participate in or benefit from the counseling process. Unfortunately, less than 6% of certified speech-language pathologists across the country can deliver clinical services in a language other than English (ASHA, 2002).

Factors Affecting Counseling with Diverse Populations

There are at least three broad categories of variables to consider in this counseling milieu: (1) socioeconomic status, (2) cultural/ethnic background, and (3) language differences. Clients of lower socioeconomic status may be primarily concerned with practical issues of daily living that revolve around making ends meet, both financially and personally. Their priority in therapy may be to seek immediate solutions. A counseling process that focuses on increasing self-awareness and insight into the personal dynamics associated with a communication disorder may not be highly valued. Recommendations and referrals that arise from the counseling process should be made with consideration of the client's financial and personal situations.

Prior to initiating the counseling process, clinicians should engage in self-reflection to identify core aspects of their own value/belief systems as they relate to intervention. Roseberry-McKibbon (2002) identified several assumptions that are common to clinicians reared in mainstream American culture. These include:

- Punctuality is an indicator of mutual respect in a therapeutic relationship.
- In meetings, value is placed on "getting to the point" quickly and directly.
- The age and gender of the clinician relative to the client are much less important than the clinician's level of competence.
- Written documentation is an integral component of all interactions with clients/families.
- The ultimate goal of intervention is independent functioning, and treatment is warranted even for individuals with no observable physical disability.
- Counseling conducted on a one-on-one basis with the client is viewed as a productive process.

These beliefs may be in substantial contrast to those held by individuals from culturally and linguistically diverse (CLD) backgrounds. Some examples of these differences are discussed below in an attempt to illustrate the scope of knowledge required to develop multicultural competence. However, it is important for clinicians to recognize that individual differences exist even within specific cultural groups. To avoid stereotyping, clincians should view clients as individuals first and members of particular ethnicities or cultures second (Battle, 2002; Kuo & Hu, 2002; Pedersen, Draguns, Lonner, & Trimble, 2002; Roseberry-McKibbon, 2002).

Members of various cultures have widely differing views regarding the nature and appropriate treatment of communication disorders. Use of professional terminology varies widely from country to country and may affect clinician-client communication during the counseling process. For example, the term "dyslexia" in Russia is confined to those with reading problems only. However, in Italy, the same term refers to writing difficulties as well (Smythe & Everatt, 2002). Even issues as fundamental as whether a disability exists or should be treated are subject to cultural interpretation. Battle (1997) highlights this point by contrasting the belief systems of Native American and Chinese cultures. Native Americans embrace a philosophy that life should be in harmony with nature. Thus, a communication disorder may be considered a part of life that should be accepted rather than changed. In contrast, Chinese cultural tradition regards a disability as an irreversible punishment for transgressions of ancestors. Members of either culture, therefore, may be reluctant to participate in the counseling component of the therapeutic process.

There are numerous other culture-specific factors that may have an influence on the clinician's approach to counseling clients with communication disorders and their families. Selected illustrations include the following (Battle, 2002):

- Islamic tradition does not permit a female client to receive therapy services from a male clinician. Extended family members may expect to participate in counseling sessions and might be offended if they are excluded.

- Hinduism allows no photographs or videotapes of female clients.

- Japanese mothers tend to use less verbal (and more nonverbal) communication behaviors than middle-class American mothers when interacting with their young children.

- Hispanic families may experience difficulty accepting disabilities that have no visible physical manifestations (e.g., language or articulation disorder, dyslexia, and so on).

In addition to socioeconomic and cultural/ethnic factors, the counseling process may be affected by language differences of clients from diverse backgrounds. These differences involve both nonverbal and verbal aspects of communication. With respect to nonverbal behaviors, beginning clinicians may assume that certain communication behaviors have universal meanings. In fact, tremendous variation exists in the interpretation of paralinguistic expressions. Three examples that are particularly relevant to counseling are eye contact, smiling, and seating arrangement. North Americans exhibit a much greater degree of eye contact as listeners than as speakers, while African Americans tend to demonstrate the opposite pattern (i.e., greater eye contact when speaking than listening). Moreover, Asian/ Pacific Islanders often perceive eye contact as an expression of hostility, while Native Americans tend to interpret direct eye contact as a sign of disrespect. Similar variation exists with respect to smiling: Western cultures assign positive meaning to this facial expression; the Japanese culture associates smiling with shyness or embarrassment; and other Asian cultures may interpret smiling as a sign of weakness or superficiality. Finally, Westerners seem to prefer a seating arrangement in which the client and clinician face each other across a table. On the other hand, Native Americans may be most comfortable with a side-by-side arrangement (Sue & Sue, 1999).

Clearly, verbal language differences are culturally determined and may influence semantic, phonologic, syntactic, and morphologic behaviors. Moreover, pragmatic language issues such as appropriate topics of conversation, turn-taking rules, and the effects of social status between communication partners are culturally bound. For specific information regarding nonverbal and verbal characteristics of three main cultural groups—African American, Hispanic, and Asian—refer to Appendix C at the end of this book.

Helpful Hints

1. The value of counseling is severely compromised if a clinician's personal feelings become a factor in the therapeutic relationship.

2. Important points can be emphasized by reiterating them in different ways at various stages of the counseling relationship.

3. The provision of a brief summary at the end of a counseling session may help the client focus on the most important points that were discussed.

4. A client's feelings and attitudes generally cannot be changed by the clinician's presentation of rational argument alone.

5. Reluctance, resentment, and opposition are predictable client reactions in the counseling process and should not evoke feelings of defensiveness on the part of the clinician.

6. A clinician's use of phrases such as "It is my impression . . ." or "I hear you saying . . ." are less likely to trigger defensive behaviors from a client than more direct statements such as "You are . . ." or "You can't . . ."

7. It is important for clinicians to realize that the overuse of positive remarks causes such reinforcers to become meaningless.

8. Counseling is more effective if it periodically acknowledges a client's strengths rather than focusing solely on weaknesses or limitations.

9. Clinicians should refrain from pressing a client for self-disclosure too early in the counseling relationship because it may actually increase a client's reluctance to confide in the clinician.

10. Sometimes conflict within a group can be a sign that the group is working well as a unit. It frequently indicates that group members have developed a sense of trust and feel secure enough to disagree openly with each other.

11. Counseling that loses its focus or purpose becomes mere conversation and accomplishes little.

Especially for Multicultural Clients:

12. Use formal titles and full names when addressing adult clients. First names or nicknames may be considered condescending or offensive.

13. Clinicians should make every effort to learn the correct pronunciation of clients' and family members' names.

14. There may be cultural inhibitions about sharing personal information. Clinicians should carefully explain the meaning and parameters of confidentiality in the clinical process.

15. When the counseling process requires information gathering about family members or personal issues, the clinician should review standardized questionnaires and omit/modify items as appropriate given a client's specific background.

16. Clinicians should inquire specifically about who the client or family wishes to be included in counseling sessions rather than making assumptions.

17. Clients from LCD backgrounds may require additional support in developing mainstream cultural knowledge (e.g., history, arts, news events) to facilitate their acquisition of reading and writing skills.

CONCLUSION

This chapter presented basic information, protocols, and procedures for counseling at an **introductory** level. This information is intended only as a starting point in the reader's clinical education and training. For more in-depth coverage of this area, the following readings are recommended:

Crowe, T. A. (1997). *Applications of counseling in speech-language pathology and audiology.* Baltimore: Williams & Wilkins.

Flasher, L. V., & Fogle, P. T. (2004). *Counseling skills for speech-language pathologists and audiologists.* Clifton Park, NY: Thomson Delmar Learning.

Luterman, D. M. (2001). *Counseling the communicatively disordered and their families.* Austin, TX: Pro-Ed.

Shipley, K. G. (1997). *Interviewing and counseling in communicative disorders: Principles and procedures.* Needham Heights, MA: Allyn & Bacon.

Especially for Multicultural Issues

Battle, D. E. (2002). *Communication disorders in multicultural populations.* Boston: Butterworth-Heinemann.

Goldstein, B. (2000). *Cultural and linguistic diversity resource guide for speech-language pathologists.* Clifton Park, NY: Singular Thomson Learning.

ADDITIONAL RESOURCES

Pro-Ed

8700 Shoal Creek Boulevard
Austin, TX 78757-6897
Phone: 800-897-3202
Fax: 800-397-7633
Web site: www.proedinc.com

Counseling Persons with Communication Disorders and Their Families
Helps professionals incorporate some of the knowledge and skills of trained counselors into their work with clients and families. Includes a free Instructor's Manual upon request.

Interviewing and Counseling in Communicative Disorders: Principles and Procedures,
 second edition
Addresses issues such as various interviewing and counseling activities, stages of interviewing and counseling, and skills and techniques for effective interviewing and counseling. Also discusses areas such as multicultural factors, professional and ethical matters, and dealing with difficult situations.

Lifespan Perspectives on the Family and Disability
Examines how families cope, adapt, and grow through the challenge of living with a child with a disability. A family-centered focus is presented within a lifespan framework: infancy/early childhood; school years; transition from school to adult life; adult years.

American Guidance Service (AGS)

4201 Woodland Road
Circle Pines, MN 55014
Phone: 800-328-2560
Fax: 800-471-8457
E-mail: agsmail@agsnet.com
Web site: www.agsnet.com

Working with Parents: Dolores Curran's Guide to Successful Parent Groups
Provides information on working with parents, listening to identify parent needs, conducting groups that empower parents, and making parent education a career.

Thomson Delmar Learning

Executive Woods
5 Maxwell Drive
Clifton Park, NY 12065-2919
Phone: 800-354-9706
Fax: 800-487-8488
Web site: www.delmarhealthcare.com

Counseling Skills for Speech-Language Pathologists and Audiologists
Written by a clinical psychologist and a speech-language pathologist, this text presents basic and advanced counseling skills as they are used by students and

professionals in the communication sciences working with individuals with communication disorders. Written in user-friendly language, this text places the theories of counseling and the therapeutic process in real-life contexts that are applicable to speech-language pathologists and audiologists.

Practical Strategies for Family-Centered Intervention
Addresses issues such as understanding family concerns, priorities, and resources; applying family-centered principles assessment and intervention planning; and day-to-day service provision.

Thinking Publications
P.O. Box 163
Eau Claire, WI 54702-0163
Phone: 800-225-4769
Fax: 800-828-8885
Web site: www.thinkingpublications.com

Daily Communication Strategies for Adolescents with Language Disorders, second
edition
Includes chapters on motivation and counseling with adolescents. Provides field-tested activities for students with language or learning disorders and focuses on strategies rather than isolated skills. Material can be incorporated into group or individual sessions.

APPENDIX A

SCOPE OF PRACTICE IN SPEECH-LANGUAGE PATHOLOGY

American
Speech-Language-Hearing
Association

2001

STATEMENT OF PURPOSE

The purpose of this document is to define the scope of practice in speech-language pathology in order to:

1. Delineate areas of speech-language pathology professional practice provided by members of the American Speech-Language-Hearing Association (ASHA) and clinical certification holders in accordance with the ASHA Code of Ethics;
2. Educate health care, education, and other professionals, consumers, payers, regulators, and members of the general public about professional services offered by speech-language pathologists as qualified providers;
3. Assist ASHA members and certificate holders in the provision of high quality and evidence-based services to individuals across the life span who present with communication, swallowing, or other upper aerodigestive concerns[1];
4. Provide guidance for education programs in speech-language pathology curriculum.

The scope of practice defined here and the areas specifically set forth describe the breadth of professional practice offered within the profession. Levels of education, experience, skill, and proficiency with respect to the activities identified within this scope of practice vary among individual providers; a speech-language pathologist does not typically practice in all areas of the field. As the ASHA Code of Ethics specifies, individuals may only practice in areas in which they are competent based on their education, training, and experience. However, speech-language pathologists may expand their current level of expertise. Certain situations may necessitate that speech-language pathologists pursue additional education or training to expand their personal scope of practice.

This scope of practice statement does not supersede existing state licensure laws or affect the interpretation or implementation of such laws. It may serve, however, as a model for the development or modification of licensure laws.

The schema in Figure A-1 (see next page) depicts the relationship of the scope of practice to practice policy documents, certification standards, and the ASHA Code of Ethics. As indicated, individuals must fulfill the speech-language pathology certification standards in order to enter the practice of the profession. Practice policy documents (i.e., preferred practice patterns, position statements, guidelines, and knowledge and skills statements), address current and emerging speech-language pathology practice areas. These documents build on the knowledge, skills, and experiences required by the certification standards. The ASHA Code of Ethics sets forth the fundamental principles and rules considered essential to the preservation of the highest standards of integrity and ethical conduct to which members of the profession of speech-language pathology are bound.

---

[1]aeromechanical events related to communication, respiration, and swallowing (e.g., speaking valve selection, respiratory retraining for paradoxical vocal fold motion, stomal stenosis management and insufflation testing after total laryngectomy).

FIGURE A-1
Conceptual framework of ASHA Standards and Policy Statements.

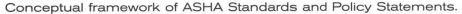

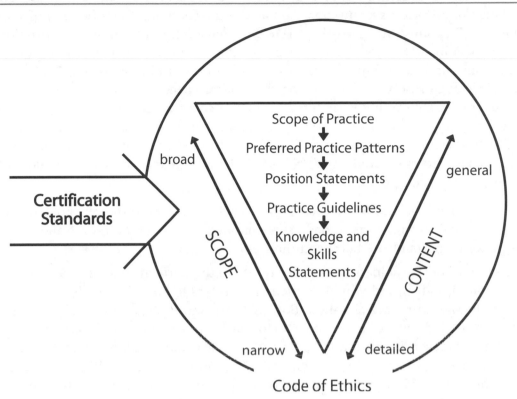

Speech-language pathology is a dynamic and continuously developing profession; listing specific areas within this scope of practice does not exclude emerging areas of practice. Although not specifically identified in this document, in certain instances speech-language pathologists may be called on to perform services (e.g., "multiskilling" in a health care setting, collaborative service delivery in schools) for the well-being of the individual(s) they are serving. In such instances it is both ethically and legally incumbent upon professionals to determine that they have the knowledge and skills necessary to conduct such tasks. Finally, it should be indicated that factors such as changes in service delivery systems, increasing numbers of people needing services, projected United States population growth of cultural and linguistic minority groups, and technological and scientific advances mandate that a scope of practice statement for the profession of speech-language pathology be dynamic in nature. For these reasons this document will undergo periodic review and possible revision.

FRAMEWORK FOR PRACTICE

The domain of speech-language pathology includes human communication behaviors and disorders as well as swallowing or other upper aerodigestive functions and disorders. The overall objective of speech-language pathology services is to optimize individuals' ability to communicate and/or swallow in natural environments, and thus improve their quality of life. This objective is best achieved through the provision of integrated services in meaningful life contexts. The World Health Organization (WHO) is in the process of finalizing a multipurpose health classification system identified as the International Classification of Functioning, Disability and Health (ICIDH-2)* that offers clinical service providers an internationally recognized conceptual framework and common language for discussing and describing human functioning and disability (WHO, 2000). This framework can be used to describe the role of speech-language pathologists in enhancing quality of life by optimizing human communication behavior, swallowing, or other upper aerodigestive functions regardless of setting. The ICIDH-2 [ICF] framework has two parts. The first is termed Functioning and Disability; the second refers to Contextual Factors. Functioning and Disability includes the following two components:

- Body Functions and Structures: Body Functions refers to the physiological or psychological functions of body systems; Body Structures refers to the anatomic parts of the body and their components.

- Activity and Participation: Activity refers to the performance of a task or action of a given individual; Participation refers to an individual's involvement in a life situation. Both Activity and Participation components are modified with Capacity and Performance qualifiers. The Capacity qualifier describes an individual's ability to execute a task or an action in a standardized or uniform environment. The Performance qualifier describes what an individual does in the current environment or actual context in which s/he lives.

Figure A-2 illustrates the components of the framework as applied to the practice of speech-language pathology. Each component can be expressed as a continuum of function. One end of the continuum indicates intact or neutral functioning; the other indicates completely compromised function or disability (e.g., impairment, activity limitation [formerly referred to as *disability* (WHO, 1980)], or participation restriction [formerly referred to as *handicap* (WHO, 1980)]). For example, the component of Body Functions and Structures has a continuum that ranges from normal variation to complete impairment; Activity ranges from no activity limitation to complete activity limitation; and Participation ranges from no participation restriction to complete participation restriction.

The second part of the ICIDH-2 [ICF] framework refers to Contextual Factors. Contextual Factors may interact with Body Functions and Structures, Activity, or Participation as facilitators or barriers to functioning. Contextual Factors include the following two components:

- Environmental Factors: defined as the physical, social, and attitudinal environment in which people live.

- Personal Factors: include such features of an individual as age, race, gender, educational background, and lifestyle. Although not formally classified in the ICIDH-2 [ICF], Personal Factors are acknowledged to be contributors to intervention outcomes.

---

*Editor's note: In 2001 the original acronym, ICIDH-2, was changed to ICF.

FIGURE A-2

Application of WHO (2000) framework to the practice of speech-language pathology.

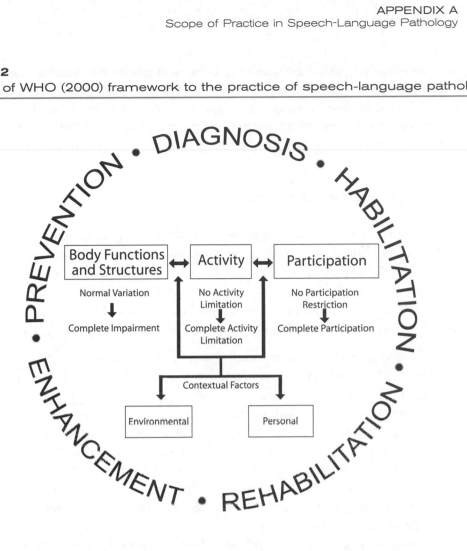

The scope of practice in speech-language pathology encompasses all components and factors identified in the WHO framework. That is, speech-language pathologists work to improve quality of life by reducing impairments of body functions and structures, activity limitations, participation restrictions, and environmental barriers of the individuals they serve. They serve individuals with known disease processes (e.g., aphasia, cleft palate) as well as those with activity limitations or participation restrictions (e.g., individuals needing classroom support services or special educational placement), including when such limitations or restrictions occur in the absence of known disease processes or impairments (e.g., individuals with differences in dialect). The role of speech-language pathologists includes prevention of communication, swallowing, or other upper aerodigestive disorders as well as diagnosis, habilitation, rehabilitation, and enhancement of these functions.

EDUCATION AND QUALIFICATIONS

Speech-language pathologists must hold a graduate degree, the Certificate of Clinical Competence (CCC-SLP) of the American Speech-Language-Hearing Association (ASHA), and where applicable, other required credentials (e.g., state licensure, teaching certification).

As primary care providers for communication, swallowing, or other upper aerodigestive disorders, speech-language pathologists are autonomous professionals; that is, their services need not be prescribed or supervised by individuals in other professions. However, in many cases individuals are best served when speech-language pathologists work collaboratively with other professionals.

SCOPE OF PRACTICE

The practice of speech-language pathology includes prevention, diagnosis, habilitation, and rehabilitation of communication, swallowing, or other upper aerodigestive disorders; elective modification of communication behaviors; and enhancement of communication. This includes services that address the dimensions of body structure and function, activity, and/or participation as proposed by the World Health Organization model (WHO, 2000). The practice of speech-language pathology involves:

1. Providing prevention, screening, consultation, assessment and diagnosis, treatment, intervention, management, counseling, and follow-up services for disorders of:
   * speech (i.e., articulation, fluency, resonance, and voice including aeromechanical components of respiration);
   * language (i.e., phonology, morphology, syntax, semantics, and pragmatic/social aspects of communication) including comprehension and expression in oral, written, graphic, and manual modalities; language processing; preliteracy and language-based literacy skills, including phonological awareness;
   * swallowing or other upper aerodigestive functions such as infant feeding and aeromechanical events (evaluation of esophageal function is for the purpose of referral to medical professionals);
   * cognitive aspects of communication (e.g., attention, memory, problem solving, executive functions).
   * sensory awareness related to communication, swallowing, or other upper aerodigestive functions.
2. Establishing augmentative and alternative communication techniques and strategies including developing, selecting, and prescribing of such systems and devices (e.g., speech generating devices).
3. Providing services to individuals with hearing loss and their families/caregivers (e.g., auditory training; speechreading; speech and language intervention secondary to hearing loss; visual inspection and listening checks of amplification devices for the purpose of troubleshooting, including verification of appropriate battery voltage).
4. Screening hearing of individuals who can participate in conventional pure-tone air conduction methods, as well as screening for middle ear pathology through screening tympanometry for the purpose of referral of individuals for further evaluation and management.
5. Using instrumentation (e.g., videofluoroscopy, EMG, nasendoscopy, stroboscopy, computer technology) to observe, collect data, and measure

parameters of communication and swallowing, or other upper aerodigestive functions in accordance with the principles of evidence-based practice.

6. Selecting, fitting, and establishing effective use of prosthetic/adaptive devices for communication, swallowing, or other upper aerodigestive functions (e.g., tracheoesophageal prostheses, speaking valves, electrolarynges). This does not include sensory devices used by individuals with hearing loss or other auditory perceptual deficits.

7. Collaborating in the assessment of central auditory processing disorders and providing intervention where there is evidence of speech, language, and/or other cognitive-communication disorders.

8. Educating and counseling individuals, families, co-workers, educators, and other persons in the community regarding acceptance, adaptation, and decision making about communication, swallowing, or other upper aerodigestive concerns.

9. Advocating for individuals through community awareness, education, and training programs to promote and facilitate access to full participation in communication, including the elimination of societal barriers.

10. Collaborating with and providing referrals and information to audiologists, educators, and health professionals as individual needs dictate.

11. Addressing behaviors (e.g., perseverative or disruptive actions) and environments (e.g., seating, positioning for swallowing safety or attention, communication opportunities) that affect communication, swallowing, or other upper aerodigestive functions.

12. Providing services to modify or enhance communication performance (e.g., accent modification, transgendered voice, care and improvement of the professional voice, personal/professional communication effectiveness).

13. Recognizing the need to provide and appropriately accommodate diagnostic and treatment services to individuals from diverse cultural backgrounds and adjust treatment and assessment services accordingly.

PROFESSIONAL ROLES AND ACTIVITIES

Speech-language pathologists serve individuals, families, groups, and the general public through a broad range of professional activities. They:

- Identify, define, and diagnose disorders of human communication and swallowing and assist in localization and diagnosis of diseases and conditions.

- Provide direct services using a variety of service delivery models to treat and/or address communication, swallowing, or other upper aerodigestive concerns.

- Conduct research related to communication sciences and disorders, swallowing, or other upper aerodigestive functions.

- Educate, supervise, and mentor future speech-language pathologists.

- Serve as case managers and service delivery coordinators.

- Administer and manage clinical and academic programs.

- Educate and provide in-service training to families, caregivers, and other professionals.

- Participate in outcomes measurement activities and use data to guide clinical decision making and determine the effectiveness of services provided in accordance with the principles of evidence-based practice.

- Train, supervise, and manage speech-language pathology assistants and other support personnel.

- Promote healthy lifestyle practices for the prevention of communication, hearing, swallowing, or other upper aerodigestive disorders.

- Foster public awareness of speech, language, hearing, and swallowing, and other upper aerodigestive disorders and their treatment.

- Advocate at the local, state, and national levels for access to and funding for services to address communication, hearing, swallowing, or other upper aerodigestive disorders.

- Serve as expert witnesses.

- Collaborate with audiologists in identifying neonates and infants at risk for hearing loss.

- Recognize the special needs of culturally diverse populations by providing services that are free of potential biases, including selection and/or adaptation of materials to ensure ethnic and linguistic sensitivity.

- Provide services using teleelectronic diagnostic measures and treatment methodologies (including remote applications).

PRACTICE SETTINGS

Speech-language pathologists provide services in a wide variety of settings, which may include but are not exclusive to:

- Public and private schools
- Health care settings (e.g., hospitals, medical rehabilitation facilities, long-term care facilities, home health agencies, community clinics, behavioral/mental health facilities)
- Private practice settings
- Universities and university clinics
- Individuals' homes
- Group homes and sheltered workshops
- Neonatal intensive care units, early intervention settings, preschools, and day care centers
- Community and state agencies and institutions
- Correctional institutions
- Research facilities
- Corporate and industrial settings

REFERENCE AND RESOURCE LIST

General

American Speech-Language-Hearing Association. (1986, May). The autonomy of speech-language pathology and audiology. *Asha, 28,* 53–57.

American Speech-Language-Hearing Association. (1992). Sedation and topical anesthetics in audiology and speech-language pathology. *Asha, 34*(Suppl. 7), 41–42.

American Speech-Language-Hearing Association. (1993). Definition of communication disorders and variations. *Asha, 35*(Suppl. 10), 40–41.

American Speech-Language-Hearing Association. (1993). Guidelines for caseload size and speech-language pathology service delivery in the school. *Asha, 35*(Suppl. 10), 33–39.

American Speech-Language-Hearing Association. (1994). *Admission/discharge criteria in speech-language pathology.* Unpublished report. Rockville, MD: Author.

American Speech-Language-Hearing Association. (1994). Code of ethics. *Asha, 36* (Suppl. 13), 1–2. under revision

American Speech-Language-Hearing Association. (1996). Inclusive practices for children and youths with communication disorders. *Asha, 38*(Suppl. 16), 35–44.

American Speech-Language-Hearing Association. (1996). Scope of practice in audiology. *Asha, 38*(Suppl. 16), 12–15.

American Speech-Language-Hearing Association. (1997). Position statement and technical report: Multiskilled personnel. *Asha, 39*(Suppl. 17), 13.

American Speech-Language-Hearing Association. (1997). *Preferred practice patterns for the profession of speech-language pathology.* Rockville, MD: Author.

American Speech-Language-Hearing Association. (1999). *Guidelines for the roles and responsibilities of the school-based speech-language pathologist.* Rockville, MD: Author.

American Speech-Language-Hearing Association. (2000). *IDEA and your caseload: A template for eligibility and dismissal criteria for students ages 3 to 21.* Rockville, MD: Author.

Council on Professional Standards in Speech-Language Pathology and Audiology. (2000). *Speech-language pathology certification standards.* Rockville, MD: Author.

World Health Organization. (2000). *International classification of functioning, disability and health: Prefinal draft.* Geneva, Switzerland: Author.

Augmentative and Alternative Communication

American Speech-Language-Hearing Association. (1989). Competencies for speech-language pathologists providing services in augmentative communication. *Asha, 31*(3), 107–110.

American Speech-Language-Hearing Association. (1991). Augmentative and alternative communication. *Asha, 33*(Suppl. 5), 8.

American Speech-Language-Hearing Association. (1991). Report: Augmentative and alternative communication. *Asha, 33*(Suppl. 5), 9–12.

American Speech-Language-Hearing Association. (1998). Maximizing the provision of appropriate technology services and devices for students in schools. *Asha, 40* (Suppl. 18), 33–42.

National Joint Committee for the Communicative Needs of Persons with Severe Disabilities. (1992). Guidelines for meeting the communication needs of persons with severe disabilities. *Asha, 34*(Suppl. 7), 1–8.

Cognitive Aspects of Communication

American Speech-Language-Hearing Association. (1982). Serving the communicatively handicapped mentally retarded individual. *Asha, 24*(8), 547–553.

American Speech-Language-Hearing Association. (1987). The role of speech-language pathologists in the habilitation and rehabilitation of cognitively impaired individuals. *Asha, 29*(6), 53–55.

American Speech-Language-Hearing Association. (1988). Mental retardation and developmental disabilities curriculum guide for speech-language pathologists and audiologists. *ASHA Desk Reference*, vol. 4, 185–189.

American Speech-Language-Hearing Association. (1988). The role of speech-language pathologists in the identification, diagnosis, and treatment of individuals with cognitive-communicative impairments. *Asha, 30*(3), 79.

American Speech-Language-Hearing Association. (1990). Interdisciplinary approaches to brain damage. *Asha, 32*(Suppl. 2), 3.

American Speech-Language-Hearing Association. (1990). The role of speech-language pathologists and audiologists in service delivery for persons with mental retardation and developmental disabilities in community settings. *Asha, 32*(Suppl. 2), 5–6.

American Speech-Language-Hearing Association. (1991). Guidelines for speech-language pathologists serving persons with language, socio-communicative and/or cognitive-communicative impairments. *Asha, 33*(Suppl. 5), 21–28.

American Speech-Language-Hearing Association. (1995). Guidelines for the structure and function of an interdisciplinary team for persons with brain injury. *Asha, 37* (Suppl. 14), 23.

Deaf and Hard of Hearing

American Speech-Language-Hearing Association. (1984). Competencies for aural rehabilitation. *Asha, 26*(5), 37–41.

American Speech-Language-Hearing Association. (1990). Aural rehabilitation: an annotated bibliography. *Asha, 32*(Suppl. 1), 1–12.

American Speech-Language-Hearing Association. (1994, August). Service provision under the Individuals with Disabilities Education Act–Part H, as Amended (IDEA–Part H) to children who are deaf and hard of hearing ages birth to 36 months. *Asha, 36*, 117–121.

Hearing Screening

American National Standards Institute. (1996). *Specifications for audiometers* (ANSI S3.6.-1996). New York: Acoustical Society of America.

American National Standards Institute. (1991). *Maximum permissible ambient noise levels for audiometric test rooms* (ANSI S3.1-1991). New York: Acoustical Society of America.

American Speech-Language-Hearing Association. (1994). Clinical practice by certificate holders in the profession in which they are not certified. *Asha, 36*(13), 11–12.

American Speech-Language-Hearing Association. (1997). *Guidelines for audiologic screening.* Rockville, MD: Author.

Joint Committee on Infant Hearing. (2000). Year 2000 position statement: Principles and guidelines for early hearing detection and intervention programs. *American Journal of Audiology, 9*, 9–29.

Language and Literacy

American Speech-Language-Hearing Association. (1982). Definition of language. *Asha*, *24*(6), 44.

American Speech-Language-Hearing Association. (1982). Position statement on language learning disorders. *Asha*, *24*(11), 937–944.

American Speech-Language-Hearing Association. (1989). Issues in determining eligibility for language intervention. *Asha*, *31*(3), 113–118.

American Speech-Language-Hearing Association. (1991). A model for collaborative service delivery for students with language-learning disorders in the public schools. *Asha*, *33*(Suppl. 5), 44–50.

American Speech-Language-Hearing Association. (1991). Guidelines for speech-language pathologists serving persons with language, socio-communicative and/or cognitive-communicative impairments. *Asha*, *33*(Suppl. 5), 21–28.

American Speech-Language-Hearing Association Task Force on Central Auditory Processing Consensus Development. (1995). *Central auditory processing: Current status of research and implications for clinical practice.* Rockville, MD: ASHA.

American Speech-Language-Hearing Association. (2000). *Guidelines on the roles and responsibilities of speech-language pathologists with respect to reading and writing in children and adolescents.* Rockville, MD: Author.

American Speech-Language-Hearing Association. (2000). *Position statement on the roles and responsibilities of speech-language pathologists with respect to reading and writing in children and adolescents.* Rockville, MD: Author.

American Speech-Language-Hearing Association. (2000). *Technical report on the roles and responsibilities of speech-language pathologists with respect to reading and writing in children and adolescents.* Rockville, MD: Author.

National Joint Committee on Learning Disabilities. (1989). Communication-based services for infants, toddlers, and their families. *ASHA Desk Reference*, vol. 3, 159–163.

Multicultural Issues

American Speech-Language-Hearing Association. (1983). Social dialects (and implications). *Asha*, *25*(9), 23–27.

American Speech-Language-Hearing Association. (1985). Clinical management of communicatively handicapped minority language populations. *Asha*, *27*(6), 29–32.

American Speech-Language-Hearing Association. (1989). Bilingual speech-language pathologists and audiologists. *Asha*, *31*, 93.

American Speech-Language-Hearing Association. (1998). Provision of English-as-a-second-language instruction by speech-language pathologists in school settings: Position statement and technical report. *Asha*, *40*(Suppl. 18), 24–27.

Prevention

American Speech-Language-Hearing Association. (1982). Prevention of speech, language, hearing problems. *Asha*, *24*, 425, 431.

American Speech-Language-Hearing Association. (1988, March). Prevention of communication disorders. *Asha*, *30*, 90.

American Speech-Language-Hearing Association. (1991). The prevention of communication disorders tutorial. *Asha*, *33*(Suppl. 6), 15–41.

Research

American Speech-Language-Hearing Association. (1992). Ethics in research and professional practice. *Asha, 34*(Suppl. 9), 11–12.

Speech: Articulation, Fluency, Voice, Resonance

American Speech-Language-Hearing Association. (1992). Position statement and guidelines for evaluation and treatment for tracheoesophageal fistulization/puncture. *Asha, 34*(Suppl. 7), 17–21.

American Speech-Language-Hearing Association. (1992). Position statement and guidelines for vocal tract visualization and imaging. *Asha, 34*(Suppl. 7), 31–40.

American Speech-Language-Hearing Association. (1993). Position statement and guidelines for oral and oropharyngeal prostheses. *Asha, 35*(Suppl. 10), 14–16.

American Speech-Language-Hearing Association. (1993). Position statement and guidelines on the use of voice prostheses in tracheotomized persons with or without ventilatory dependence. *Asha, 35*(Suppl. 10), 17–20.

American Speech-Language-Hearing Association. (1993). The role of the speech-language pathologist and teacher of voice in the remediation of singers with voice disorders. *Asha, 35*(1), 63.

American Speech-Language-Hearing Association. (1995, March). Guidelines for practice in stuttering treatment. *Asha, 37*(Suppl. 14), 26–35.

American Speech-Language-Hearing Association. (1998). Roles of otolaryngologists and speech-language pathologists in the performance and interpretation of strobovideo-laryngoscopy. *Asha, 40* (Suppl. 18), 32.

ASHA Special Interest Division 3: Voice and Voice Disorders. (1997). *Training guidelines for laryngeal videoendoscopy/stroboscopy.* Unpublished report. Rockville: MD. Author.

Supervision

American Speech-Language-Hearing Association. (1985). Clinical supervision in speech-language pathology and audiology. *Asha, 28*(6), 57–60.

American Speech-Language-Hearing Association. (1989). Preparation models for the supervisory process in speech-language pathology and audiology. *Asha, 32*(3), 97–106.

American Speech-Language-Hearing Association. (1992). Supervision of student clinicians. *Asha, 34*(Suppl. 9), 8.

American Speech-Language-Hearing Association. (1992). Clinical fellowship supervisor's responsibilities. *Asha, 34*(Suppl. 9), 16–17.

American Speech-Language-Hearing Association. (1996, Spring). Guidelines for the training, credentialing, use, and supervision of speech-language pathology assistants. *Asha, 38* (Suppl. 16), 21–34.

American Speech-Language-Hearing Association. (in preparation). Knowledge and skills for supervision of speech-language pathology assistants.

Swallowing/Upper Aerodigestive Function

American Speech-Language-Hearing Association. (1987). Ad hoc committee on dysphagia report. *Asha, 29*(4), 57–58.

American Speech-Language-Hearing Association. (1989). Report: Ad hoc committee on labial-lingual posturing function. *Asha, 31*(11), 92–94.

American Speech-Language-Hearing Association. (1990). Knowledge and skills needed by speech-language pathologists providing services to dysphagic patients/clients. *Asha, 32*(Suppl. 2), 7–12.

American Speech-Language-Hearing Association. (1991). The role of the speech-language pathologist in assessment and management of oral myofunctional disorders. *Asha, 33*(Suppl. 5), 7.

American Speech-Language-Hearing Association. (1992). Position statement and guidelines for instrumental diagnostic procedures for swallowing, *Asha, 34*(Suppl. 7), 25–33.

American Speech-Language-Hearing Association. (1993). Orofacial myofunctional disorders: knowledge and skills. *Asha, 35*(Suppl. 10), 21–23.

American Speech-Language-Hearing Association. (2000). Clinical indicators for instrumental assessment of dysphagia (guidelines): Executive summary. *ASHA Suppl. 20*, 18–19.

American Speech-Language-Hearing Association. (2000). Roles of the speech-language pathologist and otolaryngologist in the performance and interpretation of endoscopic examination of swallowing (position statement). *ASHA Suppl. 20*, 17.

ASHA Special Interest Division 13: Swallowing and Swallowing Disorders (Dysphagia). (1997). Graduate curriculum on swallowing and swallowing disorders (adult and pediatric dysphagia). *ASHA Desk Reference*, vol. 3, 248a–248n.

CODE OF ETHICS

American Speech-Language-Hearing Association

January, 2003

PREAMBLE

The preservation of the highest standards of integrity and ethical principles is vital to the responsible discharge of obligations by speech-language pathologists, audiologists, and speech, language, and hearing scientists. This Code of Ethics sets forth the fundamental principles and rules considered essential to this purpose.

Every individual who is (a) a member of the American Speech-Language-Hearing Association, whether certified or not, (b) a nonmember holding the Certificate of Clinical Competence from the Association, (c) an applicant for membership or certification, or (d) a Clinical Fellow seeking to fulfill standards for certification shall abide by this Code of Ethics.

Any violation of the spirit and purpose of this Code shall be considered unethical. Failure to specify any particular responsibility or practice in this Code of Ethics shall not be construed as denial of the existence of such responsibilities or practices.

The fundamentals of ethical conduct are described by Principles of Ethics and by Rules of Ethics as they relate to the conduct of research and scholarly activities and responsibility to persons served, the public, and speech-language pathologists, audiologists, and speech, language, and hearing scientists.

Principles of Ethics, aspirational and inspirational in nature, form the underlying moral basis for the Code of Ethics. Individuals shall observe these principles as affirmative obligations under all conditions of professional activity.

Rules of Ethics are specific statements of minimally acceptable professional conduct or of prohibitions and are applicable to all individuals.

PRINCIPLE OF ETHICS I

Individuals shall honor their responsibility to hold paramount the welfare of persons they serve professionally or participants in research and scholarly activities and shall treat animals involved in research in a humane manner.

Rules of Ethics

A. Individuals shall provide all services competently.
B. Individuals shall use every resource, including referral when appropriate, to ensure that high-quality service is provided.
C. Individuals shall not discriminate in the delivery of professional services or the conduct of research and scholarly activities on the basis of race or ethnicity, gender, age, religion, national origin, sexual orientation, or disability.
D. Individuals shall not misrepresent the credentials of assistants, technicians, or support personnel and shall inform those they serve professionally of the name and professional credentials of persons providing services.
E. Individuals who hold the Certificates of Clinical Competence shall not delegate tasks that require the unique skills, knowledge, and judgment that are within the scope of their profession to assistants, technicians, support

personnel, students, or any nonprofessionals over whom they have supervisory responsibility. An individual may delegate support services to assistants, technicians, support personnel, students, or any other persons only if those services are adequately supervised by an individual who holds the appropriate Certificate of Clinical Competence.

F. Individuals shall fully inform the persons they serve of the nature and possible effects of services rendered and products dispensed, and they shall inform participants in research about the possible effects of their participation in research conducted.

G. Individuals shall evaluate the effectiveness of services rendered and of products dispensed and shall provide services or dispense products only when benefit can reasonably be expected.

H. Individuals shall not guarantee the results of any treatment or procedure, directly or by implication; however, they may make a reasonable statement of prognosis.

I. Individuals shall not provide clinical services solely by correspondence.

J. Individuals may practice by telecommunication (for example, telehealth/ e-health), where not prohibited by law.

K. Individuals shall adequately maintain and appropriately secure records of professional services rendered, research and scholarly activities conducted, and products dispensed and shall allow access to these records only when authorized or when required by law.

L. Individuals shall not reveal, without authorization, any professional or personal information about identified persons served professionally or identified participants involved in research and scholarly activities unless required by law to do so or unless doing so is necessary to protect the welfare of the person or of the community or otherwise required by law.

M. Individuals shall not charge for services not rendered, nor shall they misrepresent services rendered, products dispensed, or research and scholarly activities conducted.

N. Individuals shall use persons in research or as subjects of teaching demonstrations only with their informed consent.

O. Individuals whose professional services are adversely affected by substance abuse or other health-related conditions shall seek professional assistance and, where appropriate, withdraw from the affected areas of practice.

PRINCIPLE OF ETHICS II

Individuals shall honor their responsibility to achieve and maintain the highest level of professional competence.

Rules of Ethics

A. Individuals shall engage in the provision of clinical services only when they hold the appropriate Certificate of Clinical Competence or when they are in the certification process and are supervised by an individual who holds the appropriate Certificate of Clinical Competence.

B. Individuals shall engage in only those aspects of the professions that are within the scope of their competence, considering their level of education, training, and experience.

C. Individuals shall continue their professional development throughout their careers.

D. Individuals shall delegate the provision of clinical services only to: (1) persons who hold the appropriate Certificate of Clinical Competence; (2) persons in the education or certification process who are appropriately supervised by an individual who holds the appropriate Certificate of Clinical Competence; or (3) assistants, technicians, or support personnel who are adequately supervised by an individual who holds the appropriate Certificate of Clinical Competence.

E. Individuals shall not require or permit their professional staff to provide services or conduct research activities that exceed the staff member's competence, level of education, training, and experience.

F. Individuals shall ensure that all equipment used in the provision of services or to conduct research and scholarly activities is in proper working order and is properly calibrated.

PRINCIPLE OF ETHICS III

Individuals shall honor their responsibility to the public by promoting public understanding of the professions, by supporting the development of services designed to fulfill the unmet needs of the public, and by providing accurate information in all communications involving any aspect of the professions, including dissemination of research findings and scholarly activities.

Rules of Ethics

A. Individuals shall not misrepresent their credentials, competence, education, training, experience, or scholarly or research contributions.

B. Individuals shall not participate in professional activities that constitute a conflict of interest.

C. Individuals shall refer those served professionally solely on the basis of the interest of those being referred and not on any personal financial interest.

D. Individuals shall not misrepresent diagnostic information, research, services rendered, or products dispensed; neither shall they engage in any scheme to defraud in connection with obtaining payment or reimbursement for such services or products.

E. Individuals' statements to the public shall provide accurate information about the nature and management of communication disorders, about the professions, about professional services, and about research and scholarly activities.

F. Individuals' statements to the public—advertising, announcing, and marketing their professional services, reporting research results, and promoting products—shall adhere to prevailing professional standards and shall not contain misrepresentations.

PRINCIPLE OF ETHICS IV

Individuals shall honor their responsibilities to the professions and their relationships with colleagues, students, and members of allied professions. Individuals shall uphold the dignity and autonomy of the professions, maintain harmonious inter-professional and intra-professional relationships, and accept the professions' self-imposed standards.

Rules of Ethics

A. Individuals shall prohibit anyone under their supervision from engaging in any practice that violates the Code of Ethics.
B. Individuals shall not engage in dishonesty, fraud, deceit, misrepresentation, sexual harassment, or any other form of conduct that adversely reflects on the professions or on the individual's fitness to serve persons professionally.
C. Individuals shall not engage in sexual activities with clients or students over whom they exercise professional authority.
D. Individuals shall assign credit only to those who have contributed to a publication, presentation, or product. Credit shall be assigned in proportion to the contribution and only with the contributor's consent.
E. Individuals shall reference the source when using other persons' ideas, research, presentations, or products in written, oral, or any other media presentation or summary.
F. Individuals' statements to colleagues about professional services, research results, and products shall adhere to prevailing professional standards and shall contain no misrepresentations.
G. Individuals shall not provide professional services without exercising independent professional judgment, regardless of referral source or prescription.
H. Individuals shall not discriminate in their relationships with colleagues, students, and members of allied professions on the basis of race or ethnicity, gender, age, religion, national origin, sexual orientation, or disability.
I. Individuals who have reason to believe that the Code of Ethics has been violated shall inform the Board of Ethics.
J. Individuals shall comply fully with the policies of the Board of Ethics in its consideration and adjudication of complaints of violations of the Code of Ethics.

MULTICULTURAL TABLES

TABLE C-1
Consonant Sound Production Characteristics of Black English

Phoneme	Description
/n/	Replaced by nasalized vowel in the final position (e.g., bin → /bɪ/)
/w, d/	Omitted in initial position for specific words (e.g., was → /əz/; don't → /ont/)
/ŋ/	Replaced by /n/ especially in final position (e.g., going → /goɪn)
/l, r/	Omitted in medial and final positions (e.g., poor → /po/)
	Replaced occasionally by /ə/ in final position (e.g., pill → /pɪə/; here → /hiə/)
/θ/	Replaced by /t/ or /f/ in initial, medial, and final positions (e.g., author → /ɔfə/; math → /mæf/)
/ð/	Replaced by /d/ in initial position and /d/ or /v/ in medial and final positions (e.g., this → /dɪs/; mother → /mʌvɚ/)
/z/	Omitted or replaced by /d/ before nasal sounds (e.g., isn't → /ɪdnt/)
Blends	
/str/	Replaced by /skr/ (e.g., street → /skrit/)
/ʃr/	Replaced by /str/ (e.g., shrill → /strɪl/)
/θr/	Replaced by /θ/ (e.g., throw → /θo/)
/pr, br, gr, kr/	Omission of /r/ (e.g., apron → /epən/; agriculture → /ægɪkəltʃɚ/)
Consonant Clusters	
/sk, nd, sp, ft, ld, dʒd, st, sd, nt/	Deletion of second consonant in final word position (e.g., left → /lɛf/; cold → /kol/; desk → /dɛs/)

Source: Adapted from Bailey & Thomas (1998); Goldstein (2000); Owens (2001); Fasold & Wolfram (1970); and Williams & Wolfram (1977).

TABLE C-2
Morphologic and Syntactic Characteristics of Black English

Structure	Description
Verbs	
Regular past -ed	Not obligatory and frequently omitted (e.g., I **talk** to him last week)
Irregular past	May remain uninflected or regularized with "-ed" (e.g., He **begin** work yesterday; She **knowed** all about it)
Regular present 3rd person singular	Not obligatory and frequently omitted (e.g., John **sleep** too much)
Irregular present 3rd person singular	Not obligatory and frequently omitted (e.g., He always **do** silly things)
Future tense	"Will" is replaced by "gonna"; "will" is omitted preceding the verb "be" (e.g., The dog **gonna** bite you; I **be** back tomorrow)
Copula and auxiliary	Not obligatory and may be omitted if contractible (e.g., He **ready**; They **eating**)
Perfect tense	"Been" is used to signify action in the distant past (e.g., He died long ago → He **been** dead)
Habitual state	Ongoing or general states are marked by uninflected "be" (e.g., She **be** funny)
Modals	Double modals are permissible with forms such as: might, could, should (e.g., They **might could** come)
Noun Phrases	
Regular plural -s	Not obligatory and frequently omitted when quantifiers are present (e.g., I see three **book** over there)
Irregular plural	May be doubly inflected (e.g., Help me find the **childrens**)
Possessive -'s	Not obligatory and frequently omitted when word order indicates possession (e.g., **Debbie** bike got wet)
Pronouns	
Apposition	Pronoun immediately follows the referent noun (e.g., My brother **he** bigger than you)
Relative pronouns	Not obligatory and frequently omitted (e.g., There's the **dog bit** me)
Reflexive pronouns	Reflexive form "-self" can be extended to possessive pronouns (e.g., **hisself**; **theirself**)
Demonstratives	Certain demonstrative/pronominal phrases are permissible (e.g., **These here** apples; **Them there** toys)

(continues)

Table C-2 Morphologic and Syntactic Characteristics of Black English (continued)

Structure	Description
Adverbs and Adjectives	
Comparatives and superlatives	The forms "-er" and "-est" can be extended to many adjectives (e.g., **worser**, **horriblest**)
	The modifiers "more" and "most" can be added to comparative and superlative forms (e.g., **more taller**; **most oldest**)
Intensifiers	Certain modifiers can be added to adverbs or adjectives for emphasis (e.g., **right** quick; **plumb** crazy)
Negation	
Ain't	"Ain't" is a permissible negative form (e.g., I **ain't** got any money)
Multiple negation	Double and triple negative markers are permissible (e.g., **Nobody don't** like me; **Nobody don't never** talk to him)
Interrogatives	
Indirect questions	The inverted form may be used for indirect questions (e.g., I wonder what **was he** singing)
	The uninverted form may be used for direct questions (e.g., What **he was** eating?)
	The conditional conjunction "if" is replaced by "do" (e.g., I wonder **do** you hear me?)

Source: Adapted from Fasold & Wolfram (1970); Goldstein (2000); Owens (2001); Roseberry-McKibbin (1995); Washington & Craig (1994); and Williams & Wolfram (1977).

TABLE C-3
Pragmatic Characteristics of Black English (BE)

- Direct eye-contact is used in the speaker role, while indirect eye contact is associated with the listener role. Speakers of other dialects may interpret this indirect eye contact as inattentiveness or disrespect.

- Interruptions during conversation are permissible and the role of speaker is yielded to the most assertive conversational partner. This interaction pattern may be interpreted by non-BE speakers as impolite or rude.

- Silence is used as a communication strategy in unfamiliar situations or to refute a speaker's statement. In other dialects, this silence may be interpreted as lack of knowledge or acceptance of the speaker's statement.

- Questions about personal matters such as family, health, and education are considered rude and discourteous when addressed to a new acquaintance.

- Humor and sarcasm are highly valued aspects of communicative interactions and are often expressed in ritualized exchanges of insults and comebacks. These interactions may be misinterpreted by non-BE speakers as instances of negative and hostile behavior.

- Conversations are considered to be private; verbal contributions from individuals outside the immediate conversational group are perceived as impolite eavesdropping behavior (even if the comments were intended to be helpful).

- Intense and demonstrative speech behavior is permissible in public conversational interactions. Speakers of other dialects may interpret this emotional display as irresponsible or in bad taste.

Source: Adapted from Kamhi, Pollack, & Harris (1996); and Paul (2001).

TABLE C-4
Speech Sound Production Characteristics of Spanish-Influenced English

Phoneme	Description
/ɪ, æ/	Do not exist in Spanish and are replaced by other vowels (e.g., mister → /mɪstɚ/)
/d/	Dentalized in medial position
/ŋ/	Replaced by /n/ in the final position (e.g., song → /sɔn/)
/j/	Replaced by /dʒ/ in initial position (e.g., you → /dʒu/)
/ʃ/	Replaced by /tʃ/ in all positions (e.g., sheet → /tʃit/; washer → /wɔtʃɚ/)
/tʃ/	Replaced by /ʃ/ in all positions (e.g., chain → /ʃen/; teacher → /tiʃɚ/)
/dʒ/	Replaced by /j/ in initial and medial positions (e.g., major → /mejɚ/)
/θ/	Replaced by /t/ in initial and final positions and omitted in medial position (e.g., think → /tɪnk/; baths → /bæs/)
/v/	Replaced by /b/ in all positions (e.g., vowel → /baʊl/; oven → /ʌbɛn/)
/z/	Replaced by /s/ in all positions (e.g., zero → /siro/; blizzard → /blɪsɚd/)
/ð/	Replaced by /d/ in initial and final positions; replaced by /d/, /v/, or /θ/ in medial position (e.g., they → /de/; brother → /brʌθɚ/)
	Consonants in the final position are usually devoiced (e.g., cab → /kæp/; bug → /bʌk/)
	A schwa or /ɛ/ is often added before consonant blends beginning with /s/ (e.g., speech → /əspitʃ/; slow → /ɛslo/)

Source: Adapted from Battle (2002); Goldstein (2000); Owens (2001); and Paul (2001).

TABLE C-5
Morphologic and Syntactic Characteristics of Spanish-Influenced English

Structure	Description
Verbs	
Regular past -**ed**	Not obligatory and frequently omitted (e.g., I **talk** to him last week)
Regular present 3rd person singular	Not obligatory and frequently omitted (e.g., John **sleep** too much)
Future	Use of "go + to" with omission of the verb "to be" as well as the progressive marker "-ing" (e.g., I **go to** store)
Copula	Occasional use of "have" instead of "be" in certain instances (e.g., I **have** fourteen years)
Noun Phrases	
Regular plural -**s**	Not obligatory and frequently omitted (e.g., I see three **book** over there)
Possessive -**'s**	Replaced by prepositional phrase following the noun (e.g., This is the shirt **of my brother**)
Articles	Not obligatory and frequently omitted (e.g., They went **to movie**)
Pronouns	
Possessive pronouns	Replaced with article in reference to body parts (e.g., I broke **the** leg)
Subject pronouns	May be omitted when subject is specified in the preceding utterance (e.g., Maria is pretty. **Got** a new dress)
Adjectives	
Comparative -**er**	Replaced by modifier "more" (e.g., That table is **more** long)
Negation	
No	"No" replaces "auxiliary + not" before a verb (e.g., He **no** drink milk)
	Replaces "don't" in imperative forms (e.g., **No** touch that)
Interrogatives	
Inversion	Not obligatory and replaced by rising intonation (e.g., **Mama is** gone?)
Do insertion	Not obligatory and frequently omitted (e.g., **You want** more soup?)

Source: Adapted from Battle (2002); Goldstein (2000); Owens (2001); and Paul (2001).

TABLE C-6
Pragmatic Characteristics of Spanish-Influenced English (SIE)

- Indirect eye contact is used in conversation to convey attentiveness or respect. Speakers of other dialects may interpret this behavior in the opposite manner.

- Distance between speakers during conversation is relatively close.

- Touching one's communication partner is common during conversations. This contact may be perceived as offensive by speakers of other cultural orientations.

- Interruptions during conversation are permissible. This pattern of interaction may be interpreted by non-SIE speakers as impolite or rude.

- Formal or business conversations are opened with personal questions and remarks, which can be extensive. Speakers of other dialects may interpret this style of conversational initiation as intrusive, a sign of procrastination, or as "a waste of time."

Source: Adapted from Kayser (1998) and Paul (2001).

TABLE C-7
Speech Sound Production Characteristics of Asian-Influenced English (AIE)

- Speakers of AIE may shorten, lengthen, or otherwise distort English vowels. For example, native speakers of Mandarin may produce *bead* as /bɪd/, or *fit* as /fit/.

- AIE speakers tend to omit or distort final consonants because the rule systems of many Asian languages highly restrict or eliminate consonant sounds in the final position, e.g., *did* → /dɪ/.

- In many Asian languages, /r/ and /l/ are not categorized as distinctly separate phonemes. As a result, these sounds may be used interchangeably in English, e.g., *rice* → /laɪs/.

- Consonant blends are uncommon in many Asian languages. AIE speakers tend to simplify clusters either by inserting a /ə/ into the blend (e.g., Chinese and Japanese) or by omitting the entire cluster (e.g., Vietnamese).

- Several Asian languages are predominantly monosyllabic in nature. AIE speakers may shorten or misplace stress on multisyllabic words (i.e., sepa'rately).

- Asian languages such as Chinese, Vietnamese, or Laotian use changes in "tone" (prosody) to signify changes in word meaning. In contrast, tonal changes in English are used to differentiate declarative from interrogative utterances and to convey communicative intent (e.g., sarcasm, humor, protest). AIE speakers may experience difficulty acquiring English intonation patterns and their messages frequently may be misinterpreted.

Source: Adapted from Cheng (1987a, 1987b) and Owens (2001).

TABLE C-8
Morphologic and Syntactic Characteristics of Asian-Influenced English

Structure	Description
Verbs	
Regular past -**ed**	Not obligatory and frequently omitted (e.g., He **walk** home yesterday)
Irregular past	May be regularized with "-ed" or doubly inflected, even in perfect tense (e.g., He **sleeped** in the bed; He **didn't ran** home; He **had wented**)
Singular present	Not obligatory and frequently omitted in 3rd person; overly inflected in 2nd person (e.g., He usually **walk** to school; You **talks** too loud)
Auxiliary	"Be" and "do" may be omitted or remain uninflected (e.g., He **eating** dinner now; He **do** not know her)
Perfect tense	Marker "-en" is not obligatory and frequently omitted (e.g., I **have speak** to her)
Noun Phrases	
Regular plural -s	Not obligatory and frequently omitted when quantifiers are present (e.g., I have **three shirt**)
Irregular plural	May be doubly inflected and overregularized (e.g., She brushed her **teeths**)
Possessive -'s	Not obligatory and frequently omitted (e.g., That my **mom** hat)
Pronouns	
Possessive	Pronoun usage may be confused (e.g., I see **she** car)
Case	Subject and object pronouns may be confused (e.g., **Him** coming soon)
Gender	Male and female pronouns may be confused (e.g., I meet **her** wife)
Demonstratives	Singular and plural pronouns may be confused (e.g., He own **that** cars)
Adjectives	
Comparatives	The former "-er" may be extended to many adjectives (e.g., **gooder**, **honester**)
	The modifier "more" may be added to comparative forms (e.g., She is **more shorter** than me)
Negation	
Multiple negation	Double negative markers are permissible (e.g., He **didn't** have **none**)
No	"No" replaces "auxiliary + not" (e.g., He **no** live here)

(continues)

Table C-8 Morphologic and Syntactic Characteristics of Asian-Influenced English (continued)

Structure	Description
Interrogatives	
Inversion	Not obligatory and replaced by rising intonation (e.g., **You are** coming home?)
Do insertion	Not obligatory and frequently omitted (e.g., **You see** her today?)
Prepositions	May be omitted or confused (e.g., I put **it drawer**; I am **at** kitchen)
Conjunctions	Not obligatory and frequently omitted (e.g., **Brother sister** went home)
Articles	May be omitted or overused (e.g., I saw **boy**; I go to **the school**)
Word Order	Changes in word order frequently occur (e.g., I have **car new**; **Book mine** got lost; He put **down it**)

Source: Adapted from Cheng (1987b) and Owens (2001).

TABLE C-9
Pragmatic Characteristics of Asian-Influenced English (AIE)

- Direct eye contact is avoided; indirect eye contact is used in conversation to convey respect. Speakers of other dialects may interpret this behavior unfavorably.

- Interruptions during conversations are considered impolite. Children who ask questions or interrupt teachers during classroom lectures are considered disobedient. Western cultures may perceive this behavior as passive and nonparticipatory.

- Third party introductions are preferred to informal self-introductions, especially when interacting with individuals of high status. Non-AIE speakers may regard this preference for formal introductions as unfriendly or aloof behavior.

- Questions about age, marital status, or employment are considered appropriate even of new acquaintances in order to establish proper social distance between or among the speakers. Western cultures may regard such queries as inappropriate or "nosy," especially in initial conversations.

- Professionals are automatically treated with respect and are regarded as authorities.

- Kinship terms may be used with elders who are not family members as an indication of respect.

- Embarrassment is a common reaction to praise; humility is emphasized and highly valued.

- Feelings are not openly exhibited; public affection is not displayed. The facial expressions of AIE speakers may remain impassive even when being provoked or reprimanded. Western speakers may perceive this affect as indifference or insensitivity.

- Giggling may reflect shyness or embarrassment rather than amusement.

- Direct and open disagreement is infrequent, particularly with individuals regarded as high status professionals or authorities. Speakers in Western cultures may misinterpret this behavior as an indication of agreement.

Source: Adapted from Cheng (1987a, 1987b) and Langdon & Cheng (2002).

INTERNATIONAL PHONETIC ALPHABET SYMBOLS

TABLE D-1

International Phonetic Alphabet Symbols for English Vowels

Phonetic Symbol	Example	Phonetic Transcription
i	wheel	[wil]
ɪ	this	[ðɪs]
e	plane	[pleɪn], [plen]
ɛ	bed	[bɛd]
æ	matches	[mætʃɪz]
ɑ	hot	[hɑt]
ɔ	clause	[klɔz]
o	stove	[stov]
ʊ	put	[pʊt]
u	blue	[blu]
ʌ	cup	[kʌp] (stressed)
ə	umbrella	[əmbrɛlə] (unstressed)
aɪ	knife	[naɪf]
aʊ	shout	[ʃaʊt]
ɔɪ	boy	[bɔɪ]
ɝ	squirrel	[skwɝl] (stressed)
ɚ	zipper	[zɪpɚ] (unstressed)

TABLE D-2
International Phonetic Alphabet Symbols for English Consonants

Phonetic Symbol	Example	Phonetic Transcription
p	plane	[plen]
b	bed	[bɛd]
t	toy	[tɔi]
d	dot	[dɑt]
k	cup	[kʌp] (stressed)
g	glue	[glu]
h	hot	[hɑt]
ʔ	mitten	[mɪʔn]
m	matches	[mætʃɪz]
n	knife	[naif]
ŋ	swing	[swɪŋ]
f	fast	[fæst]
v	voice	[vɔis]
θ	thick	[θɪk]
ð	this	[ðɪs]
s	squirrel	[skwɝl] (stressed)
z	zipper	[zɪpɚ] (unstressed)
ʃ	shovel	[ʃʌvəl]
ʒ	measure	[mɛʒɚ]
tʃ	chicken	[tʃɪkɪn]
l	lamp	[læmp]
r	rabbit	[ræbɪt]
j	yellow	[jɛlo]
w	wagon	[wægən]
dʒ	jumping	[dʒʌmpɪŋ]

REFERENCES

Adams, M. J., Foorman, B. R., Lundberg, I., & Beeler, T. (1998). *Phonemic awareness in young children.* Baltimore: Paul H. Brookes.

Albert, M., Sparks, R., & Helm, N., (1973). Melodic intonation therapy for aphasia. *Archives of Neurology, 29,* 130–131.

Alexander, R., Boehme, R., & Cupps, B. (1998). *Normal development of functional motor skills: The first year of life.* Tucson, AZ: Therapy Skill Builders.

Ambrose, N. G., & Yairi, E. (1999). Normative disfluency data for early childhood stuttering. *Journal of Speech, Language, and Hearing Research, 42,* 895–909.

American Speech Language Hearing Association (2000). *Technical Assistance Series: Part II.* Rockville, MD: ASHA.

American Speech-Language-Hearing Association (2000). *Roles and responsibilities of speech-language pathologists with respect to reading and writing in children and adolescents: Position statement, technical report, and guidelines.* Rockville, MD: ASHA.

American Speech-Language-Hearing Association (2002). Roles of speech-language pathologists in swallowing and feeding disorders: Position statement. *ASHA Leader, 7*(Suppl. 22), 73.

American Speech-Language-Hearing Association (2002). *Communication development and disorders in multicultural populations: Readings and related materials.* Rockville, MD: ASHA.

American Speech-Language-Hearing Association (2003). Survey reveals parents' reactions to children who stutter. *ASHA Leader, 8* (May 27), 21.

American Speech-Language-Hearing Association (2004). Evaluation and treatment for tracheoesophageal puncture and prosthesis: Technical report. *ASHA Supplement, 24,* in press. Rockville, MD: ASHA.

Andrew, M., & Summers, A. (2002). *Voice treatment for children and adolescents.* Clifton Park, NY: Thomson Delmar Learning.

Andrews, G., & Cutler, J. (1974). Stuttering therapy: The relation between changes in symptom level and attitudes. *Journal of Speech and Hearing Disorders, 39,* 312–319.

Andrews, G., & Harris, M. (1964). *The syndrome of stuttering.* Clinics in Developmental Medicine, no. 17. London: Spastics Society Medical Education and Information Unit in Association with Heinemann Medical Books.

Andrews, G., & Ingham, R. (1971). Stuttering: Considerations in the evaluation of treatment. *British Journal of Communication Disorders, 6,* 129–138.

Aronson, A. E. (1990). *Clinical voice disorders.* New York: Thieme Medical Publishers.

Bahr, D. C. (2001). *Oral motor assessment and treatment: Ages and stages.* Boston: Allyn & Bacon.

Bailey, G., & Thomas, E. (1998). Some aspects of African-American vernacular English phonology. In S. Mufwene, J. Rickford, G. Bailey, & J. Baugh (Eds.), *African-American English: History and use* (pp. 85–109). London: Routledge.

Baker, S. K., Simmons, D. C., & Kameenui, E. J. (1998). Vocabulary acquisition: Reading bases. In D. C. Simmons & E. J. Kameenui (Eds.), *What reading research tells us about children with diverse learning needs: Bases and basics* (pp. 183–217). Mahwah, NJ: Lawrence Earlbaum.

Ballard, K. J. (2001). Response generalization in apraxia of speech treatments: Taking another look. *Journal of Communication Disorders, 34,* 3–20.

Barkley, R. A. (1996). Linkages between attention and executive functions. In G. R. Lyon & N. A. Krasnegor (Eds.), *Attention, memory, and executive function* (pp. 307–325). Baltimore: Paul H. Brookes.

Bates, E., Camaioni, L., & Volterra, V. (1975). The acquisition of performatives prior to speech. *Merrill-Palmer Quarterly, 21,* 205–224.

Bates, E., & MacWhinney, B. (1987). Competition, variation, and language learning. In B. MacWhinney (Ed.), *Mechanisms of language learning* (pp. 157–194). Hillsdale, NJ: Erlbaum.

Battle, D. E. (1997). Multicultural considerations in counseling communicatively disordered persons and their families. In T. A. Crowe (Ed.), *Applications of counseling in speech-language pathology and audiology* (pp. 118–141). Baltimore: Williams & Wilkins.

Battle, D. E. (2002). *Communication disorders in multicultural populations.* Boston: Butterworth-Heinemann.

Bauman-Waengler, J. (2004). *Articulatory and phonological impairments: A clinical focus.* Boston: Allyn & Bacon.

Bear, D., & Templeton, S. (1998). Explorations in spelling: Foundations for learning and teaching phonics, spelling, and vocabulary. *The Reading Teacher, 52,* 222–242.

Begun, A. L. (1996). Family systems and family-centered care. In P. Rosin, A. D. Whitehead, L. I. Tuchman, G. S. Jesien, A. L. Begun, & L. Irwin (Eds.), *Partnerships in family-centered care: A guide to collabo-rative early intervention* (pp. 33–63). Baltimore: Paul H. Brookes.

Benedict, H. (1979). Early lexical development: Comprehension and production. *Journal of Child Language, 6,* 183–200.

Benson, V., & Marano, M. A. (1994). Current estimates from the National Health Interview Survey, 1993. *Vital and Health Statistics Series, 10,* Hyattsville, MD: National Center for Health Statistics.

Bentler, R. A. (2000). Amplification for the hearing-impaired child. In J. G. Alpiner & P. A. McCarthy (Eds.). *Rehabilitative audiology* (pp. 106–139). New York: Lippincott Williams & Wilkins.

Berke, G. S., Blackwell, K. E., Gerratt, B. R., Verneil, A., Jackson, K. S., & Sercarz, J. A. (1999). Selective laryngeal adductor denervation-reinervation: A new surgical treatment for adductor spasmodic dysphonia. *Annals of Otology, Rhinology, and Laryngology, 108,* 227–231.

Berndt, R. S., Mitchum, C. C., & Wayland, S. (1997). Patterns of sentence comprehension in aphasia: A consideration of three hypotheses. *Brain and Language, 60,* 197–221.

Bernthal, J. E., & Bankson, N. W. (1993). *Articulation and phonological disorders.* Needham Heights, MA: Allyn & Bacon.

Bernthal, J. E., & Bankson, N. W. (2004). *Articulation and phonological disorders.* Boston: Allyn & Bacon.

Biggs, D., & Blocher, D. (1987). *Foundations of ethical counseling.* New York: Springer.

Blachman, B. A., Ball, E. W., Black, R., & Tangel, D. N. (2000). *Rode to the code: A phonological awareness program for young children.* Baltimore: Paul H. Brookes.

Blitzer, A., Brin, M. F., Fahn, S., & Lovelace, R. E. (1988). Localized injections of botulinum toxin for the treatment of focal laryngeal dystonia (spastic dysphonia). *Laryngoscope, 98,* 193–197.

Blitzer, A., Brin, M. F., & Stewart, C. (1998). Botulinum toxin management of spasmodic dysphonia (laryngeal dystonia): A 12-year experience in more than 900 patients. *Laryngoscope, 108*, 1435–1441.

Blom, E. D, Singer, M. I., & Hamaker, R. C. (1998). *Tracheoesophageal voice restoration following total laryngectomy.* San Diego, CA: Singular Publishing Group.

Blood, G. W. (1995). POWER^2: Relapse management with adolescents who stutter. *Language, Speech, and Hearing Services in Schools, 26*, 169–179.

Blood, G. W., & Conture, E. G. (1998). Outcomes measurement issues in fluency disorders. In C. M. Frattali (Ed.), *Measuring outcomes in speech-language pathology* (pp. 387–405). New York: Thieme.

Bloodstein, O. (1960). The development of stuttering: II. Development phases. *Journal of Speech and Hearing Disorders, 25*, 366–376.

Bloodstein, O. (1975). Stuttering as tension and fragmentation. In J. Eisenson (Ed.), *Stuttering: A second symposium.* New York: Harper & Row.

Bloodstein, O. (1987). *A handbook on stuttering.* Chicago: National Easter Seals Society.

Bloodstein, O. (1995). *A handbook on stuttering.* San Diego, CA: Singular Publishing Group.

Bloom, L. (1973). *One word at a time: The use of single-word utterances before syntax.* New York: The Hague Mouton.

Blosser, J. L. (2003). *Pediatric traumatic brain injury: Proactive intervention* (2nd ed.). Clifton Park, NY: Singular Thomson Learning.

Boone, D. R., & McFarlane, S. C. (2000). *The voice and voice therapy.* Englewood Cliffs, NJ: Prentice Hall.

Borkowksi, J. G., & Burke, J. E. (1996). Theories, models, and measurements of executive functioning: An information processing perspective. In G. R. Lyon and N. A. Krasnegor (Eds.), *Attention, memory, and executive function* (pp. 235–261). Baltimore: Paul H. Brookes.

Boutsen, F. R., Cannito, M. P., Taylor, M., & Bender, B. K. (2002). Botox treatment in adductor spasmodic dysphonia: A meta-analysis. *Journal of Speech, Language, and Hearing Research, 45*, 469–481.

Brammer, L. M., & MacDonald, G. (1999). *The helping relationship: Process and skills.* Boston: Allyn & Bacon.

Brockman, L. M., Morgan, G. A., & Harmon, R. J. (1988). Mastery motivation and developmental delay. In T. D. Wachs & R. Sheehan (Eds.), *Assessment of young developmentally disabled children.* New York: Plenum.

Brookshire, R. H. (2002). *An introduction to neurogenic communication disorders.* St. Louis, MO: Mosby-Year Book.

Brown, R. (1968). *Words and things.* New York: The Free Press.

Brown, R. (1973). *A first language.* Cambridge, MA: Harvard University Press.

Bruner, J. (1974). The organization of early skilled action. In M. P. M. Richards (Ed.), *The integration of a child into a social world.* London: Cambridge University Press.

Bruner, J (1977). Early social interaction and language acquisition. In R. Schafter (Ed.), *Studies in mother-infant interaction.* New York: Academic Press.

Burns, S. M., Griffin, P., & Snow, C. E. (1999). *Starting out right: A guide to promoting children's reading success.* Washington, DC: National Academy Press.

Byng, S., Pound, C., & Parr, S. (2000). Living with aphasia: A framework for therapy interventions. In I. Papathanasiou (Ed.), *Acquired neurological communication disorders: A clinical perspective* (pp. 49–75). London: Whurr.

Calandrella, A. M., & Wilcox, M. J. (2000). Predicting language outcomes for prelinguistic children with developmental delay. *Journal of Speech, Language, and Hearing, 43*, 1061–1071.

Calvert, D. R., & Silverman, S. R. (1983). *Speech and deafness.* Washington, DC:

Alexander Graham Bell Association for the Deaf.

Campbell, C. R., & Jackson, S. T. (1995). Transparency of one-handed Amer-Ind hand signals to nonfamiliar viewers. *Journal of Speech and Hearing Research, 38,* 1284–1289.

Carlomagno, S., Losanno, N., Emanuelli, S. & Casadio, P. (1991). Expressive language recovery or improved communication skills: Effects of P.A.C.E. therapy on aphasics' referential communication and story retelling. *Aphasiology, 5,* 419–424.

Carrow, E. (1973). *Test of auditory comprehension of language.* Austin, TX: Urban Research Group.

Casper, J. K., & Colton, R. H. (1998). *Clinical manual for laryngectomy and head/neck cancer rehabilitation.* San Diego, CA: Singular Thomson Learning.

Casper, J. K., & Murry, T. (2000). Voice therapy methods in dsyphonia. *Otolaryngologic Clinics of North America, 33,* 983–1002.

Chapey, R. (2001). *Language intervention strategies in aphasia and related neurogenic communication disorders.* Baltimore: Lippincott, Williams & Wilkins.

Chappell, G. E. (1973). Childhood verbal apraxia and its treatment. *Journal of Hearing and Speech Disorders, 38,* 362–368.

Cheng, L. L. (1987a). *Assessing Asian language performance: Guidelines for assessing limited-English-proficient students.* Gaithersburg, MD: Aspen Publishers.

Cheng, L. L. (1987b). Cross-cultural and linguistic considerations in working with Asian populations. *Asha, 29,* 33–38.

Chomsky, N. (1965). *Aspects of a theory of syntax.* Cambridge, MA: MIT Press.

Chomsky, N., & Halle, M. (1968). *The sound pattern of English.* New York: Harper & Row.

Clark, J. G. (1981). Uses and abuses of hearing loss classification. *Asha, 23,* 493–500.

Coelho, C. A. (1990). Acquisition and generalization of simple manual sign grammars by aphasic subjects. *Journal of Communication Disorders, 23,* 383–400.

Coggins, T. E., & Carpenter, R. L. (1981). The Communicative Intention Inventory: A system for coding children's early intentional communication. *Applied Psycholinguistics, 2,* 235–252.

Conture, E. G. (1996). Treatment efficacy: Stuttering. *Journal of Speech and Hearing Research, 39,* S18–S26.

Cooper, E., & Cooper, C. (1985). *Cooper Personalized Fluency Control Therapy—Revised.* Allen, TX: DLM Teaching Resources.

Cordes, A. K., & Ingam, R. J. (1998). *Treatment efficacy for stuttering: A search for empirical bases.* San Diego, CA: Singular Publishing Group.

Cormier, L. S. & Hackney, H. (1999). *Counseling strategies and interventions.* Needham Heights, MA: Allyn & Bacon.

Cornett, R. O. (1967). Cued speech. *American Annals of the Deaf, 112,* 3–13.

Cornett, B. S. & Chabon, S. S. (1988). *The clinical practice of speech-language pathology.* New York: Merrill.

Crary, M., & Groher, M. (2003). *Introduction to adult swallowing disorders.* Little Rock, AR: Elsevier.

Creaghead, N. A., Newman, P. W., & Secord, W. A. (1989). *Assessment and remediation of articulatory and phonological disorders.* Columbus, OH: Charles E. Merrill.

Croot, K. (2002). Diagnosis of AOS: Definition and criteria. *Seminars in Speech and Language, 23,* 267–279.

Crowe, T. A. (1997). *Applications of counseling in speech-language pathology and audiology.* Baltimore: Williams & Wilkins.

Cuadrado, E. M., & Weber-Fox, C. M. (2003). Atypical syntactic processing in individuals who stutter: Evidence from event-related brain potentials and behavioral measures.

Journal of Speech, Language, and Hearing Research, 46, 960–976.

Dale, P. S. (1980). Is early pragmatic development measurable? *Journal of Child Language, 8,* 1–12.

Daly, D. A., & Burnett, M. L. (1999). Cluttering: Traditional views and new perspectives. In R. Curlee (Ed.), *Stuttering and related disorders of fluency* (pp. 222–254). New York: Thieme.

Darley, F. L., Aronson, A. E., & Brown, J. R. (1969a). Clusters of deviant speech dimensions in the dysarthrias. *Journal of Speech and Hearing Research, 12,* 462–496.

Darley, F. L., Aronson, A. E., & Brown, J. R. (1969b). Differential diagnostic patterns of dysarthria. *Journal of Speech and Hearing Research, 12,* 246–269.

Darley, F. L., & Spriestersbach, D. C. (1978). *Diagnostic methods in speech pathology.* New York: Harper & Row.

Davis, G. A. (1993). *A survey of adult aphasia and related language disorders.* Englewood Cliffs, NJ: Prentice Hall.

Davis, G. A., & Wilcox, M. J. (1981). Incorporating parameters of natural conversation in aphasia treatment. In R. Chapey (Ed.), *Language intervention strategies in adult aphasia.* Baltimore: Williams & Wilkins.

Dedo, H. H., & Izdebski, K. (1983). Inter mediate results of 306 laryngeal nerve sections for spastic dysphonia. *Laryngoscope, 93,* 9–15.

Deem, J. F., & Miller, L. (2000). *Manual of voice therapy.* Austin, TX: Pro-Ed.

De Nil, L. F. (1999). Stuttering: A neurophysiological perspective. In N. B. Ratner & E. C. Healey (Eds.), *Stuttering research and practice: Bridging the gap* (pp. 85–102). Mahwah, NJ: Earlbaum.

Dore, J. (1974). A pragmatic description of early language development. *Journal of Psycholinguistic Research, 3,* 343–350.

Duffy, J. R. (1995). *Motor speech disorders: Substrates, differential diagnosis, and management.* St. Louis, MO: Mosby-Year Book.

Duffy, J. R., & Coelho, C. A. (2001). Schuell's stimulation approach to rehabilitation. In R. Chapey (Ed.), *Language intervention strategies in aphasia and related neurogenic communication disorders* (pp. 341–382). Baltimore: Lippincott Williams & Wilkins.

Dworkin, J. P. (1991). *Motor speech disorders: A treatment guide.* St. Louis, MO: Mosby-Year Book.

Edgar, J. D. (2003). Respiration and swallowing in healthy adults and infants. *Perspectives on Swallowing and Swallowing Disorders, 12,* 2–6.

Elbert, M., & Gierut, J. (1991). *Handbook of clinical phonology: Approaches to assessment and treatment.* Austin, TX: Pro-Ed.

Ellis, A. (1977). The basic clinical theory of rational-emotive therapy. In A. Ellis & R. Grieger (Eds.), *Handbook of rational-emotive therapy.* New York: Springer.

Elman, R. J. (1999). *Group treatment of neurogenic communication disorders: The expert clinician's approach.* Boston: Butterworth-Heinemann.

Elman, R. J., & Bernstein-Ellis, E. (1999). The efficacy of group communication treatment in adults with chronic aphasia. *Journal of Speech, Language, and Hearing Research, 42,* 411–419.

Erikson, E. H. (1968). *Identity, youth, and crises.* New York: W. W. Norton.

Escalona, S. (1973). Basic modes of social interaction: Their emergence and patterning during the first two years of life. *Merrill-Palmer Quarterly, 19,* 205–232.

Fasold, R., & Wolfram, W. (1970). Some linguistic features of Negro dialect. In R. Fasold & R. Shuy (Eds.), *Teaching standard English in the inner city* (pp. 41–86). Washington, DC: Center for Applied Linguistics.

Ferrier, L. J. (1978). Some observations of errors in context. In N. Waterson & C.

Snow (Eds.), *The development of communication* (pp. 301–309). New York: John Wiley & Sons.

Fey, M. E. (1986). *Language intervention with young children*. San Diego, CA: College Hill Press.

Finn, P. (2003). Evidence-based treatment of stuttering: II. Clinical significance of behavioral stuttering treatments. *Journal of Fluency Disorders, 28,* 209–218.

Flasher, L. V., & Fogle, P. T. (2004). *Counseling skills for speech-language pathologists and audiologists*. Clifton Park, NY: Thomson Delmar Learning.

Fletcher, S. G. (1972). Time-by-count measurement of diadochokinetic syllable rate. *Journal of Speech and Hearing Research, 15,* 763–770.

Forrest, K. (2002). Are oral-motor exercises useful in the treatment of phonological/articulatory disorders? *Seminars in Speech and Language, 23,* 15–26.

Frattali, C. M., Thompson, C. K., Holland, A. I., Wohl, C. B., & Ferketic, M. M. (1995). *Functional Assessment of Communication Skills for Adults (FACS)*. Rockville, MD: ASHA.

Freed, D. (2000). *Motor speech disorders: Diagnosis and treatment*. San Diego, CA: Singular Publishing Group.

Freeman, S. B., & Hamaker, R. C. (1998). Tracheoesophageal voice restoration at time of laryngectomy. In E. D. Blom, M. I. Singer, & R. C. Hamaker (Eds.), *Tracheoesophageal voice restoration following total laryngectomy* (pp. 19–25). San Diego, CA: Singular Publishing Group.

Froeschels, E. (1952). Chewing method as therapy. *Archives of Otolaryngology, 56,* 427–434.

Froeschels, E., Kastein, S., & Weiss, D. A. (1955). A method of therapy for paralytic conditions of the mechanisms of phonation, respiration and glutination. *Journal of Speech and Hearing Disorders, 20,* 365–370.

Gebers, J. L. (1990). *Books are for talking too!* Tucson, AZ: Communication Skill Builders.

Geers, A. E. (2002). Factors affecting the development of speech, language, and literacy in children with early cochlear implantation. *Language, Speech and Hearing Services in Schools, 33,* 172–183.

Gentry, J. R., (2000). A retrospective on invented spelling and a look forward. *The Reading Teacher, 54,* 318–332.

Goebel, M. (1986). *A computer-aided fluency establishment trainer*. Annandale, VA: Annandale Fluency Clinic.

Goldman-Eisler, F. (1961). The significance of changes in the rate of articulation. *Language and Speech, 4,* 171.

Goldman-Eisler, F. (1968). *Psycholinguistics: Experiments in spontaneous speech*. New York: Academic Press.

Goldstein, B. (2000). *Cultural and linguistic diversity resource guide for speech-language pathologists*. Clifton Park, NY: Singular Thomson Learning.

Goodglass, H., & Wingfield, A. (1998). The changing relationship between anatomic and cognitive explanation in the neuropsychology of language. *Journal of Psycholinguistic Research, 27,* 147–165.

Goodglass, H., Kaplan, E., & Barresi, B. (2000). *The assessment of aphasia and related disorders*. Philadelphia: Lippincott Williams & Wilkins.

Graves, M. F. (1986). Vocabulary learning and instruction. In E. Z. Rothkopk & L. C. Ehri (Eds.), *Review of research in education* (pp. 49–89). Washington, DC: American Educational Research Association.

Greenfield, P. M., & Smith, J. (1976). *The structure of communication in early language development*. New York: Academic Press.

Gregory, H. H. (1979). Controversial issues: Statement and review of the literature. In H. H. Gregory (Ed.), *Controversies about stuttering therapy* (pp. 1–62). Baltimore: University Park Press.

Gregory, H. H. (2003). *Stuttering therapy: Rationale and procedures.* Boston: Allyn & Bacon.

Gregory, H., & Hill, D. (1993). Differential evaluation and differential therapy for stuttering children. In R. Curlee (Ed.), *Stuttering and related disorders of fluency* (pp. 23–44). New York: Thieme-Stratton.

Groher, M. E. (1997). *Dysphagia: Diagnosis and management.* Little Rock, AR: Elsevier.

Guitar, B. (1998). *Stuttering: An integrated approach to its nature and treatment.* Baltimore: Williams & Wilkins.

Guitar, B., & Marchinkowski, L. (2001). Influence of mothers' slower speech on their children's speech rate. *Journal of Speech, Language, and Hearing Research, 44,* 853–861.

Hall, P. K. (2000a). A letter to the parent(s) of a child with developmental apraxia of speech. Part I: Speech characteristics of the disorder. *Language, Speech and Hearing Services in Schools, 31,* 169–172.

Hall, C., & Golding-Kushner, K. J. (1989). *Long-term follow-up of 500 patients after palate repair performed prior to 18 months of age.* Presented at the Sixth International Congress on Cleft Palate and Related Craniofacial Anomalies, Israel.

Hall, P. K. (2000b). A letter to the parent(s) of a child with developmental apraxia of speech. Part II: The nature and causes of DAS. *Language, Speech, and Hearing Services in Schools, 31,* 173–175.

Hall, P. K. (2000c). A letter to the parent(s) of a child with developmental apraxia of speech. Part III: Other problems often associated with the disorders. *Language, Speech and Hearing Services in Schools, 31,* 176–178.

Hall, P. K. (2000d). A letter to the parent(s) of a child with developmental apraxia of speech. Part IV: Treatment of DAS. *Language, Speech and Hearing Services in Schools, 31,* 179–181.

Hall, P. K., Jordan, L. S., & Robin, D. A. (1993). *Developmental apraxia of speech:*

Theory and clinical practice. Austin, TX: Pro-Ed.

Halliday, M. A. K. (1975). *Learning how to mean: Explorations in the development of language.* London: Edward Arnold.

Halliday, M. A. K., & Hasan, R. (1975). *Cohesion in English.* London: Longman.

Halper, A. S. (1996). *Clinical management of right hemisphere dysfunction.* Gaithersburg, MD: Aspen Publishers.

Ham, R. (1990). *Therapy of stuttering: Preschool through adolescence.* Englewood Cliffs, NJ: Prentice Hall.

Ham, R. E. (1999). *Clinical management of stuttering in older children and adults.* Austin, TX: Pro-Ed.

Harris, K. R., & Graham, S. (1996). *Making the writing process work: Strategies for composition and self-regulation.* Cambridge, MA: Brookline Books.

Hartley, L. L. (1995). *Cognitive-communicative abilities following brain injury: A functional approach.* San Diego, CA: Singular Publishing Group.

Hayes, J., & Flower, L. (1987). On the structure of the writing process. *Topics in Language Disorders, 7,* 19–30.

Hegde, M. N. (1998). *Treatment procedures in communicative disorders.* Austin, TX: Pro-Ed.

Hegde, M. N. (1995). *Introduction to communicative disorders.* Austin, TX: Pro-Ed.

Hegde, M. N., & Davis, D. (1999). *Clinical methods and practicum in speech-language pathology.* San Diego, CA: Singular Thomson Learning.

Helm, N. A. (1979). Management of palilalia with a pacing board. *Journal of Speech and Hearing Disorders, 44,* 350–353.

Helm-Estabrooks, N., & Holland, A. (1998). *Approaches to the treatment of aphasia.* San Diego, CA: Singular.

Helm-Estabrooks, N., & Albert, M. L. (2004). *Manual of aphasia and aphasia therapy.* Austin, TX: Pro-Ed.

Hillis, A. E. (2001). Cognitive neuropsychological approaches to rehabilitation of language disorders: Introduction. In R. Chapey (Ed.), *Language intervention strategies in aphasia and related neurogenic communication disorders* (pp. 513–523). Baltimore: Lippincott Williams & Wilkins.

Hodson, B. W. (1986). *Assessment of phonological processes* (Rev. ed.). Danville, IL: Interstate Printers & Publishers.

Hodson, B. W., & Paden, E. P. (1981). Phonological processes which characterize unintelligible and intelligible speech in early childhood. *Journal of Speech and Hearing Disorders, 46,* 369–373.

Hodson, B. W., & Paden, E. P. (1991). *Targeting intelligible speech* (2nd ed.). Austin, TX: Pro-Ed.

Holland, A. (1995). *Current realities of aphasia rehabilitation: Time constraints, documentation demands, and functional outcomes.* Paper presented at Mid-America Rehabilitation Hospital, Overland Park, KS.

Holland, A. L., Fromm, D. S., DeRuyter, F., & Stein, M. (1996). Treatment efficacy: Aphasia. *Journal of Speech and Hearing Research, 39,* 27–39.

Hollien, H., & Shipp, T. (1972). Speaking fundamental frequency and chronologic age in males. *Journal of Speech and Hearing Research, 15,* 155–159.

Hudgins, C. V., & Numbers, F. C. (1942). An investigation of the intelligibility of speech of the deaf. *Genetic Psychology Monographs, 25,* 289–392.

Hull, R. (2001). *Aural rehabilitation: Serving children and adults.* Clifton Park, NY: Singular Thomson Learning.

Ingham, J. C. (2003). Evidence-based treatment of stuttering: I. Definition and application. *Journal of Fluency Disorders, 28,* 197–207.

Ingham, J. C., & Riley, G. (1998). Guidelines for documentation of treatment efficacy for young children who stutter. *Journal of Speech, Language, and Hearing Research, 41,* 753–770.

Ingham, R. J., & Bothe, A. K. (2001). Recovery from early stuttering: Additional issues within the Onslow & Packman-Yairi & Ambrose (1999) exchange. *Journal of Speech, Language, and Hearing Research 44,* 862–867.

Jacobson, E. (1938). *Progressive relaxation.* Chicago: University of Chicago Press.

Jakobson, R. (1964). Toward a linguistic typology of aphasic impairments. In A. DeReuck & M. O'Connor (Eds.), *Disorders of language* (pp. 21–46). London: Churchill.

Jakobson, R. (1968). *Child language: Aphasia and phonological universals.* The Hague: Mouton.

Johnson, J., Christie, J., & Yawkey, T. (1987). *Play and early childhood development.* Glenville, IL: Scott, Foresman.

Kamhi, A., Pollock, K., & Harris, J. (1996). *Communication development and disorders in African-American children.* Baltimore: Paul H. Brookes.

Katz, J. R. (2001). Playing at home: The talk of pretend play. In D. K. Dickinson & P. O. Tabors (Eds.), *Beginning literacy with language* (pp. 53–73). Baltimore: Paul H. Brookes.

Kayser, H. (1998). *Assessment and intervention resource for Hispanic children.* San Diego, CA: Singular Publishing.

Kelley, A. (1977). *Fundamental frequency measurements of female voices from twenty to ninety years of age.* Unpublished manuscript, University of North Carolina at Greensboro.

Kent, R. D. (1984). Stuttering as a temporal programming disorder. In R. F. Curlee & W. H. Perkins (Eds.), *Nature and treatment of stuttering: New directions* (pp. 283–301). San Diego, CA: College-Hill Press.

Kent, R. D. (2000). Research on speech motor control and its disorders: A review and prospective. *Journal of Communication Disorders, 33,* 391–427.

Kent, R. D., Kent, J. F., & Rosenbek, J. C. (1987). Maximum performance tests of speech production. *Journal of Speech and Hearing Disorders, 52,* 367–387.

Kertesz, A. (1979). *Aphasia and associated disorders: Taxonomy, localization and recovery.* New York: Grune & Stratton.

Kertesz, A., & McCabe, P. (1977). Recovery patterns and prognosis in aphasia. *Brain, 100,* 1–18.

Khan, L., & Lewis, N. (2002). *Khan-Lewis phonological analysis.* Circle Pines, MN: American Guidance Service.

Knepflar, K. J., & May, A. A. (1989). *Report writing in the field of communication disorders: A handbook for students and clinicians.* Rockville, MD: National Student Speech-Language-Hearing Association.

Kolk, H. H. J. (1991). Is stuttering a symptom of adaption or of impairment? In H. F. M. Peters, W. Hulstijn, & C. W. Starkweather (Eds.), *Speech motor control and stuttering.* Amsterdam: Elsevier Science Publishers.

Kolk, H. H. J., & Postma, A. (1997). Stuttering as a covert repair phenomenon. In R. F. Curlee & G. M. Siegel (Eds.), *Nature and treatment of stuttering* (pp. 182–203). Needham Heights, MA: Allyn & Bacon.

Kubler-Ross, E. (1969). *On death and dying.* New York: Macmillan.

Kuehn, D., & Moller, K. (2000). State of the art: Speech and language issues in the cleft palate population. *Cleft Palate Craniofacial Journal, 37,* 348.

Kuo, J., & Hu, X. (2002). Counseling Asian American adults with speech, language, and swallowing disorders. *Contemporary Issues in Communication Sciences and Disorders, 29,* 35–42.

Lahey, M. (1988). *Language disorders and language development.* New York: Macmillan.

Langdon, H. W., & Cheng, L. R. (2002). *Collaborating with interpreters and translators.* Eau Claire, WI: Thinking Publications.

Langeveld, T. P., van Rossum, M., Houtman, E. H., Zwinderman, A. H., Briaire, J. J., &

Baatenburg de Jong, R. J. (2001). Evaluation of voice quality in adductor spasmodic dysphonia before and after botulinum toxin treatment. *Annals of Otology, Rhinology, and Laryngology, 110,* 627–634.

Langevin, M., & Kully, D. (2003). Evidence-based treatment of stuttering: III. Evidence-based practice in a clinical setting. *Journal of Fluency Disorders, 28,* 219–236.

LaPointe, L. L. (1985). Aphasia therapy: Some principles and strategies for treatment. In D. Johns (Ed.), *Clinical management of neurogenic communicative disorders* (pp. 179–241). Boston: Little, Brown.

LaPointe, L. L., & Katz, R. C. (2002). Neurogenic disorders of speech. In G. H. Shames & N. B. Anderson (Eds.), *Human communication disorders* (6th ed., pp. 472–509). Boston: Allyn & Bacon.

Leinonen-Davis, E. (1988). Assessing the functional adequacy of children's phonological systems. *Clinical Linguistics and Phonetics, 2,* 257–270.

Leonard, R., & Kendall, K. (1997). *Dysphagia assessment and treatment planning: A team approach.* San Diego, CA: Singular Publishing Group.

Leopold, N. A., & Kagel, M. A. (1996). Prepharyngeal dysphagia in Parkinson's disease. *Dysphagia, 11,* 14–22.

Lieberth, A. K. (1990). Rehabilitative issues in the bilingual education of deaf children. *Journal of the Academy of Rehabilitative Audiology, 23,* 53–61.

Logemann, J. A. (1998). *Evaluation and treatment of swallowing disorders.* Austin, TX: Pro-Ed.

Love, R. J., & Webb, W. G. (1996). *Neurology for the speech-language pathologist.* Woburn, MA: Butterworth-Heinemann.

Lundberg, I., Olofsson, A., & Wall, S. (1980). Reading and spelling skills in the first school years predicted from phonemic awareness skills in kindergarten. *Scandinavian Journal of Psychology, 21,* 159–173.

Luria, A. R. (1970). *Traumatic aphasia: Its syndromes, psychology and treatment.* The Hague: Mouton.

Luterman, D. M. (2001). *Counseling the communicatively disordered and their families.* Austin, TX: Pro-Ed.

Lyon, J. G. (1998). Treating real-life functionality in a couple coping with severe aphasia. In N. Helm-Estabrooks & A. Holland (Eds.), *Approaches to the treatment of aphasia* (pp. 203–239). San Diego, CA: Singular.

Mackie, E. (1996). *Oral-motor activities for young children.* East Moline, IL: Lingui-Systems.

Magill, R. A. (1998). *Motor learning: Concepts and applications.* Boston: MacGraw Hill.

Manning, W. H. (2001). *Clinical decision making in fluency disorders.* Clifton Park, NY: Singular Thomson Learning.

Martin, F. N., & Clark, J. G. (1996). *Hearing care for children.* Boston: Allyn & Bacon.

Martin, F. N., & Clark, J. G. (2002). Considerations and implications for habilitation of hearing-impaired children. In D. K. Berstein & E. Tiegerman-Farber (Eds.), *Language and communication disorders in children* (pp. 565–598). Boston: Allyn & Bacon.

Marshall, R. C. (1998). *Introduction to group treatment for aphasia: Design and management.* San Diego, CA: Elsevier.

Marshalla, P. R. (1985). The role of reflexes in oral-motor learning: Techniques for improved articulation. *Seminars in Speech and Language, 6,* 317–335.

McCrory, E. (2001). Voice therapy outcomes in vocal fold nodules: A retrospective audit. *International Journal of Communication Disorders, 36,* 19–24.

McCullough, G., Pelletier, D., & Steele, C. (2003). National Dysphagia Diet: What to swallow. *ASHA Leader, 8,* 16.

McDonald, P. A., & Haney, M. (1997). *Counseling the older adult: A training manual in clinical gerontology.* San Francisco: Jossey-Bass.

McKeown, M. G., & Curtis, M. E. (Eds.). (1987). *The nature of vocabulary acquisition.* Hillsdale, NJ: Erlbaum.

McNeil, M. R. (1997). *Clinical management of sensorimotor speech disorders.* New York: Thieme.

McNeil, M. R., Robin, D. A., & Schmidt, R. A. (1997). Apraxia of speech: Definition, differentiation, and treatment. In M. R. McNeil (Ed.), *Clinical management of sensorimotor speech disorders* (pp. 311–344). New York: Thieme.

McWilliams, B. J., Morris, H. L., & Shelton, R. L. (1990). *Cleft palate speech.* Philadelphia: B. C. Decker.

Melnick, K. S., Conture, E. G., & Ohde, R. N. (2003). Phonological priming in picture naming in young children who stutter. *Journal of Speech, Language, and Hearing Research, 46,* 1428–1443.

Miccio, A. W., Elbert, M., & Forrest, K. (1991). The relationship between stimulability and phonological acquisition in children with normally developing and disordered phonologies. *Amercian Journal of Speech-Language Pathology, 8,* 347–363.

Milisen, R. (1954). A rationale for articulation disorders. *Journal of Speech and Hearing Disorders, 4,* 5–17.

Mitchum, C. C., & Berndt, R. S. (2001). Cognitive neuropsychological approaches to diagnosing and treating language disorders: Production and comprehension of sentences. In R. Chapey (Ed.), *Language intervention strategies in aphasia and related neurogenic communication disorders* (pp. 551–571). Baltimore: Lippincott Williams & Wilkins.

Moore, C. A., & Ruark, J. L. (1996). Does speech emerge from earlier appearing motor behaviors? *Journal of Speech and Hearing Research, 39,* 1034–1047.

Morris, S. E., & Klein, M. D. (1987). *Pre-feeding skills: A comprehensive resource for feeding development.* Tucson, AZ: Therapy Skill Builders.

Mowrer, D. E. (1982). *Methods of modifying speech behaviors.* Columbus, OH: Charles E. Merrill.

Murdoch, B., & Theodoros, D. G. (2001). *Traumatic brain injury: Associated speech, language, and swallowing disorders.* Clifton Park, NY: Singular Thomson Learning.

Myers, P. S., (1999). *Right hemisphere damage: Disorders of communication and cognition.* San Diego, CA: Singular Thomson Learning.

Myers, P. S. (2001). Communication disorders associated with right hemisphere damage. In R. Chapey (Ed.), *Language intervention strategies in aphasia and related neurogenic communication disorders* (pp. 809–828). Baltimore: Lippincott Williams & Wilkins.

Nagy, W. E., & Herman, P. A. (1987). Breadth and depth of vocabulary knowledge: Implications for acquisition and instruction. In M. G. McKeown & M. E. Curtis (Eds.), *The nature of vocabulary acquisition* (pp. 19–35). Hillsdale, NJ: Erlbaum.

Neidecker, E. A. (1987). *School programs in speech-language: Organization and management.* Englewood Cliffs, NJ: Prentice Hall.

Nelson, K. (1973). Structure and strategy in learning to talk. *Monographs of the Society for Research in Child Development, 38.*

Nelson, N. W. (1998). *Childhood language disorders in context: Infancy through adolescence.* Boston: Allyn & Bacon.

Newhoff, M., & Apel, K. (1990). Impairments in pragmatics. In L. L. LaPointe (Ed.), *Aphasia and related neurogenic language disorders* (pp. 221–233). New York: Thieme Medical Publishers.

Newson, J. (1979). The growth of shared understanding between infant and caregiver. In M. Bullowa (Ed.), *Before speech* (pp. 207–243). New York: Cambridge University Press.

Nicholich, L. (1977). Beyond sensorimotor intelligence: Assessment of symbolic play through analysis of pretend play. *Merrill-Palmer Quarterly, 23,* 89–101.

Ninio, A., & Bruner, J. (1978). The achievement and antecedents of labeling. *Journal of Child Language, 5,* 1–14.

Nippold, M. A. (1991). Evaluating and enhancing idiom comprehension in language-disordered children. *Language, Speech and Hearing Services in Schools, 22,* 100–106.

Nippold, M. A., Leonard, L. B., & Kail, R. (1984). Syntactic and conceptual factors in children's understanding of metaphors. *Journal of Speech and Hearing Research, 27,* 197–205.

Nittrouer, S. (1993). The emergence of mature gestural patterns is not uniform: Evidence from an acoustic study. *Journal of Speech and Hearing Research, 36,* 959–972.

Nober, E. H. (1967). Articulation of the deaf. *Exceptional Child, 33,* 611–621.

Norris, J. A., & Hoffman, P. R. (1990). Language intervention within naturalistic environments. *Language, Speech, and Hearing Services in Schools, 21,* 72–84.

Northern, J., & Downs, M. (1991). *Hearing in children.* Baltimore: Williams & Wilkins.

Oller, D. K. (1975). Simplification as the goal of phonological processes in child speech. *Language Learning, 24,* 299–303.

Oller, D. (1980). The emergence of the sounds of speech in infancy. In G. Yeni-Komshian, J. Cavanaugh, & C. Ferguson (Eds.), *Child Phonology: Vol. 1. Production.* New York: Academic Press.

Oller, D. K., & Kelly, C. A. (1974). Phonological substitution processes of a hard-of-hearing child. *Journal of Speech and Hearing Disorders, 39,* 65–74.

Onslow, M., & Andrews, C. (1994). A control/experimental trial of an operant treatment for early stuttering. *Journal of Speech and Hearing Research, 37,* 1244–1260.

Onslow, M., & Packman, A. (1999). The Lidcombe program of early stuttering intervention. In N. B. Ratner & E. C. Healy (Eds.), *Stuttering research and practice: Bridging the gap* (pp. 193–210). Mahwah, NJ: Lawrence Erlbaum.

Onslow, M., & Packman, A. (1999). Treatment recovery and spontaneous recovery from early stuttering: The need for consistent methods in collecting and interpreting data. *Journal of Speech, Language, and Hearing Research, 42,* 398–401.

Osborn, J. M., & Kelleher, J. C. (1983). A survey of cleft lip and palate surgery taught in plastic surgery training programs. *Cleft Palate Journal, 20,* 166.

Owens, R. E. (2001). *Language development: An introduction.* Needham Heights, MA: Allyn & Bacon.

Owens, R. E. (2004). *Language disorders: A functional approach to assessment and intervention.* Needham Heights, MA: Allyn & Bacon.

Paul, P. (2000). *Language and deafness.* Clifton Park, NY: Delmar Thomson Learning.

Paul, R. (2001). *Language disorders from infancy to adolescence: Assessment and intervention.* Boston: C. V. Mosby.

Paul, R. (2002). *Introduction to clinical methods in communication disorders.* Baltimore: Paul H. Brookes.

Pedersen, P., Draguns, J., Lonner, W., & Trimble, J. (2002). *Counseling across cultures.* Thousand Oaks, CA: SAGE Publications.

Pellowski, M. W., & Conture, E. G. (2002). Characteristics of speech disfluency and stuttering behaviors in 3- and 4-year-old children. *Journal of Speech, Language, and Hearing Research, 45,* 20–34.

Peterson-Falzone, S. J., Hardin-Jones, M. S., & Karnell, M. (2001). *Cleft palate speech.* St. Louis, MO: Mosby.

Piaget, Jean (1951). *Plays, dreams and imitation in childhood.* London: Heinnemann.

Piaget, J. (1954). *Origins of intelligence.* New York: Basic Books.

Pindzola, R. H., Jenkins, M. M., & Lokken, K. J. (1989). Speaking rates of young children. *Language, Speech and Hearing Services in Schools, 20,* 133–138.

Pinker, S. (1996). *Language learnability and language development.* Cambridge, MA: Harvard University Press.

Pinker, S. (1989). *Learnability and cognition: The acquisition of argument structure.* Cambridge, MA: MIT Press.

Poole, E. (1934). Genetic development of articulation of consonant sounds in speech. *Elementary English Review, 11,* 159–161.

Powell, T. W., Elbert, M., & Dinnsen, D. A. (1991). Stimulability as a factor in the phonological generalization of misarticulating preschool children. *Journal of Speech and Hearing Research, 34,* 1318–1328.

Prather, E., Hedrick, D., & Kern, C. (1975). Articulation development in children aged two to four years. *Journal of Speech and Hearing Disorders, 40,* 179–191.

Pulvermuller, F., & Roth, V. M. (1991). Communicative aphasia treatment as a further development of PACE therapy. *Aphasiology, 5,* 39–50.

Purcell, R. M., & Runyan, C. M. (1980). Normative study of speech rates of children. *Journal of the Speech and Hearing Association of Virginia, 21,* 6–14.

Quigley, S. P., & Kretschmer, R. E. (1982). *The education of deaf children.* Baltimore: University Park Press.

Ramig, L. O. (1998). Speech and voice disorders in Parkinson disease and their treatment. In L. Chernery (Ed.), *Topics in geriatric rehabilitation.* Gaithersburg, MD: Aspen Publishers.

Ramig, L. O., Pawlas, A., & Countryman, S. (1995). *The Lee Silverman Voice Treatment.* Iowa City, IA: National Center for Voice and Speech.

Ramig, L. O., Sapir, S., Countryman, S., Pawlas, A. A., O'Brien, C., Hoehn, M., & Thompson, L. L. (2001). Intensive voice treatment (LSVT) for patients with

Parkinson's disease: A 2 year follow up. *Journal of Neurology, Neurosurgery, and Psychiatry, 71*, 493–498.

Ramig, L. O., & Verdolini, K. (1998). Treatment efficacy: Voice disorders. *Journal of Speech, Language, and Hearing Research, 41*, 101–116.

Rao, P. R. (1994). Use of Amer-Ind code by persons with aphasia. In R. Chapey (Ed.), *Language intervention strategies in adult aphasia* (pp. 358–367). Baltimore: Williams & Wilkins.

Rao, P. R. (2001). Use of Amer-Ind code by persons with severe aphasia. In R. Chapey (Ed.), *Language intervention strategies in aphasia and related neurogenic communication disorders* (pp. 688–702). Baltimore: Lippincott Williams & Wilkins.

Ratner, N. (1995). Treating the stuttering child with concomitant grammatical or phonological disorders. *Language, Speech and Hearing Services in Schools, 26*, 180–186.

Ratner, N., & Bruner, J. (1978). Games, social exchange and the acquisition of language. *Journal of Child Language, 5*, 391–402.

Renner, M. J. (1995). Counseling laryngectomees and families. *Seminars in Speech and Language, 12*, 215–220.

Rivkin, M. (1986). The teacher's place in children's play. In G. Fein & M. Rivkin (Eds.), *The young child at play*. Washington, DC: National Association for the Education of Young Children.

Robey, R. R. (1998). A meta-analysis of clinical outcomes in the treatment of aphasia. *Journal of Speech, Language, and Hearing Research, 41*, 172–187.

Robin, D. A., Somodi, L. B., & Luschei, E. S. (1991). Measurement of tongue strength and endurance in normal and articulation disordered subjects. In C. A. Moore, K. M. Yorkston, & D. R. Beukelman (Eds.), *Dysarthria and apraxia of speech: Perspectives on management* (pp. 173–184). Baltimore: Paul H. Brookes.

Rogers, C. R. (1951). *Client-centered therapy.* Boston: Houghton Mifflin.

Rogers, C., & Sawyers, J. (1988). *Play in the lives of children*. Washington, DC: National Association for the Education of Young Children.

Rollin, W. (2000). *Counseling individuals with communication disorders: Pyschodynamic and family aspects*. Boston: Butterworth-Heinemann.

Roseberry-McKibbin, C. (1995). *Multicultural students with special language needs*. Oceanside, CA: Academic Communication Associates.

Roseberry-McKibbin, C. (2002). *Multicultural students with special language needs: Practical strategies for assessment and intervention*. Oceanside, CA: Academic Communication Associates.

Rosenbek, J. C. (1985). Treating apraxia of speech. In D. Johns (Ed.), *Clinical management of neurogenic communicative disorders* (pp. 267–312). Boston: Little, Brown.

Rosenbek, J. C., & Wertz, R. T. (1972). Review of 50 cases of developmental apraxia of speech. *Language, Speech and Hearing Services in Schools, 3*, 23–33.

Rossotti, L. M. (2001). *Communication intervention: Birth to three*. Clifton Park, NY: Singular Thomson Learning.

Roth, F. P., & Baden, B. (2001). Investing in emergent literacy intervention: A key role for speech-language pathologists. *Seminars in Speech and Language 22*, 163–174.

Roth, F. P., & Spekman, N. J. (1984). Intervention strategies for learning disabled children with oral communication disorders. *Learning Disability Quarterly, 2*, 7–18.

Ruark, J. L., & Moore, C.A. (1997). Coordination of lip muscle activity by 2-year-old children during speech and nonspeech tasks. *Journal of Speech and Hearing Research, 40*, 1373–1385.

Rvachew, S., & Nowak, M. (2001). The effect of target-selection strategy on phonological learning. *Journal of Speech, Language, and Hearing Research, 44*, 610–623.

Rvachew, S., Rafaat, S., & Martin, M. (1999). Stimulability, speech perception skills, and the treatment of phonological disorders. *American Journal of Speech-Language Pathology, 8*, 33–43.

Ryan, B. P. (1974). *Programmed therapy of stuttering in children and adults.* Springfield, IL: Charles C. Thomas.

Salinger, T. (2001). Assessing the literacy of young children: The case for multiple forms of evidence. In S. B. Neuman & D. K. Dickinson (Eds.), *Handbook of early literacy research* (pp. 390–418). New York: Guilford Press.

Sarno, M. T., & Levita, E. (1971). Natural course of recovery in severe aphasia. *Archives of Physical Medicine and Rehabilitation, 52*, 175–178.

Sarno, M. T., Silverman, M., & Sands, E. (1970). Speech therapy and language recovery in severe aphasia. *Journal of Speech and Hearing Research, 13*, 607–623.

Scarborough, H. (1989). Index of productive syntax. *Applied Psycholinguistics, 11*, 1–22.

Scarborough, H. S. (1998). Early identification of children at risk for reading disabilities. In B. K. Shapiro, P. J. Accardo, & A. J. Capute (Eds.), *Specific reading disabilities: A view of the spectrum* (pp. 75–119). Timonium, MD: York Press.

Scarborough, H., & Dobrich, W. (1990). Development of children with early language delay. *Journal of Speech and Hearing Research, 33*, 70–83.

Scheetz, N. (2001). *Orientation to deafness.* Boston: Allyn & Bacon.

Schlesinger, I. (1971). Production of utterances and language acquisition. In D. Slobin (Ed.), *The ontogenesis of grammar* (pp. 63–101). New York: Academic Press.

Schow, R. L. (2001). A standardized AR battery for dispensers. *Hearing Journal, 54*, 10–20.

Schuell, H., Jenkins, J. H., & Jimenez-Pabon, E. (1964). *Aphasia in adults: Diagnosis, prognosis and treatment.* New York: Hober-Harper.

Schulz, G. M., Greer, M., & Friedman, W. (2000). Changes in vocal intensity in Parkinson's disease following pallidotomy surgery. *Journal of Voice, 14*, 589–606.

Schulz, G. M., Peterson, T., Sapienza, C., Greer, M., & Friedman, W. (1999). Voice and speech characteristics of persons with Parkinson's disease pre- and post-pallidotomy surgery: Preliminary findings. *Journal of Speech, Language, and Hearing Research, 42*, 1176–1195.

Schumaker, J., Deshler, D., Alley, G., Warner, M., Clark, F., & Nolan, S. (1982). Error monitoring: A learning strategy for improving adolescent performance. In W. Cruickshank & J. Lerner (Eds.), *Best of ACLD* (pp. 179–183). Syracuse, NY: Syracuse University Press.

Schwartz, S., & Miller, J. E. (1996). *The new language of toys: Teaching communication skills to special-needs children.* Rockville, MD: Woodbine House.

Schweigert, W. A. (1986). The comprehension of familiar and less familiar idioms. *Journal of Psychological Research, 15*, 33–45.

Seikel, A. J., & Drumwright, D. G. (2004). *Essential Anatomy and Physiology for Communicative Disorders.* Clifton Park, NY: Thomson Delmar Learning.

Senturia, B. H., & Wilson, F. B. (1968). Otorhinolaryngologic findings in children with voice deviations. *Annals of Otology, Rhinology, and Laryngology, 77*, 1027–1042.

Shames, G. H., & Florance, C. L. (1980). *Stutter-free speech: A goal for therapy.* Columbus, OH: Charles E. Merrill.

Shames, G. H., & Wiig, E. (1998). *Human communication disorders: An introduction.* Needham Heights, MA: Allyn & Bacon.

Shapiro, D. (1999). *Stuttering intervention: A collaborative journey to fluency freedom.* Austin, TX: Pro-Ed.

Sharp, H. M., & Bryant, K. M. (2003). Ethical issues in dysphagia: When patients refuse assessment or treatment. *Seminars in Speech and Language, 24*, 285–299.

Sheehan, J. G. (1968). Stuttering as a self-role conflict. In H. H. Gregory (Ed.), *Learning theory and stuttering therapy* (pp. 72–83). Evanston, IL: Northwestern University Press.

Shelton, R. L., Hahn, E., & Morris, H. L. (1968). Diagnosis and therapy. In D. C. Spriestersbach & D. Sherman (Eds.), *Cleft palate and communication* (pp. 225–269). New York: Academic Press.

Shine, R. E. (1980). Direct management of the beginning stutterer. *Seminars in Speech, Language and Hearing, 1,* 339–350.

Shipley, K. G. (1997). *Interviewing and counseling in communicative disorders: Principles and procedures.* Needham Heights, MA: Allyn & Bacon.

Shprintzen, R. J., & Bardach, J. (1995). *Cleft palate speech management: A multidisciplinary approach.* St. Louis, MO: Mosby.

Shprintzen, R. J., McCall, R. N., & Skolnick, M. L. (1975). A new therapeutic technique for the treatment of velopharyngeal incompetence. *Journal of Speech and Hearing Disorders, 40,* 69.

Shriberg, L., Aram, D., & Kwiatkowski, J. (1997a). Developmental apraxia of speech: I. Descriptive and theoretical perspectives. *Journal of Speech, Language, and Hearing Research, 40,* 273–285.

Shriberg, L., Aram, D., & Kwiatkowski, J. (1997b). Developmental apraxia of speech: II. Toward a diagnostic marker. *Journal of Speech, Language, and Hearing Research, 40,* 286–312.

Shriberg, L., Aram, D., & Kwiatkowski, J. (1997c). Developmental apraxia of speech: III. A subtype marked by inappropriate stress. *Journal of Speech, Language, and Hearing Research, 40,* 313–337.

Shriberg, L. D., & Kwiatkowski, J. (1980). *Natural process analysis.* New York: Wiley.

Shriberg, L. D., & Kwiatkowski, J. (1983). Computer-assisted natural process analysis (NPA): Recent issues and data. *Seminars in Speech and Language, 4,* 11.

Silverman, E. M., & Zimmer, C. H. (1975). Incidence of chronic hoarseness among school-age children. *Journal of Speech and Hearing Disorders, 40,* 211–215.

Simmons-Mackie, N. (2000). Social approaches to the management of aphasia. In L. Worrall & C. Frattali (Eds.), *Neurogenic communication disorders: A functional approach* (pp. 162–187). New York: Thieme.

Simmons-Mackie, N. (2001). Social approaches to aphasia intervention. In R. Chapey, (Ed.), *Language intervention strategies in aphasia and related neurogenic communication disorders* (pp. 246–268). Baltimore: Lippincott Williams & Wilkins.

Sisskin, V. (2002). Therapy planning for school-age children who stutter. *Seminars in Speech and Language, 23,* 173–180.

Skelly, M. (1975). Aphasia patients talk back. *American Journal of Nursing, 75,* 1140–1142.

Skelly, M. (1979). *Amer-Ind gestural code based on universal American Indian hand talk.* New York: Elsevier.

Skelly, M., Schinsky, L., Smith, R. W., & Fust, R. S. (1974). American Indian sign (Amerind) as a facilitator of verbalization for oral verbal apraxia. *Journal of Speech and Hearing Disorders, 39,* 445–456.

Skinner, B. F. (1953). *Science and human behavior.* New York: Macmillan.

Skinner, B. F. (1957). *Verbal behavior.* New York: Appleton-Century-Crofts.

Smit, A. B., Hand, L., Freilinger, J., Bernthal, J., & Bird, A. (1990). The Iowa Articulation Norms Project and its Nebraska replication. *Journal of Speech and Hearing Disorders, 55,* 779–798.

Smith, A. (1999). Stuttering: A unified approach to a mulitfactorial, dynamic disorder. In N. B. Ratner & E. C. Healey (Eds.), *Stuttering research and practice: Bridging the gap* (pp. 27–44). Mahwah, NJ: Earlbaum.

Smith, A., & Kelly, E. (1997). Stuttering: A dynamic, multifactorial model. In R. F.

Curlee & G.M. Siegel (Eds.), *Nature and treatment of stuttering: New directions* (pp. 204–217). Needham Heights, MA.

Smythe, I., & Everatt, J. (2002). Dyslexia and the multicultural child: Policy into practice. *Topics in Language Disorders, 22*, 71–80.

Snow, C. (1978). The conversational context of language acquisition. In R. Campbell & P. Smith (Eds.), *Recent advances in the psychology of language* (Vol. 4a, pp. 253–269). New York: Plenum Press.

Snow, C. (1981). Social interaction and language acquisition. In P. Dale & D. Ingram (Eds.), *Child language: An international perspective* (pp. 195–214). Baltimore: University Park Press.

Sparks, R. W. (2001). Melodic intonation therapy. In R. Chapey (Ed.), *Language intervention strategies in aphasia and related communication disorders* (pp. 703–717). Baltimore: Lippincott Williams & Wilkins.

Sparks, R. W., Helm, N., & Albert, M. (1974). Aphasia rehabilitation resulting from melodic intonation therapy. *Cortex, 10*, 303.

Sparks, R. W., & Holland, A. L. (1976). Method: Melodic intonation therapy for aphasia. *Journal of Speech and Hearing Disorders, 41*, 287–297.

Spekman, N. J., & Roth, F. P. (1984). Intervention strategies for learning disabled children with oral communication disorders. *Learning Disability Quarterly, 7*, 7–18.

Speyer, R., Weineke, G., Hosseini, E. G., Kempen, P. A., Kersing, W., & Dejonckere, P. H. (2002). Effects of voice therapy as objectively evaluated by digitized laryngeal stroboscopic imaging. *Annals of Otology, Rhinology, and Laryngology, 111*, 902–908.

St. Louis, K. O. (1996). Research and opinion on cluttering: State of the art and science. *Journal of Fluency Disorders, 21*, 171–371.

Stanovich, K. E. (1986). Matthew effects in reading: Some consequences of individual differences in the acquisition of literacy. *Reading Research Quarterly, 21*, 360–406.

Stark, R. (1980). Stages of speech development in the first year of life. In G. Yeni-Komshian, J. Cavanaugh, & C. Ferguson (Eds.), *Child Phonology: Vol. 1. Production*. New York: Academic Press.

Starkweather, C. W. (1985). The development of fluency in normal children. In H. H. Gregory (Ed.), *Stuttering therapy: Prevention and intervention with children* (pp. 67–100). Memphis: Speech Foundation of America.

Starkweather, C. W. (1987). *Fluency and stuttering*. Englewood Cliffs, NJ: Prentice Hall.

Stein, N. L., & Glenn, C. G. (1979). An analysis of story comprehension in elementary school children. In R. O. Freedle (Ed.), *New directions in discourse processing* (Vol. 2, pp. 53–120). Norwood, NJ: Ablex.

Stemple, J. C., Glaze, L. E., & Klaben, B. G. (2000). *Clinical voice pathology: Theory and management*. Clifton Park, NY: Singular Thomson Learning.

Stone, C. A., Silliman, E. R., Ehren, B. J., & Apel, K. (2004). *Handbook of language and literacy: Development and disorders*. NY: Guilford.

Stone, J. R., & Olswang, L. B. (1989). The hidden challenge in counseling. *Asha, 31*, 27–31.

Stone, J., Shapiro, J., & Pasino, J. (1990). *The boundaries of counseling: Strategies for habilitation/rehabilitation professionals*. Conference, Reno, NV.

Sue, D. W., & Sue, D. (1999). *Counseling the culturally different: Theory and practice*. New York: John Wiley & Sons.

Sulica, L., Blitzer, A., Brin, M., & Stewart, C. (2003). Botulinum toxin management of adductor spasmodic dysphonia after failed recurrent laryngeal nerve section. *Annals of Otology, Rhinology, and Laryngology, 112*, 499–505.

Sullivan, H. (1953). *The interpersonal theory of psychiatry*. New York: Norton.

Swank, L. K., & Catts, H. W. (1994). Phonological awareness and written word decoding. *Language, Speech and Hearing Services in Schools, 25*, 9–14.

Tanner, D. C. (1999). *The family guide to surviving stroke and communication disorders.* Needham Heights, MA: Allyn & Bacon.

Tanner, D. C. (2003). *The psychology of neurogenic communication disorders: A primer for health care professionals.* Boston: Allyn & Bacon.

Templin, M. C. (1957). *Certain language skills in children.* Minneapolis, MN: University of Minnesota Press.

Thelen, E., & Smith, L. B. (1994). *A dynamic systems approach to the development of cognition and action.* Cambridge, MA: MIT Press.

Thomas, P. (1971). "Stand back, said the elephant. I'm going to sneeze." New York: Lothrop, Lee and Shepard Company.

Thompson, C. K., Shapiro, L. P., Kiran, S., & Sobecks, J. (2003). The role of syntactic complexity in treatment of sentence deficits in agrammatic aphasia: The complexity account of treatment efficacy (CATE). *Journal of Speech, Language, and Hearing Research, 46,* 591–608.

Throneburg, R. N., & Yairi, E. (2001). Durational, proportionate, and absolute frequency characteristics of disfluencies: A longitudinal study regarding persistence and recovery. *Journal of Speech, Language, and Hearing Research, 44,* 38–52.

Thurber, J. (1964). *The Thurber carnival.* New York: Dell.

Tobey, E. A., Geers, A. E., Brenner, C., Altuna, D., & Gabbert, G. (2003). Factors associated with development of speech production skills in children implanted by age five. *Ear & Hearing, 24,* 36S–45S.

Tompkins, C. A. (1995). *Right hemisphere communication disorders: Theory and management.* San Diego, CA: Singular Publishing Group.

Torgesen, J. K., & Davis, C. (1996). Individual difference variables that predict response to training in phonological awareness. *Journal of Experimental Child Psychology, 63,* 1–21.

Torgesen, J. K., Wagner, R. K., & Rashotte, C. A. (1994). Longitudinal studies of phonological processing and reading. *Journal of Learning Disabilities, 27,* 276–286.

Travis, L. E. (1931). *Speech pathology.* New York: Appleton-Century.

Troia, G. A., Roth, F. P., & Graham, S. (1998). An educator's guide to phonological awareness: Assessment measures and intervention activities for children. *Focus on Exceptional Children, 31,* 1–12.

Tucker, H. M. (1993). *The larynx.* New York: Thieme Medical Publishers.

U.S. Bureau of the Census. (2000). *Statistical abstract of the United States* (119th ed.). Washington, DC: U.S. Department of Commerce.

U.S. Department of Health and Human Services. (1995). *Recovering after a stroke.* Washington, DC: U.S. Government Printing Office.

Van Heugten, C. M., Dekker, J., Deelman, B. G., Stehmann-Saris, J. C., & Kinebanian, A. (2002). Rehabilitation of stroke patients with apraxia: The role of additional cognitive and motor impairments. *Disability and Rehabilitation, 22,* 547–554.

van Kleeck, A., & Schuele, C. M. (1987). Precursors to literacy. *Topics in Language Disorders, 7,* 13–31.

Van Riper, C. (1973). *The treatment of stuttering.* Englewood Cliffs, NJ: Prentice Hall.

Van Riper, C. (1982). *The nature of stuttering* (2nd ed.). Englewood Cliffs, NJ: Prentice Hall.

Verdolini, K. (1998). *NCVS guide to vocology.* Iowa City, IA: University of Iowa, National Center for Voice and Speech.

Verdolini, K. (2000). Voice disorders. In J. B. Tomblin, H. L. Morris, & D. C. Spriestersbach (Eds.), *Diagnosis in speech-language pathology* (pp. 233–280). San Diego, CA: Singular Thomson Learning.

Vygotsky, L. S. (1962). *Thought and language.* Cambridge, MA: MIT Press.

Wagner, R. K., & Torgesen, J. K. (1987). The nature of phonological processing and its causal role in the acquisition of reading skills. *Psychological Bulletin, 101,* 192–212.

Wagner, R. K., Torgesen, J. K., & Rashotte, C. A. (1994). Development of reading-related phonological processing abilities: New evidence of bidirectional causality from a latent variable longitudinal study. *Developmental Psychology, 30,* 73–87.

Waldron, C. M. (1998). Comments regarding the investigation of developmental apraxia of speech: Response to Shriberg, Aram, and Kwiatkowski. *Journal of Speech, Language, and Hearing Research, 41,* 958–963.

Wall, M., & Myers, F. (1995). *Clinical management of childhood stuttering.* Austin, TX: Pro-Ed.

Ward, E. C., Koh, S. K., Frisby, J., & Hodge, R. (2003). Differential modes of alaryngeal communication and long-term voice outcomes following pharyngeolaryngectomy and laryngectomy. *Folio Phoniatrica and Logopedics, 55,* 39–49.

Washington, J., & Craig, H. (1994). Dialect forms during discourse of poor, urban African-American preschoolers. *Journal of Speech and Hearing Research, 37,* 816–823.

Weber, R. S., Berkey, B. A., Forastiere, A., Cooper, J., Maor, M., Goepfert, H., Morrison, W., Glisson, B., Trotti, A., Ridge, J. A., Chao, K. S., Peters, G., Lee, D. J., Leaf, A., & Ensley, J. (2003). Outcome of salvage total laryngectomy following organ preservation therapy: The radiation therapy oncology group trial 91-11. *Archives of Otolaryngology, Head & Neck Surgery, 129,* 44–49.

Webster, R., Schumacher, S., & Lubker, B. (1970). Changes in stuttering frequency as a function of various intervals of DAF. *Journal of Abnormal Psychology, 75,* 45–49.

Weiner, A. E. (1984). Vocal control therapy for stutterers. In M. Peins (Ed.), *Contemporary approaches to stuttering therapy* (pp. 217–269). Boston: Little, Brown.

Wertz, R. T. (1981). Veteran's Administration cooperative study on aphasia: A comparison of individual and group treatment. *Journal of Speech and Hearing Research, 24,* 580–594.

Wertz, R. T., Collins, M. J., Weiss, D. G., Kurtzke, J. F., Friden, T., Brookshire, R. H., Pierce, J., Holzapple, P., Hubbard, D. J., Porch, B. E., West, J. A., Davis, L., Matovich, V., Morley, G. K., & Resurreccion, E. (1981). Veteran's Administration cooperative study on aphasia: A comparison of individual and group treatment. *Journal of Speech and Hearing Research, 24,* 580–594.

Wertz, R. T., LaPointe, L. L., & Rosenbek, J. C. (1984). *Apraxia of speech: The disorder and its management.* Orlando, FL: Grune & Stratton.

Wertz, R. T., LaPointe, L. L., & Rosenbek, J. C. (1991). *Apraxia of speech in adults: The disorder and its management.* Clifton Park, NY: Thomson Delmar Learning.

Wertz, R. T., Weiss, D. G., Aten, J. L., Brookshire, R. H., Garcia-Bunuel, L., Holland, A. L., Kurtzke, J. F., LaPointe, L. L., Milianti, F. J., Brannegan, R., Greenbaum, H., Marshall, R. C., Vogel, D., Carter, B., Barnes, N. S., & Goodman, R. (1986). Comparison of clinic, home, and deferred language treatment for aphasia: A Veteran's Administration cooperative study. *Archives of Neurology, 43,* 653–658.

Westby, C. E. (1999). Assessing and facilitating text comprehension problems. In H. W. Catts & A. G. Kahmi (Eds.), *Language and reading disabilities* (pp.154–223). Boston: Allyn & Bacon.

Wetherby, A., Cain, D., Yonclas, D., & Walker, V. (1988). Analysis of intentional communication of normal children from the prelinguistic to the multi-word stage. *Journal of Speech and Hearing Research, 31,* 240–252.

Whitehurst, G., Fischel, J., Lonigan, C., Valdez-Menchaca, M., Arnold, D., & Smith, M. (1991). Treatment of early expressive language delay: If, when, and how. *Topics in Language Disorders, 11,* 55–68.

Whitehurst, G. J. (2002). *Evidence-based education.* Presented to the Institute of Education Sciences. Washington, DC: U.S. Department of Education.

Williams, R., Ingham, R. J., & Rosenthal, R. (1981). A further analysis for developmental apraxia of speech in children with defective articulation. *Journal of Speech and Hearing Research, 24,* 496–505.

Williams, R., & Wolfram, W. (1977). *Social dialects: Differences vs. disorders.* Washington, DC: American Speech-Language-Hearing Association.

Wilson, B. S. (2000). Cochlear implant technology. In J. Niparko, K. I. Kirk, A. M. Robbins, D. L. Tucci, & B. S. Wilson (Eds.), *Cochlear implants: Principles and practices* (pp. 109–127). Philadelphia: Lippincott Williams & Wilkins.

Winefield, R. (1987). *Never the twain shall meet: Bell, Gallaudet, and the communications debate.* Washington, DC: Gallaudet University Press.

Wingate, M. E. (1964). Recovery from stuttering. *Journal of Speech and Hearing Disorders, 29,* 312–321.

Wingate, M. E. (1976). *Stuttering: Theory and treatment.* New York: Irvington Publishers.

Witzel, M. A. (1995). Communicative impairment associated with clefting. In R. J. Shprintzen & J. Bardach (Eds.), *Cleft palate speech management: A multidisciplinary approach.* St. Louis, MO: Mosby.

Wolf, M. (1984). Naming, reading, and the dyslexias: A longitudinal overview. *Annals of Dyslexia, 34,* 87–136.

Wolf, M. (1991). Naming speed and reading: The contribution of the cognitive neurosciences. *Reading Research Quarterly, 26,* 123–141.

Yairi, E., & Ambrose, N. (1992). A longitudinal study of stuttering in children: A preliminary report. *Journal of Speech and Hearing Research, 35,* 755–768.

Yairi, E., & Ambrose, N. G. (1999). Early childhood stuttering I: Persistency and recovery rates. *Journal of Speech, Language, and Hearing Research, 42,* 1097–1112.

Yairi, E., & Ambrose, N. G. (2001). Longitudinal studies of childhood stuttering:

Evaluation of critiques. *Journal of Speech, Language, and Hearing Research 44,* 867–872.

Yairi, E., Currin, L. H., Bulian, N., & Yairi, J. (1974). Incidence of hoarseness in school children over a 1 year period. *Journal of Communication Disorders, 7,* 321–328.

Yalom, I. (1980). *Existential psychotherapy.* New York: Basic Books.

Yaruss, J. S. (1998). Describing the consequences of disorders: Stuttering and the International Classification of Impairments, Disabilities, and Handicaps. *Journal of Speech, Language, and Hearing Research, 49,* 249–257.

Yavas, M., & Lamprecht, R. (1988). Processes and intelligibility in disordered phonology. *Clinical Linguistics and Phonetics, 2,* 329–345.

Ylvisaker, M. (1985). *Head injury rehabilitation: Children and adolescents.* San Diego, CA: College-Hill Press.

Ylvisaker, M., & Feeney, T. (1998). *Collaborative brain injury intervention: Positive everyday routines.* San Diego, CA: Singular Thomson Learning.

Yopp, H. K., & Yopp, R. H. (2000). Supporting phonemic awareness in the classroom. *The Reading Teacher, 54,* 130–143.

Yorkston, K. M. (1996). Treatment efficacy: Dysarthria. *Journal of Speech and Hearing Research, 39,* S46–S57.

Yorkston, K. M., Beukelman, D. R., & Bell, K. R. (1988). *Clinical management of dysarthric speakers.* Boston: Little, Brown.

Yorkston, K. M., Miller, R. M., & Strand, E. A. (2004). *Management of speech and swallowing in degenerative diseases.* Austin, TX: Pro-Ed.

Yoss, K. A., & Darley, F. L. (1974). Developmental apraxia of speech in children. *Journal of Speech and Hearing Research, 17,* 399–416.

Zebrowski, P. M. (1994). Stuttering. In J. B. Tomblin, H. L. Morris, & D. C. Spriestersbach (Eds.), *Diagnosis in Speech-Language Pathology* (pp. 215–245). San Diego, CA: Singular Publishing Group.

Zemlin, W. R. (1998). *Speech and hearing science*. Needham Heights, MA: Allyn & Bacon.

INDEX